Your *Clinics* subscription just got better!

You can now access the FULL TEXT of this publication online at no additional cost! Activate your online subscription today and receive...

- Full text of all issues from 2002 to the present
- Photographs, tables, illustrations, and references
- Comprehensive search capabilities
- Links to MEDLINE and Elsevier journals

Activate Your Online Access Today!

Plus, you can also sign up for E-alerts of upcoming issues or articles that interest you, and take advantage of exclusive access to bonus features!

To activate your individual online subscription:

1. Visit our website at **www.TheClinics.com**.
2. Click on "Register" at the top of the page, and follow the instructions.
3. To activate your account, you will need your subscriber account number, which you can find on your mailing label (note: the number of digits in your subscriber account number varies from six to ten digits). See the sample below where the subscriber account number has been circled.

This is your subscriber account number

```
**********************************************3-DIGIT 001
FEB00   J0167   C7   123456-89   10/00   Q: 1

J.H. DOE, MD
531 MAIN ST
CENTER CITY, NY  10001-001
```

4. That's it! Your online access to the most trusted source for clinical reviews is now available.

theclinics.com

ELSEVIER

theclinics.com

INFECTIOUS DISEASE CLINICS OF NORTH AMERICA

Sexually Transmitted Infections

GUEST EDITOR
Jonathan M. Zenilman, MD

CONSULTING EDITOR
Robert C. Moellering, Jr, MD

June 2005 • Volume 19 • Number 2

SAUNDERS

An Imprint of Elsevier, Inc.
PHILADELPHIA   LONDON   TORONTO   MONTREAL   SYDNEY   TOKYO

W.B. SAUNDERS COMPANY
A Division of Elsevier Inc.

Elsevier, Inc., 1600 John F. Kennedy Blvd., Suite 1800, Philadelphia, PA 19103-2899.

http://www.theclinics.com

INFECTIOUS DISEASE CLINICS OF NORTH AMERICA
June 2005
Editor: Carin Davis

Volume 19, Number 2
ISSN 0891–5520
ISBN 1-4160-2668-1

Copyright © 2005 by Elsevier Inc. All rights reserved. No part of this publication may be reproduced or transmitted in any form or by any means, electronic or mechanical, including photocopy, recording, or any information retrieval system, without written permission from the Publisher.

Single photocopies of single articles may be made for personal use as allowed by national copyright laws. Permission of the publisher and payment of a fee is required for all other photocopying, including multiple or systematic copying, copying for advertising or promotional purposes, resale, and all forms of document delivery. Special rates are available for educational institutions that wish to make photocopies for non-profit educational classroom use. Permissions may be sought directly from Elsevier's Rights Department in Philadelphia, PA, USA: phone: (+1) 215 239 3804, fax: (+1) 215 239 3805, e-mail: healthpermissions @elsevier.com. Requests may also be completed on-line via the Elsevier homepage (http://www.elsevier.com/locate/permissions). In the USA, users may clear permissions and make payments through the Copyright Clearance Center, Inc., 222 Rosewood Drive, Danvers, MA 01923, USA; phone: (978) 750-8400, fax: (978) 750-4744, and in the UK through the Copyright Licensing Agency Rapid Clearance Service (CLARCS), 90 Tottenham Court Road, London WIP 0LP, UK; phone: (+44) 171 436 5931; fax: (+44) 171 436 3986. Other countries may have a local reprographic rights agency for payments.

The ideas and opinions expressed in *Infectious Disease Clinics of North America* do not necessarily reflect those of the Publisher. The Publisher does not assume any responsibility for any injury and/or damage to persons or property arising out of or related to any use of the material contained in this periodical. The reader is advised to check the appropriate medical literature and the product information currently provided by the manufacturer of each drug to be administered to verify the dosage, the method and duration of administration, or contraindications. It is the responsibility of the treating physician or other health care professional, relying on independent experience and knowledge of the patient, to determine drug dosages and the best treatment for the patient. Mention of any product in this issue should not be construed as endorsement by the contributors, editors, or the Publisher of the product or manufacturers' claims.

Infectious Disease Clinics of North America (ISSN 0891–5520) is published in March, June, September, and December (For Post Office use only: volume 19 issue 2 of 4) by Elsevier, Inc. Corporate and editorial offices: Elsevier, Inc., 1600 John F. Kennedy Blvd., Suite 1800, Philadelphia, PA 19103-2899. Accounting and circulation offices: 6277 Sea Harbor Drive, Orlando, FL 32887-4800. Periodicals postage paid at Orlando, FL 32862, and additional mailing offices. Subscription prices are $165.00 per year for US individuals, $272.00 per year for US institutions, $83.00 per year for US students, $196.00 per year for Canadian individuals, $328.00 per year for Canadian institutions, $215.00 per year for international individuals, $328.00 per year for international institutions, and $108.00 per year for Canadian and foreign students. To receive student rate, orders must be accompanied by name of affiliated institution, date of term, and the *signature* of program/residency coordinator on institution letterhead. Orders will be billed at individual rate until proof of status is received. Foreign air speed delivery is included in all *Clinics* subscription prices. All prices are subject to change without notice. POSTMASTER: Send address changes to *Infectious Disease Clinics of North America*, W.B. Saunders Company, Periodicals Fulfillment, Orlando, FL 32887-4800. **Customer Service: 1-800-654-2452 (US). From outside of the US, call 1-407-345-4000. E-mail: hhspcs@wbsaunders.com**

Infectious Disease Clinics of North America is also published in Spanish by Editorial Inter-Médica, Junin 917, 1er A 1113, Buenos Aires, Argentina.

Reprints. For copies of 100 or more, of articles in this publication, please contact the Commercial Reprints Department, Elsevier Inc., 360 Park Avenue South, New York, New York 10010-1710. Tel. (212) 633-3813, Fax: (212) 462-1935, email: reprints@elsevier.com

Infectious Disease Clinics of North America is covered in *Index Medicus, Current Contents/Clinical Medicine, Science Citation Alert, SCISEARCH, and Research Alert.*

Printed in the United States of America.

SEXUALLY TRANSMITTED INFECTIONS

CONSULTING EDITOR

ROBERT C. MOELLERING, Jr, MD, Herrman L. Blumgart Professor of Medical Research, Harvard Medical School; and Physician-in-Chief and Chairman, Department of Medicine, Beth Israel Deaconess Medical Center, Boston, Massachusetts

GUEST EDITOR

JONATHAN M. ZENILMAN, MD, Professor of Medicine, Infectious Diseases Division, Johns Hopkins University School of Medicine, Baltimore, Maryland

CONTRIBUTORS

SEVGI O. ARAL, PhD, MSc, MA, Associate Director for Science, Division of STD Prevention, Centers for Disease Control and Prevention, Atlanta, Georgia

CHARLES EBEL, BA, Vice President, Health Program Resources, American Social Health Association, Research Triangle Park, North Carolina

KEVIN A. FENTON, MD, PhD, Division of STD Prevention, National Centers for HIV, STD and TB Prevention, Centers for Disease Control and Prevention (CDC), Atlanta, Georgia; HIV/STI Department, Health Protection Agency Centre for Infections, London, United Kingdom

CHARLOTTE A. GAYDOS, MS, MPH, DrPH, Associate Professor, Division of Infectious Diseases, Medicine, Johns Hopkins University School of Medicine, Baltimore, Maryland

KHALIL G. GHANEM, MD, Assistant Professor, Division of Infectious Diseases, Johns Hopkins University Bayview Medical Center, Baltimore, Maryland

JULIE A. GILES, MS, Senior Laboratory Technician, Division of Infectious Diseases, Johns Hopkins University Bayview Medical Center, Baltimore, Maryland

MATTHEW R. GOLDEN, MD, MPH, Assistant Professor of Medicine, Division of Infectious Diseases, University of Washington; Acting Director, Public Health—Seattle & King County, Seattle, Washington

PATTI E. GRAVITT, PhD, Assistant Professor of Epidemiology and Molecular Microbiology and Immunology, Johns Hopkins Bloomberg School of Public Heath, Baltimore, Maryland

ZSAKEBA HENDERSON, MD, EIS Officer, Health Services Research & Evaluation Branch, Division of STD Prevention, Centers for Disease Control and Prevention, Atlanta, Georgia

JOHN IMRIE, PhD, Centre for Sexual Health and HIV Research, Royal Free & University College Medical School, University College London, London, United Kingdom

KATHLEEN IRWIN, MD, MPH, Chief, Health Services Research and Evaluation Branch, Division of STD Prevention, Centers for Disease Control and Prevention, Atlanta, Georgia

ROXANNE JAMSHIDI, MD, Assistant Professor of Obstetrics and Gynecology, Johns Hopkins School of Medicine, Baltimore, Maryland

LISA E. MANHART, PhD, Assistant Professor, Department of Epidemiology, University of Washington, Seattle, Washington

JEANNE M. MARRAZZO, MD, MPH, Associate Professor of Medicine, Division of Allergy and Infectious Diseases, University of Washington; Medical Director, Seattle STD/HIV Prevention Training Center, Seattle, Washington

WILLIAM C. MILLER, MD, PhD, MPH, Assistant Professor, Division of Infectious Diseases, Department of Medicine, School of Medicine; Department of Epidemiology, School of Public Health, University of North Carolina at Chapel Hill, Chapel Hill, North Carolina

RAJ PATEL, MD, Consultant, Department of Genitourinary Medicine, Royal South Hampshire Hospital, Southhampton, Hants, United Kingdom

THOMAS C. QUINN, MD, MSc, Professor of Medicine and International Health, Division of Infectious Diseases, Johns Hopkins University School of Medicine, Baltimore; Laboratory of Immunoregulation, National Institute of Allergy and Infectious Diseases, National Institutes of Health, Bethesda, Maryland

STEVEN J. REYNOLDS, MD, MPH, FRCP(C), Asssistant Professor of Medicine, Division of Infectious Diseases, Johns Hopkins University School of Medicine, Baltimore; Laboratory of Immunoregulation, National Institute of Allergy and Infectious Diseases, National Institutes of Health, Bethesda, Maryland

ANNE ROMPALO, MD, Professor of Medicine, Johns Hopkins University School of Medicine, Baltimore, Maryland

SUSAN L. ROSENTHAL, PhD, Professor, Department of Pediatrics and the Sealy Center for Vaccine Development, University of Texas Medical Branch, Galveston, Texas

JONATHAN D. C. ROSS, MB, ChB, MD, FRCP, Professor of Sexual Health and HIV, Whittall Street Clinic, Birmingham, United Kingdom

JACK D. SOBEL, MD, Chief, Division of Infectious Diseases: Professor of Medicine, Wayne State University School of Medicine, Detroit, Michigan

LAWRENCE R. STANBERRY, MD, PhD, John Sealy Distinguished Professor and Chair, Department of Pediatrics and the Sealy Center for Vaccine Development, University of Texas Medical Branch, Galveston, Texas

GUOYU TAO, PhD, Health Scientist, Health Services Research and Evaluation Branch, Division of STD Prevention, Centers for Disease Control and Prevention, Atlanta, Georgia

HELEN WARD, MB CHB, FFPHM, MSc, Clinical Senior Lecturer in Epidemiology and Public Health, Honorary Consultant in Genitourinary Medicine, School of Medicine, Imperial College of Science Technology and Medicine, London, United Kingdom

TERRI WARREN, RN, ANP, Westover Heights Clinic, Portland, Oregon

JONATHAN M. ZENILMAN, MD, Professor of Medicine, Infectious Diseases Division, Johns Hopkins University School of Medicine, Baltimore, Maryland

SEXUALLY TRANSMITTED INFECTIONS

CONTENTS

Preface   xv
Jonathan M. Zenilman

Epidemiology of Chlamydial Infection, Gonorrhea, and Trichomoniasis in the United States—2005   281
William C. Miller and Jonathan M. Zenilman

>Chlamydial infection, gonorrhea, and trichomoniasis are the most common nonviral sexually transmitted infections (STIs) in the United States. Prevalence and incidence estimates are derived from several sources, including reported cases, clinic-based estimates, and community-based estimates. The combination of nucleic acid amplification tests and survey sampling techniques have led to the availability of true population-based estimates of the prevalence of these infections. This article reviews the estimates of prevalence and incidence, excluding purely clinic-based estimates, for these STIs. The strengths and limitations of each type of estimate also are discussed.

Modern Day Influences on Sexual Behavior   297
Sevgi O. Aral and Helen Ward

>Understanding sexual behavior is key to the effective prevention of sexually transmitted diseases (STDs) and developing effective intervention programs. As a social activity, sex and the activities that surround it, are linked intimately to the society and the context in which they occur. Sexual partnerships, and the factors that are related to their creation and dissolution, have received particular interest as a key determinant of STD risk. Sexual risk and partnership development patterns respond to societal economic, sociologic, political, and technologic change. This article explores these patterns and relationships.

Increasing Rates of Sexually Transmitted Diseases in Homosexual Men in Western Europe and the United States: Why? 311
Kevin A. Fenton and John Imrie

> STDs among homosexual and other men who have sex with men (MSM) are again on the increase. This is a finding that is consistent across Western Europe and the United States and, given the increasingly global interconnectedness of this community, is likely to have an impact on other geographic regions. The reasons for the increase are multifaceted, including substantial demographic shifts in MSM populations in industrialized countries; biologic factors such as epidemiologic synergy between HIV and other STDs; the possible transmission of drug-resistant STDs; and expansions in the sexual marketplace, which involves social and sexual networks that facilitate sex partner acquisition, with the Internet adding to, or in some cases replacing, more traditional meeting venues. Although evidence related to changing psychosocial contexts is emerging, a better understanding of the associations between high-risk sexual behavior and mental ill health, recreational drug use, socioeconomic deprivation, discrimination, and homophobia is required. In considering the strategic response to this issue, holistic approaches to improving sexual health among MSM within the "post-AIDS" context are urgently needed, alongside targeted interventions for HIV-positive MSM, the health care providers who care for them, and the custodians of social establishments directed at MSM.

Mucopurulent Cervicitis: No Longer Ignored, but Still Misunderstood 333
Jeanne M. Marrazzo

> The last decade has produced considerable advances in the diagnosis of the common etiologies of mucopurulent cervicitis (MPC), including *Chlamydia trachomatis* and *Neisseria gonorrhoeae*, and in the delineation of key aspects of their pathogenesis. Despite this, clear understanding of why these bacteria cause cervical inflammation in a minority of women who is infected with either organism is limited. Furthermore, many women who have MPC have neither of these infections detected, even when highly sensitive diagnostic tests are used. This article describes current data regarding this common condition, and charts new developments that might inform a more comprehensive understanding of MPC and its management, and of the more subtle signs of cervical inflammation that may impact women's susceptibility to a variety of infectious diseases, including HIV-1.

Fluoroquinolone-resistant *Neisseria gonorrhoeae*: the Inevitable Epidemic 351
Khalil G. Ghanem, Julie A. Giles, and Jonathan M. Zenilman

> The worldwide incidence of fluoroquinolone-resistant *Neisseria gonorrhoeae* has increased dramatically in the last few years.

Single doses of fluoroquinolones can no longer be used to treat *N gonorrhoeae* infections acquired in the Far East, parts of the Middle East, the Pacific Islands, and parts of Western Europe and the United States. Although California and Hawaii account for most of the current United States cases, the increased incidence of fluoroquinolone resistance in some high-risk groups independent of geography heralds an imminent spread of drug-resistant strains throughout the rest of the population.

Nucleic Acid Amplification Tests for Gonorrhea and Chlamydia: Practice and Applications 367
Charlotte A. Gaydos

Nucleic acid amplification tests (NAATs), which are highly sensitive and specific, have provided the ability to use alternative sample types for the diagnosis of sexually transmitted infections (STIs). Self-collected genital specimens, such as urine or even vaginal swabs, can now be accurately used to diagnose gonorrhea or chlamydia infections. In many cases, use of these sample types can decrease the necessity for a clinician to perform a pelvic examination on women or to collect a urethral swab from men, thus extending the diagnostic capability for detecting these infections to nonclinic screening venues. As most chlamydia infections and many gonorrhea infections are asymptomatic, the use of NAATs for self-collected samples greatly increases the types and numbers of patients that can be screened outside of clinic settings. Self-sampling also allows clinicians to easily screen patients in the clinic for STIs who are not presenting for pelvic or urogenital examinations. The application of NAATs to self-collected specimens has the potential to augment public health programs designed to control the epidemic of STIs in the community.

What's New in Bacterial Vaginosis and Trichomoniasis? 387
Jack D. Sobel

With worldwide occurrence and no evidence of decreased prevalence, trichomoniasis and bacterial vaginosis continue to serve as major challenges to the development of new diagnostic and therapeutic modalities. Major complications of these so-called "nuisance infections" are being increasingly recognized. Symptomatic and asymptomatic types of vaginitis facilitate HIV transmission, and therefore their eradication may offer a potential solution to reducing heterosexual spread.

Is *Mycoplasma genitalium* a Cause of Pelvic Inflammatory Disease? 407
Jonathan D. C. Ross

Although *Neisseria gonorrhoeae* and *Chlamydia trachomatis* are well recognized causes of pelvic inflammatory disease, they only account for 30 to 50% of cases. *Mycoplasma genitalium* can cause urthritis in men, but its role in female infection has been less well studied. The available evidence does suggest however that *M genitalium* is a sexually transmitted agent in women, which can cause cervicitis, urethritis, and occasionally salpingitis. Serologic studies and animal studies also support a role for *M genitalium* in causing upper genital tract infection and in the pathogenesis of tubular infertility.

Developments in STD/HIV Interactions: The Intertwining Epidemics of HIV and HSV-2   415
Steven J. Reynolds and Thomas C. Quinn

More than 75 million people worldwide have been infected with HIV over the past 2 decades despite ambitious global prevention programs. Currently 40 million people are living with HIV and over 35 million have died from AIDS. The spread of HIV has been primarily through sexual intercourse with a lesser proportion of cases attributable to intravenous drug use and contaminated blood transfusions. The alarming numbers camouflage the fact that the HIV virus is spread inefficiently through sexual intercourse, perhaps as infrequently as 1 out of 1000 sexual exposures. Sexually transmitted diseases, particularly ulcerative genital diseases, increase infectiousness and susceptibility to HIV infections. Data from international and domestic studies point increasingly to the role of herpes simplex virus type 2 (HSV-2) as a primary cofactor in facilitating the spread of HIV infection. This article reviews the recent developments in this important interaction and the potential impact of different intervention strategies targeting HSV-2.

Managing Patients with Genital Herpes and their Sexual Partners   427
Raj Patel and Anne Rompalo

There is increasing recognition of the growing size and significance of the genital herpes epidemic. Recent developments in the widescale availability of type-specific herpes simplex virus (HSV) serologic assays have meant that many previously undiagnosed mild, atypical, and subclinical infections may now be diagnosed with some degree of confidence without the use of Western blots. The value of such diagnostics is controversial. However, the importance of HSV with its facilitation of HIV transmission and acquisition, the availability of various preventative strategies for limiting vertical HSV transmission, and the growing evidence that condoms, some educational and counseling interventions, and antiviral therapies may limit sexual transmission, have challenged many of the arguments against wider testing of the population.

Diagnosis and Management of Oncogenic Cervical Human Papillomavirus Infection   439
Patti E. Gravitt and Roxanne Jamshidi

Because of the strong association of human papillomavirus (HPV) with invasive cervical cancer, research on HPV infection has targeted women. This article focuses primarily on the natural history and management of cervical HPV infection. A large body of epidemiologic research has allowed the development of a model of the natural history of HPV-associated cervical cancer whereby HPV is acquired by sexual transmission and is largely transient. Persistent infection with high-risk HPV confers a high risk for developing high-grade neoplasia and cancer.

Counseling the Patient who has Genital Herpes or Genital Human Papillomavirus Infection 459
Terri Warren and Charles Ebel

Educational counseling has an important role in managing patients who have viral sexually transmitted infections, such as genital herpes and genital human papillomavirus infections. Given the lack of a curative therapy for both, patients may require long-term management and may need to be attentive to recurring symptoms. In addition, both diagnoses may raise issues of persisting infectiousness along with a need for patient counseling about potential risk to partners and risk-reduction strategies. Lastly, dozens of published papers over the years describe potential psychosocial sequelae for patients who have genital herpes, and there is a growing psychosocial literature on genital HPV. Educational counseling may play a role in minimizing these sequelae.

Progress in Vaccines for Sexually Transmitted Diseases 477
Lawrence R. Stanberry and Susan L. Rosenthal

The development pipeline for vaccines to control sexually transmitted infections holds greater promise than ever before. Preclinical studies are encouraging in the development of chlamydia and gonococcal vaccines, and for the first time, recent clinical trials have shown the feasibility of creating vaccines to control genital herpes and cervical human papillomavirus infections. Behavioral research suggests that these vaccines will likely find acceptance among health care providers and consumers.

Sexually Transmitted Disease Care in Managed Care Organizations 491
Zsakeba Henderson, Guoyu Tao, and Kathleen Irwin

Clinicians affiliated with managed care organizations (MCOs) provide most of the care for sexually transmitted disease (STD) in the United States. A search of the medical literature since 1990 to find information on the burden of bacterial STD and quality of care in commercial and Medicaid MCO enrollees revealed that chlamydial infections are far more common in MCO enrollees than gonorrhea and syphilis. Although treatment and case reporting appear adequate in the MCOs studied, there is considerable room for improvement in sexual risk assessment, STD screening, risk-reduction counseling, patient education, and services for exposed sex partners. Many of the interventions that have been implemented in MCOs to improve STD care have addressed chlamydia control, with several showing promising results.

Innovative Approaches to the Prevention and Control of Bacterial Sexually Transmitted Infections 513
Matthew R. Golden and Lisa E. Manhart

Rate of gonorrhea and syphilis in the United States and Europe have declined dramatically in the last 30 years and are now at or near their lowest levels since World War II, while the prevalence of *chlamydia trachomatis* appears to be stable in areas with long-standing chlamydial screening programs. Further progress in the control of bacterial sexually transmitted infections (STI) is likely to require new approaches to prevention. This article summarizes recent, clinical and public health innovations in the control of STI.

Behavioral Interventions—Rationale, Measurement, and Effectiveness 541
Jonathan M. Zenilman

This article provides an overview for clinicians on the development and implementation of behavioral interventions for sexually transmitted diseases (STDs) and HIV infection. It includes a brief discussion of behavioral models and how these are used to develop intervention strategies, providing some examples in specific populations. The subject of bias and outcome evaluation in behavioral research is comprehensively addressed. Case studies of population-based STD/HIV intervention programs are presented, emphasizing settings where societal-level behavior change occurred. The article concludes by addressing important political and structural challenges to STD/HIV prevention efforts. This article interdigitates with Dr. Aral's article on sexual behavior and Dr. Golden's article on new approaches to STD intervention.

Index 563

FORTHCOMING ISSUES

September 2005
Pediatric Infectious Diseases
Jeffrey Blumer, MD, PhD, and
Philip Toltzis, MD, *Guest Editors*

December 2005
Musculoskeletal Infections
John James Ross, MD, *Guest Editor*

RECENT ISSUES

March 2005
Travel and Tropical Medicine
Frank J. Bia, MD, MPH, and
David R. Hill, MD, DTM&H
Guest Editors

December 2004
Lower Respiratory Tract Infections
Thomas M. File, Jr, MD, *Guest Editor*

September 2004
Antibacterial Therapy and Newer Agents
Donald Kaye, MD, *Guest Editor*

The Clinics are now available online!

Access your subscription at:
www.theclinics.com

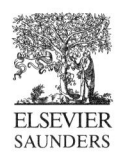

Preface

Sexually Transmitted Infections

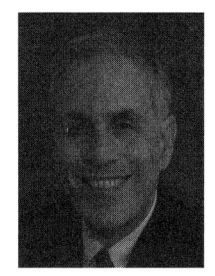

Jonathan M. Zenilman, MD
Guest Editor

It has been a privilege to edit this issue of *Infectious Disease Clinics of North America*. The field of sexually transmitted infections has been characterized by newly emerging epidemiological trends, an increased appreciation of behavioral risks, rapid advances in diagnostic testing, and new clinical syndromes. In this volume, contributors who are epidemiologists, behavioral scientists, clinicians, and laboratory scientists have contributed articles illustrating the highlights in these areas. We have developed the articles which would be of interest to the practicing clinician as well as the clinician who has an interest in public health, with the intent of providing an overall background to STDs and also imparting some useful clinical skills and information. Our authors are expert clinicians and epidemiologists from the United States and the United Kingdom.

In the first article, Bill Miller reviews the epidemiology of sexually transmitted diseases (STDs) in the United States, focusing on recent large-scale population-based behavioral surveys, which have the potential to provide accurate population-based information on STD incidence and prevalence. Sevgi Aral, a well known behavioral researcher from the Centers for Disease Control and Prevention (CDC) writes on important demographic trends which have the tremendous potential to impact STD risks, especially changes in society which impacts sexuality and therefore risk of STDs. She has done so in a very digestible format for busy clinicians who often don't have the opportunity to see this type of information in print. Kevin Fenton, an international expert on public health surveillance and on STDs in gay men, discusses the recent troubling increased rates of syphilis and other STDs in gay men, and compares the Western Europe and the United States experience. In the clinical realm, Jeannie Marrazzo discusses the current approaches to the diagnoses and management of mucopurulent cervicitis, an often vexing clinical problem because many cases do not have an easily indentifiable cause. Khalil Ghanem reviews the current and rapidly moving epidemiology of quinelone resistant gonorrhea and its implications for public health and for therapy. Charlotte Gaydos reviews the new diagnostic tests which have emerged in the past decade for a diagnosis of gonorrhea and chlamydia and its impact on clinical practice, focusing on the movement of diagnostic testing from the clinician's office into field settings. Jack Sobel reviews bacterial vaginosis and trichomonas, building on his incredible wealth of knowledge in this area and providing a format for clinicians to evaluate vaginal discharge in a logical and consistent manner. Jonathan Ross, from the United Kingdom, reviews the role of *Mycoplasma genitalium* in the pathogenesis of non gonococcal, urethritis, and proposes that this may be an organism in pelvic inflammatory disease.

Steve Reynolds and Thomas Quinn review the STD–HIV interaction, focusing on recent data which implicates herpes as an important issue in that interaction. Drs. Raj Patel and Anne Rompalo review recent data and clinical trials in the most effective ways of managing patients who have clinical genital herpes and their partners, emphasizing the new data that suggest that treatment of infected individuals may be an approach to preventing infection in their partners. Pattie Gravitt, a human papillomavirus (HPV) basic scientist and epidemiologist, and Roxanne Jamshidi, who is a gynecologist, reviewed the clinical approach to managing cervical HPV infection and the role of new diagnostic testing, such as the sensitive HPV assays for HPV and their role in clinical management. Charlie Ebel and Terry Warren, both experts in counseling provide a structured counseling approach for patients with herpes and HPV infection. Counseling in particular has been a clinical conundrum, because counseling patients about a chronic viral infection in an office setting can be quite challenging.

The last part of the volume deals with selected programmatic and scientific advances. Larry Stanberry and Susan Rosenthal review progress in STD vaccines, focusing mostly on new viral vaccines, specifically HPV and herpes simplex. Kathleen Irwin and Zsakeba Henderson from the CDC review the approach to STDs in managed care environments, and how to utilize the managed care environment for the most effective patient-based STD control as well as population-based STD control issues. Matthew Golden from the University of Washington reviews outreach approaches partner management issues related to STD. He builds on his having tremendous experience in developing innovative partner approaches, including partner delivered therapy, and the enlistment of pharmacies to provide STD treatment to potentially infected partners. Finally, I review the behavioral intervention literature on what works and what does not work, with a critical evaluation of how to approach behavioral interventions from the standpoint of the clinician and trying to understand the advantages and limits of the behavioral intervention approach.

Because of space constraints, we could not address other current and important topics. For example, we did not discuss the current clinical management of pelvic inflammatory disease or nongonococcal urethritis. These topics will potentially be addressed in a future volume.

This project would not have happened without my assistants Lin McGrogan and Marci Fenloch, and Carin Davis, from Elsevier, who continually provided encouragement.

I hope you enjoy this volume and that it helps you in clinical practice and in the public health management of your patients.

Jonathan M. Zenilman, MD
Infectious Diseases Division
Johns Hopkins Bayview Medical Center
4940 Eastern Avenue B-3 North
Baltimore, MD 21224, USA

E-mail address: jzenilm1@jhmi.edu

Epidemiology of Chlamydial Infection, Gonorrhea, and Trichomoniasis in the United States—2005

William C. Miller, MD, PhD, MPH[a,b,*], Jonathan M. Zenilman, MD[c]

[a]*Department of Epidemiology, School of Public Health, University of North Carolina at Chapel Hill, CB#7435, 2105F McGavran-Greenberg, Chapel Hill, NC 27599-7435, USA*
[b]*Division of Infectious Diseases, Department of Medicine, School of Medicine, University of North Carolina at Chapel Hill, Chapel Hill, NC 27599, USA*
[c]*Infectious Diseases Division, Johns Hopkins Bayview Medical Center, 4940 Eastern Avenue B-3 North, Baltimore, MD*

The mucosal sexually transmitted infections (STIs), including chlamydial infection, gonorrhea, and trichomoniasis, cause substantial morbidity in the United States. Chlamydial infection and gonorrhea cause lower and upper genital tract infections, including salpingitis and endometritis. Long-term complications include tubal infertility, ectopic pregnancy, and chronic pelvic pain [1,2]. Infertility in men who have chlamydial infection has been suggested, but is controversial [3]. All three infections seem to increase the risk for acquisition of HIV infection and also may increase transmissibility of HIV [4]. These important consequences, coupled with the fact that these infections are preventable and easily treatable, necessitate an accurate understanding of the epidemiology of these STIs.

Traditionally, much of the information available regarding the epidemiology of STIs has come from the passive surveillance system that was established by the Centers for Disease Control and Prevention (CDC) and states. Of the mucosal STIs, chlamydial infection, gonorrhea, and, in some cases, nongonococcal urethritis, are reportable diseases. Clinicians or laboratories that make diagnoses of these STIs are required to report

---

* Corresponding author. Department of Epidemiology, School of Public Health, University of North Carolina at Chapel Hill, CB#7435, 2105F McGavran-Greenberg, Chapel Hill, NC 27599-7435, USA.
   E-mail address: bill_miller@unc.edu (W.C. Miller).

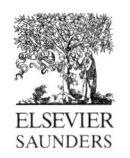

0891-5520/05/$ - see front matter © 2005 Elsevier Inc. All rights reserved.
doi:10.1016/j.idc.2005.04.001   *id.theclinics.com*

them to the local public health authorities. Although the addition of laboratory reporting is believed to increase the yield of reporting, underreporting of cases is a well-recognized limitation of estimates that are derived from surveillance [5]. These estimates also are criticized often because of the potential for reporting bias. Publicly funded clinics, with high proportions of economically disadvantaged persons, generally are more likely to submit reports than private clinicians [6,7]. Private physicians also are less likely to report the race/ethnicity of diagnosed patients [7].

In the past decade, technologic advances have provided the opportunity to obtain new insights into the epidemiology of STIs. In particular, the development of nucleic acid amplification tests (NAATs), such as polymerase chain reaction (PCR) assays, has provided a new set of tools for epidemiologic studies. The advantage of these new assays is amplified by their use with specimens that do not require a physical examination, such as urine or self-collected vaginal swabs. Consequently, for the first time, the prevalence and incidence of these infections may be examined in populations that are not actively seeking health care. These estimates provide the first glimpses of the epidemiology of these STIs in the general population.

Combining the new NAAT technology with population-based surveys provides new insights into the burden of these STIs in the general population. Population-based surveys use complex sampling methods to identify a study sample that is representative of a larger target population. For example, the National Longitudinal Study of Adolescent Health (Add Health) used a stratified, multistage sample of schools and students to develop a sample of adolescents that yields estimates that are representative of the United States [8,9]. The participants in Add Health are now young adults. Another example was a survey in Baltimore that provided estimates that were representative of adults who were living in the city who were between the ages of 18 and 35 years [10]. The National Survey of Adolescent Males (NSAM), which was conducted in 1988 and 1995, provided a representative sample of adolescent and young men in the United States [11].

Studies in special populations also have provided new and important insights into the epidemiology of STIs. Examples of special populations that were evaluated in STI research include the military and high school students. Although commonly referred to as "population-based" because these studies are conducted outside of clinics, studies in special populations are not truly population-based, but rather are "community-based." This difference may seem subtle, but it is important. Population-based implies that the estimates are generalizable to the general population. The self-selection involved in many special populations substantially limits the generalizability of these studies. For example, the population of military recruits is unlikely to be representative of all young adults in the United States.

To provide an overview of the epidemiology of these three infections, this article examines recent studies that assessed their prevalence and incidence. It also examines population-based studies, special populations studied outside of clinics or under special circumstances, and considers recent developments in surveillance and reporting. The advantages and disadvantages of each approach are highlighted. The purpose is not to provide an exhaustive review of all available studies, but rather to highlight demonstrative and insightful studies.

Chlamydial infection

Microbiologic and clinical overview

Chlamydia trachomatis (Ct) is an obligate intracellular pathogen with a unique two-phase growth cycle [12]. The organism cannot be cultured on standard artificial media. To survive, the organism must attach and penetrate the host cell. Ct cannot synthesize ATP or GTP and must rely on the host for these energy sources. There seems to be a significant immune response to chlamydial infections, with detectable levels of circulating antibodies. After the acute phase of infection, many persons seem to experience a long duration, presumably lower grade infection.

Clinically, Ct causes urethritis, epididymitis, and prostatitis in men [13]. Proctitis is common in men who have sex with men; however, more than 50% of infections in men may be asymptomatic. In women, cervicitis and urethritis are common. Acute infectious complications may include pelvic inflammatory disease and perihepatitis. Asymptomatic disease is common in women and occurs in more than 70% of infections. The high prevalence of asymptomatic disease and the potential to prevent complications has led to recommendations for screening of asymptomatic women [14–20].

Challenges to the epidemiologic assessment of chlamydial infection

The high prevalence of asymptomatic infections presents a major challenge to estimating the burden of chlamydial infection. Asymptomatic persons will not seek health care for the infection. Consequently, clinic-based estimates tend to underestimate the disease burden. The establishment of screening programs in women has improved estimates to some degree, because screening captures infections among asymptomatic women; however, these estimates are still suboptimal. Women must present to a health care provider and that provider must perform screening, to be included in any estimates. Furthermore, because screening is not performed routinely in men, the degree of bias differs substantially between the genders. Supplementation of estimates with information about syndromic diagnoses, such as nongonococcal urethritis or mucopurulent cervicitis, is problematic because numerous organisms other than chlamydia may cause these syndromes.

Population-based estimates of the prevalence of chlamydial infection

A major advantage of population-based estimates of the prevalence of chlamydial infection is that these estimates provide the most accurate assessment of disease burden. Clinic-based estimates and reported cases require presentation to a health care provider, testing, and in the case of reporting, the submission of the surveillance report card. Prevalence estimates that are obtained in special populations, such as schools and military personnel, may not be representative of the general population, and often are selectively representative of higher prevalence populations. True population-based estimates avoid these biases by sampling schemes that provide representation of the general population. These sampling schemes often are complex. The adequacy of the representation of the target population depends on the appropriateness of the sample and the sampling scheme.

Add Health has provided one of the most comprehensive and generalizable estimates of chlamydial infection in the United States (Table 1) [8,9]. Add Health is a complex longitudinal survey that began in 1994. In the initial wave of data collection, a stratified random sample of junior and senior high schools was selected. Students in grades 7 through 12 were selected randomly and interviewed. In 2001, the persons were recontacted during the third wave of data collection. At the time of this interview, the former school students were now young adults, aged 18 to 26 years. Urine specimens were collected and tested for Ct, *Neisseria gonorrhoeae* (GC), and *Trichomonas vaginalis* (Tv) using NAATs.

Based on a sample of more than 12,000 persons, the overall prevalence of chlamydial infection in the United States was estimated to be 4.2% [21].

Table 1
Population-based or special national sample studies of chlamydia and gonococcal infections in the United States

Study	Population	Year	Age range	CT-M	CT-F	GC-M	GC-F
Add Health [21]	National sample of adolescents recruited in high school-follow-up visits	2001	18–26	3.7%	4.7%	0.4%	0.4%
National Survey of Adolescent Males [11]	National population-based survey of adolescents	1995	18–19	3.1%			
Baltimore Sexual Behavior Survey [10]	Population-based sample of Baltimore City residents	1998–9	18–35	2.2%	4.3%	3.8%	6.7%
Military recruits [22–24]	U.S. military recruits in 1996–9 (women); 1998–9 (men)	1996–9	18–39	5.3%	9.5%	0.6%	—
Job Corp [25]	Entrants to Job Corps training programs	2003	16–24	8.0%	9.9%		

Abbreviations: F, female; M, male.

Regional differences were evident with the South having the highest prevalence (5.4%). The prevalence was higher among women (4.7%) than men (3.7%). Substantial differences were observed by race/ethnicity. Among African American women, the prevalence was approximately 14% and among African American men, 11%. Latino women (4.4%) and men (7.2%) had intermediate prevalences of chlamydial infection. The prevalence among white women (2.5%) and men (1.4%) was lower.

NSAM provided a similar estimate of chlamydial infection. Based on a survey that was conducted in 1995 among approximately 500 men ages 18 and 19 and 1000 men ages 22 to 26 years, the prevalence of chlamydial infection was 3.1% and 4.5%, respectively; these were comparable to the Add Health estimate.

Other population-based studies have provided geographically-restricted estimates of the prevalence of chlamydial infection in the United States. The Baltimore STD and Behavior Survey, conducted in Baltimore in 1998, used the Baltimore Real Estate Property Registry to sample households and identify participants in the households [10]. This method ensured that virtually anyone living in the city, whether they owned their property or rented, was eligible for inclusion in the sample. Persons at greater risk were oversampled to increase precision. The oversampling was accounted for by applying appropriate sampling weights during analyses. The technique of oversampling is an important tool in survey research, and should not be misunderstood as introducing or increasing the likelihood of bias. In fact, oversampling of specific target groups often improves the estimates that are obtained in the surveys by increasing the precision of the estimates or the efficiency of conducting the study. Appropriate analytic methods must be used to account for the oversampling.

In the Baltimore study, the prevalence of chlamydial infection overall was 3.0% in adults who were aged 18 to 35 years [10]. The prevalence ranged from 8% in 19- and 20-year-olds to 0.5% in 33- to 35-year-olds. This gradient by age is expected, based on clinic studies. Many persons who had chlamydial infection did not report recent high-risk behaviors; this suggests the possibility that the duration of many infections was long [26].

Estimates of chlamydial infection in special populations

Testing for chlamydial infection in the high school setting was shown to be feasible in several studies that were conducted in Louisiana, Maryland, and Pennsylvania [27–31]. These studies can be considered in two general categories: school-wide screening and school-based health centers. In school-wide screening, the program was offered to all students who attended the selected high schools [28,29,31]. In contrast, school-based health center studies are essentially clinic-based, and require the presentation of a student to the clinic for care [27,30]. Typically, screening was conducted among students who presented for any condition, regardless of STI-related symptoms. Nevertheless, the clinic-based studies are less comprehensive than studies that use school-wide screening.

The demonstration projects in Louisiana schools have been among the most successful [28,29,31]. In eight Louisiana high schools, among boys, the prevalence of chlamydial infection ranged from 4.3% in 9th grade to 11.4% in 12th grade. Among girls, the prevalence was 8.7% in 9th grade and increased to 14.1% in 12th grade.

School-based studies have provided some of the first assessments of the incidence of chlamydial infection in defined cohorts of adolescents. In the Louisiana program, the incidence of chlamydial infection was consistently higher among girls and ranged from 6.6 to 11.4 cases/1000 persons-months, as compared with 2.1 to 4.5 cases/1000 person-months among boys. The study of adolescent girls in Baltimore schools also provided evidence of high incidence of chlamydial infection. In this group, the estimated incidence was 28.0 cases/1000 person-months. The median duration to a new infection was 6.3 months. The high incidence of chlamydial infection in these studies led to a slight change in the CDC recommendations for chlamydia screening. In 1998, the recommendations were for annual screening of female adolescents [16]; in 2002, the wording was changed slightly to "at least annually" to account for the high frequency of repeat infections in female adolescents [15].

Military recruits are another population that highlights the importance of testing asymptomatic populations and provides insight into the prevalence of chlamydial infection. In a series of papers, the prevalence of chlamydial infection among women and men was assessed [22–24,32]. Among more than 13,000 female military recruits who were older than 17 years of age, the prevalence of chlamydial infection varied dramatically by age; it decreased from 12% among 17-year-olds to less than 2.5% for women who were older than 33 years of age [22]. In these female Army recruits, the prevalence was 14.9% in African Americans and 5.5% among whites. Similar results were observed in a more recent sample of military recruits [23]. In this study, recruits from the South had the highest prevalence of chlamydial infection [23]. Among male recruits, the prevalence of chlamydial infection was considerably lower (5.3%). The prevalence was considerably higher among African Americans (11.9%) than whites (2.8%) [24].

Since 1990, the CDC and Department of Labor have monitored the prevalence of chlamydial infection among young persons who enter the National Job Training Program [25,33]. Most of the youth who enter this program are from socioeconomically disadvantaged families [33]. From 1990 to 1997, the prevalence of chlamydial infection among the young women who entered this program decreased from 14.9% in 1990 to 10.0% in 1997 [33]. In 2003, among the approximately 20,000 youth who entered the program, the prevalence of chlamydial infection was 9.9% among young women and 8.0% among young men.

Reported cases and surveillance for chlamydial infection

As of the year 2000, all 50 states and the District of Columbia must report all cases of chlamydial infection to the CDC. In addition to the issues of bias with reported cases, interpretation of reported incidence data for chlamydial infection is complicated further by the gradual implementation of reporting regulations by different states and the use of multiple tests with differing performance characteristics. The impact of changing tests (eg, from an enzyme immunoassay to an NAAT) can increase incidence estimates substantially [34].

In 2003, 877,478 cases of chlamydial infection were reported to the CDC [35]. The estimated incidence for chlamydial infection based on reported cases was 466.9 cases per 100,000 person-years among women and 134.3 cases per 100,000 person-years among men. The highest rates were among 15- to 19-year-old women (2687.3 per 100,000 person-years; 2.2 cases per 1000 person-months).

Women who attend family planning clinics represent a special population for chlamydial infection surveillance [25]. Among women who attended family planning clinics in all 50 states, the positivity proportion (or approximately the prevalence) was 5.9%.

Symptoms and chlamydial infection

An important observation of these studies is the infrequency of symptoms among persons who live with prevalent infections. The asymptomatic nature of chlamydial infection is especially prominent in the population-based studies, but also is evident in the studies among special populations. In Add Health, less than 5% of persons who had chlamydial infection were symptomatic [21]. Low frequencies of symptoms also were observed in other population-based surveys [10,11].

Generally, chlamydial infection is recognized to have a low intensity of symptoms, but the high frequency of asymptomatic infections that are detected in the general population has several implications. It suggests that a large pool of undetected and undiagnosed chlamydial infection is present in the general population. It seems highly unlikely that relying solely on clinic-based screening is adequate to reach many of these persons, because many young adults do not access health care regularly [36,37]. The high frequency of asymptomatic infections in the general population also leads to several unanswered research questions, such as the transmissibility of these infections and the long-term clinical consequences. These questions are the subject of ongoing investigations.

Chlamydial infection summary

The prevalence of chlamydial infection is unacceptably high among adolescents and young adults in the United States. Population estimates suggest a prevalence of 3% to 4% in the U.S. general population, with higher prevalences in certain regions, especially the South. The prevalence is undoubtedly higher among certain racial and ethnic groups, and in selected populations. The high frequency of asymptomatic disease contributes to the high prevalence.

Gonorrhea

Microbiologic and clinical overview

GC are gram-negative diplococci with several mechanisms to survive in the human host [38]. Gonococci frequently adhere to the surface of polymorphonuclear cells, but often seem to be resistant to phagocytosis. Most gonococci are killed after phagocytosis, but a small percentage can survive intracellularly. Because reinfection with gonococci is common, the immune response is incompletely protective, in part, as a result of the high frequency of changes in the cell-surface antigens of this organism.

The clinical syndromes that are caused by GC are similar to those of Ct, but typically are associated with more purulence. In men, the most common infections include urethritis, proctitis, epididymitis, and prostatitis [39]. Among women, cervicitis and urethritis are the most common manifestations, and may be complicated by salpingitis or endometritis. Disseminated gonococcal infection is a potentially severe and life-threatening complication that can occur in men or women, but more commonly in women. Asymptomatic infection is common, especially among women.

Population-based estimates of the prevalence of gonorrhea

As with chlamydial infection, the advent of NAAT for gonococcal infection led to the first population-based estimates of prevalence. Several of the studies that examined the prevalence of chlamydial infection also reported the prevalence of gonorrhea.

In Add Health, the nationally representative estimate of the prevalence of gonococcal infection was 0.4% (or 4 per 1000 persons) among young adults ages 18 to 26 years [21]. The highest prevalence (0.6%) was in the South. The prevalence among men and women was the same (0.4%). The prevalence of gonococcal infection was substantially higher among African American men (2.4%) and women (1.9%), as compared with whites (0.1% in men and women).

In a population-based survey in Baltimore, the estimated prevalence was considerably higher than most other population-based estimates [10]. Overall, the prevalence was 5.3% among adults aged 18 to 35 years. Among African American women and men, the prevalence was 9.3% and 5.3%, respectively. The prevalence was 1.3% in white men and women.

Estimates of gonorrhea in special populations

The estimates of the prevalence of gonococcal infection in special populations are largely consistent with the national estimate that was obtained in Add Health. Among predominately African American high school students, the prevalence of gonococcal infection was 1.2% in boys and 2.5% in girls [21]. The overall incidence of gonorrhea in this population was 0.7 cases/1000 person-months among boys and 3.6 cases/1000 person-months among girls. In male military recruits, the overall prevalence of gonorrhea was 0.6% [24].

Reported cases and surveillance for gonorrhea

The CDC has monitored the incidence of gonorrhea for several decades. The bias that is associated with reported cases of gonorrhea is likely to be less than for corresponding surveillance for chlamydial infection. One important reason is that gonorrhea is more likely to be symptomatic, especially among men; this leads most persons who have infection to seek health care. Consequently, most infections are likely to be captured as incident infections during a health care visit, rather than become long duration prevalent infections. The potential for bias, however, especially with regard to underreporting, remains because physicians may not complete report cards, and public health clinics may be more likely to report diagnosed infections.

The incidence of gonorrhea has decreased dramatically from a peak of approximately 450 cases/100,000 person-years in the mid-1970s [35]. The rate of decline decreased in the mid-1990s when the rate leveled off at approximately 120 cases/100,000 person-years. The incidence has not decreased significantly since.

In 2003, 335,104 cases of gonorrhea were reported to the CDC; this corresponded to an incidence of 116.2 cases per 100,000 person-years [35]. The incidence was highest in the South (149.8 cases/100,000 person-years). Rates of reported cases were similar among men (113.0 cases/100,000 person-years) and women (118.8 cases/100,000 person-years). The incidence among African Americans was 655.8 cases per 100,000 person-years. Among whites, the rate was 32.7 cases/100,000 person-years; this reflects an increase in the incidence. Since 1999, the incidence has been decreasing consistently among African Americans and increasing among whites.

An interesting use of reported case data for gonorrhea is the spatial representation of cases using geographic information systems. To assess the distribution of cases in a city or county, the addresses of patients who have gonorrhea, their partners, or the venues at which partners were met are "geocoded," or placed on a map using coordinates. The cases are aggregated to a larger geographical unit, such as the zip code or census block. The distribution of disease can be represented as case counts, case density (number of cases over the area), or incidence (number of cases over the number of persons living in the area). Application of these techniques in Baltimore, Maryland [40–42] and in Wake County, North Carolina [43] has provided useful information regarding the core areas of gonorrhea transmission. Such information can be used to target interventions to specific areas with high incidence of disease.

Trichomoniasis

Microbiologic and clinical overview

Tv is a flagellated protozoan that requires culture in liquid or semisolid media. The most common methods for diagnosing trichomoniasis are wet preparation or culture of a urethral or vaginal swab. Although routinely available culture represents a significant advance over wet preparation, these tests have low sensitivity. The recent development of PCR assays for Tv represents a significant advance over culture and wet preparation [44–47]. The ability of the PCR assays to detect Tv in urine or self-collected vaginal swabs has allowed the first assessments of the prevalence of this organism outside of a clinic setting. Unlike Ct and GC, however, the PCR assays for Tv are not approved by the U.S. Food and Drug Administration and have not been standardized.

Clinically, most emphasis has been placed on the vaginitis that is observed in women who have trichomoniasis; however, the difficult to diagnose urethritis that occurs in men is underrecognized. In some clinic-based studies, the prevalence of Tv among men who have symptoms of urethritis rivals the prevalence of gonorrhea or chlamydial infection [48,49]. Tv has been associated strongly with nongonococcal urethritis [49]. Prostatitis may occur as a complication.

In men and women, asymptomatic infections are common [50,51]; however, our understanding of the frequency of asymptomatic trichomoniasis is limited by the use of wet preparation and culture in most clinic-based studies. The low sensitivity of these tests increases the likelihood that infections will not be detected.

Although trichomoniasis often has been considered to be a nuisance infection, recent developments have indicated that it is not a minor STI [52]. Trichomoniasis has been associated with adverse birth outcomes, such as premature rupture of membranes and premature birth [53–56]. Tv also may cause pelvic inflammatory disease [57,58], although the evidence for this association is considerably weaker than with Ct or GC. Tv also may influence the transmission of, and susceptibility to, HIV. Among men who have Tv, the HIV RNA concentration in semen is increased, which suggests an increased risk of transmission [59]. Among women, trichomoniasis increases the number of HIV-receptive cells in the genital tract [60].

Population-based estimates of the prevalence of trichomoniasis

In contrast to chlamydial infection and gonorrhea, few studies of the epidemiology of trichomoniasis have been conducted in settings other than sexually transmitted diseases or other clinic settings. Furthermore, trichomoniasis is not reported to the CDC. Consequently, estimates of incidence that are based on reported cases are not available.

To date, Add Health provides the only population-based estimate of trichomoniasis [61]. Using a PCR assay, the overall prevalence of trichomoniasis in young adults in the United States was 2.3%. The prevalence was slightly higher in women (2.8%) than in men (1.7%). As with the other STIs in this report, the prevalence varied substantially by race/ethnicity. Among African Americans, the prevalence was 10.5% in women and 3.3% in men. Among whites, the prevalence was 1.1% and 1.3% in women and men, respectively.

Estimates of trichomoniasis in special populations

One study in Alabama recruited adolescent women from clinic settings and school health classes to participate in a HIV prevention intervention study [62]. At baseline and at 6-month intervals over the course of the study, Tv was detected using culture of self-collected vaginal swabs. At baseline, the prevalence of Tv was approximately 13% in this cohort of African American female adolescents. The cumulative incidence was 10% over a 12-month period. The frequency of repeat infections was high in this cohort, and occurred in nearly 5% of the girls who returned for follow-up.

Discussion

Estimates of the population burden of STIs are available from several sources. Each source has its advantages and disadvantages, which influence the interpretation and application of the estimates. Recent technologic advances provide new opportunities to assess the epidemiology of STIs.

Historically, reported cases and surveillance activities have provided the primary estimates of the burden of chlamydial infection and gonorrhea, but not trichomoniasis, because trichomoniasis has not been a reportable infection. Although these estimates have some value for monitoring rates over time, several factors affect the validity of the estimates. With chlamydial infection and gonorrhea, reported cases reflect a combination of symptomatic cases, asymptomatic cases detected by screening, and cases detected by contract tracing and referral. Depending on the clinic setting, symptomatic cases may be treated empirically, rather than tested and reported. The policies of clinics and public health agencies for asymptomatic screening and contact referral vary widely, and thereby, influence the likelihood of detecting cases. Furthermore, the specific tests that are used may differ over time. Varying sensitivity is a problem, particularly for Ct, where the common inexpensive assays, such as enzyme immunoassay, are much less sensitive than the NAATs. The influence of the sensitivity of the test on the reported estimates is well-recognized by the CDC [34], and adjustments to reports are made often [25].

The passive surveillance methods that are used for chlamydial infection and gonorrhea depend upon presentation to a medical setting, detection of the infection, and reporting of the infection. Presentation to a medical setting is more complete for symptomatic infections. Consequently, estimates for gonorrhea in men are probably more complete than gonorrhea in women or chlamydial infection overall. In contrast, screening recommendations are in place for chlamydial infection in women, but not in men, so chlamydial infection in men will be underestimated. Finally, a common observation has been that private providers tend to complete reports less commonly than public providers [5]. Implementation of laboratory reporting reduces this disparity to some extent.

Population-based studies overcome most of the biases that are associated with reported case estimates. By developing an appropriate sampling strategy to represent the target population, these studies can provide accurate estimates of the prevalence of STIs in the general population. National estimates require large samples from across the country. Often, the sample size that is needed for a precise estimate (eg, within a specific subgroup) may not be available because the cost to obtain the appropriate sample would be exorbitant. Population-based estimates in more restricted geographic areas have the potential to provide more precise estimates, and potentially greater insight into the local dynamics of the STI epidemiology.

It is important to recognize that population-based studies, and, more generally, community-based studies, are likely to detect predominately asymptomatic and preferentially long-duration infections. Persons who have significant symptoms typically seek care within a few days of onset, which leads to treatment and resolution of the infection. Consequently, those persons who have not been treated are likely to have minimal or no symptoms, and because they did not have a cue to seek care, the duration could be substantially longer.

Prevalence and incidence estimates obtained from special populations are valuable, but require careful interpretation. For example, although military recruits may come from the entire country, they are a highly self-selected group. It is highly unlikely that this group is comparable to a simple random sample of the general population in the same age range. School-based estimates that are obtained in a single geographic area apply to that school, and possibly to other schools in the area; however, it is difficult to conceive an appropriate target population beyond the local area. Overall, it often is difficult to know to whom estimates that are obtained in a special population apply; however, these data are extremely useful in terms of providing information regarding the burden of disease in a specific population and the potential benefit of programs that are targeted to that group.

Summary

The prevalence and incidence of chlamydial infection, gonorrhea, and trichomoniasis are unacceptably high in the United States. The prevalence of gonorrhea is substantially lower than chlamydial infection and trichomoniasis; in part, this is presumably due to the greater frequency of symptomatic disease. The disparity between racial/ethnic groups is considerable for each of these infections. Greater effort must be devoted to reducing this disparity and to understanding the underlying mechanisms of disease persistence in the United States.

Acknowledgments

Support was provided, in part, by the UNC STD Cooperative Research Center (National Institute of Allergy and Infectious Diseases UO131496) and NICHD RO1-39633.

References

[1] Westrom L, Eschenbach D. Pelvic inflammatory disease. In: Holmes KK, Mardh PA, Sparling PF, et al, editors. Sexually transmitted diseases. 3rd edition. New York: McGraw-Hill; 1999. p. 783–809.
[2] Cates W Jr, Wasserheit JN. Genital chlamydial infections: epidemiology and reproductive sequelae. Am J Obstet Gynecol 1991;164:1771–81.
[3] Gonzales GF, Munoz G, Sanchez R, et al. Update on the impact of *Chlamydia trachomatis* infection on male fertility. Andrologia 2004;36:1–23.
[4] Fleming DT, Wasserheit JN. From epidemiological synergy to public health policy and practice: the contribution of other sexually transmitted diseases to sexual transmission of HIV infection. Sex Transm Infect 1999;75:3–17.
[5] St. Lawrence JS, Montano DE, Kasprzyk D, et al. STD screening, testing, case reporting, and clinical and partner notification practices: a national survey of US physicians. Am J Public Health 2002;92:1784–8.
[6] Smucker DR, Thomas JC. Evidence of thorough reporting of sexually transmitted diseases in a southern rural county. Sex Transm Dis 1995;22:149–54.
[7] Ross MW, Courtney P, Dennison J, et al. Incomplete reporting of race and ethnicity in gonorrhoea cases and potential bias in disease reporting by private and public sector providers. Int J STD AIDS 2004;15:778.
[8] Bearman PS, Jones J, Udry JR. The National Longitudinal Study of Adolescent Health: research design. Available at: http://www.cpc.unc.edu/projects/addhealth/design.html. Accessed July 30, 2002.
[9] Resnick MD, Bearman PS, Blum RW, et al. Protecting adolescents from harm: findings from the National Longitudinal Study of Adolescent Health. JAMA 1997;278: 823–32.
[10] Turner CF, Rogers SM, Miller HG, et al. Untreated gonococcal and chlamydial infection in a probability sample of adults. JAMA 2002;287:726–33.

[11] Ku L, Louis MS, Farshy C, et al. Risk behaviors, medical care, and chlamydia infection among young men in the United States. Am J Public Health 2002;92:1140–3.
[12] Schachter J. Biology of *Chlamydia trachomatis*. In: Holmes KK, Sparling PF, Mardh PA, et al, editors. Sexually transmitted diseases. 3rd edition. New York: McGraw-Hill; 1999. p. 391–7.
[13] Stamm WE. *Chlamydia trachomatis* infections of the adult. In: Holmes KK, Sparling PF, Mardh PA, et al, editors. Sexually transmitted diseases. 3rd edition. New York: McGraw-Hill; 1999. p. 407–22.
[14] Centers for Disease Control and Prevention. Recommendations for prevention and management of *Chlamydia trachomatis* infections, 1993. MMWR Morb Mortal Wkly Rep 1993;42(RR-12):1–39.
[15] Centers for Disease Control and Prevention. Sexually transmitted diseases treatment guidelines—2002. MMWR Morb Mortal Wkly Rep 2002;51(RR-6):1–77.
[16] Centers for Disease Control and Prevention. 1998 Guidelines for treatment of sexually transmitted disease. MMWR Morb Mortal Wkly Rep 1998;47(RR-1):1–118.
[17] Hollblad-Fadiman K, Goldman SM. American College of Preventive Medicine Practice Policy Statement: Screening for *Chlamydia trachomatis*. Am J Prev Med 2003;24:287–92.
[18] Nelson HD, Helfand M. Screening for chlamydial infection. Am J Prev Med 2001;20:95–107.
[19] Committee on Practice and Ambulatory Medicine. Recommendations for preventive pediatric health care. Pediatrics 2000;105:645.
[20] American Academy of Family Physicians. Recommendations for periodic health examinations. August 2003. Available at: http://www.aafp.org/PreBuilt/PHErev54.pdf. Accessed October 25, 2003.
[21] Miller WC, Ford CA, Morris M, et al. Prevalence of chlamydial and gonococcal infections among young adults in the United States. JAMA 2004;291:2229–36.
[22] Gaydos CA, Howell MR, Pare B, et al. *Chlamydia trachomatis* infections in female military recruits. N Engl J Med 1998;339:739–44.
[23] Gaydos CA, Howell MR, Quinn TC, et al. Sustained high prevalence of *Chlamydia trachomatis* infections in female army recruits. Sex Transm Dis 2003;30:539–44.
[24] Cecil JA, Howell MR, Tawes JJ, et al. Features of *Chlamydia trachomatis* and *Neisseria gonorrhoeae* infection in male Army recruits. J Infect Dis 2001;184:1216–9.
[25] Centers for Disease Control and Prevention. Sexually transmitted disease surveillance 2003 supplement: Chlamydia Prevalence Monitoring Project. Atlanta (GA): Department of Health and Human Services, Centers for Disease Control and Prevention; 2004.
[26] Rogers SM, Miller HG, Miller WC, et al. NAAT-identified and self-reported gonorrhea and chlamydial infections: different at-risk population subgroups? Sex Transm Dis 2002;29:588–96.
[27] Burstein GR, Waterfield G, Joffe A, et al. Screening for gonorrhea and chlamydia by DNA amplification in adolescents attending middle school health centers: opportunity for early intervention. Sex Transm Dis 1998;25:395–402.
[28] Cohen DA, Nsuami M, Etame RB, et al. A school-based chlamydia control program using DNA amplification technology. Pediatrics 1998;101:E1.
[29] Cohen DA, Nsuami M, Martin DH, et al. Repeated school-based screening for sexually transmitted diseases: a feasible strategy for reaching adolescents. Pediatrics 1999;104:1281–5.
[30] Wiesenfeld HC, Lowry DL, Heine RP, et al. Self-collection of vaginal swabs for the detection of chlamydia, gonorrhea, and trichomoniasis: opportunity to encourage sexually transmitted disease testing among adolescents. Sex Transm Dis 2001;28:321–5.
[31] Nsuami M, Cohen DA. Participation in a school-based sexually transmitted disease screening program. Sex Transm Dis 2000;27:473–9.
[32] Arcari CM, Gaydos JC, Howell MR, et al. Feasibility and short-term impact of linked education and urine screening interventions for chlamydia and gonorrhea in male army recruits. Sex Transm Dis 2004;31:443–7.

[33] Mertz KJ, Ransom RL, St Louis ME, et al. Prevalence of genital chlamydial infection in young women entering a national job training program, 1990–1997. Am J Public Health 2001;91:1287–90.
[34] Dicker LW, Mosure DJ, Levine WC, et al. Impact of switching laboratory tests on reported trends in *Chlamydia trachomatis* infections. Am J Epidemiol 2000;151:430–5.
[35] Centers for Disease Control and Prevention. Sexually transmitted disease surveillance, 2003. Atlanta (GA): US Department of Health and Human Services, Centers for Disease Control and Prevention; 2004.
[36] Quinn K, Schoen C, Buatti L. On their own, young adults living without health insurance. Available at: http://www.cmwf.org/usr_doc/quinn_ya_391.pdf. Accessed December 15, 2004.
[37] Sandman D, Simantov E, An C. Out of touch: American men and the health care system—Commonwealth Fund men's and women's health survey findings. Available at: http://www.cmwf.org/usr_doc/sandman_outoftouch_374.pdf. Accessed December 15, 2004.
[38] Sparling PF. Biology of *Neisseria gonorrhoeae*. In: Holmes KK, Sparling PF, Mardh PA, et al, editors. Sexually transmitted diseases. 3rd edition. New York: McGraw-Hill; 1999. p. 433–49.
[39] Hook EW III, Handsfield HH. Gonococcal infections in the adult. In: Holmes KK, Sparling PF, Mardh PA, et al, editors. Sexually Transmitted Diseases. 3rd edition. New York: McGraw-Hill; 1999. p. 451–66.
[40] Bernstein KT, Curriero FC, Jennings JM, et al. Defining core gonorrhea transmission utilizing spatial data. Am J Epidemiol 2004;160:51–8.
[41] Zenilman JM, Ellish N, Fresia A, et al. The geography of sexual partnerships in Baltimore: applications of core theory dynamics using a geographic information system. Sex Transm Dis 1999;26:75–81.
[42] Becker KM, Glass GE, Brathwaite W, et al. Geographic epidemiology of gonorrhea in Baltimore, Maryland, using a geographic information system. Am J Epidemiol 1998;147:709–16.
[43] Law DC, Serre ML, Christakos G, et al. Spatial analysis and mapping of sexually transmitted diseases to optimise intervention and prevention strategies. Sex Transm Infect 2004;80:294–9.
[44] Kaydos SC, Swygard H, Wise SL, et al. Development and validation of a PCR enzyme-linked immunosorbent assay with urine for use in clinical research settings to detect *Trichomonas vaginalis* in women. J Clin Microbiol 2002;40:89–95.
[45] Kaydos-Daniels SC, Miller WC, Hoffman I, et al. Validation of a urine-based PCR-enzyme-linked immunosorbent assay for use in clinical research settings to detect *Trichomonas vaginalis* in men. J Clin Microbiol 2003;41:318–23.
[46] Hardick J, Yang S, Lin S, et al. Use of the Roche LightCycler instrument in a real-time PCR for *Trichomonas vaginalis* in urine samples from females and males. J Clin Microbiol 2003;41:5619–22.
[47] Wendel KA, Erbelding EJ, Gaydos CA, et al. *Trichomonas vaginalis* polymerase chain reaction compared with standard diagnostic and therapeutic protocols for detection and treatment of vaginal trichomoniasis. Clin Infect Dis 2002;35:576–80.
[48] Joyner JL, Douglas JM, Ragsdale S, et al. Comparative prevalence of infection with *Trichomonas vaginalis* among men attending a sexually transmitted diseases clinic. 2000. Sex Transm Dis 2000;27:236–40.
[49] Krieger JN, Jenny C, Verdon M, et al. Clinical manifestations of trichomoniasis in men. Ann Intern Med 1993;118:844–9.
[50] Jackson DJ, Rakwar JP, Bwayo JJ, et al. Urethral *Trichomonas vaginalis* infection and HIV-1 transmission [letter]. Lancet 1997;350:1076.
[51] Paxton LA, Sewankambo N, Gray R, et al. Asymptomatic non-ulcerative genital tract infections in a rural Ugandan population. Sex Transm Infect 1998;74:421–5.

[52] Hook EW III. Trichomonas vaginalis–no longer a minor STD [letter]. Sex Transm Dis 1999; 26:388–9.
[53] Minkoff H, Grunebaum A, Schwarz R, et al. Risk factors for prematurity and premature rupture of membranes: a prospective study of the vaginal flora in pregnancy. Am J Obstet Gynecol 1984;150:965–72.
[54] Cotch MF, Pastorek JG II, Nugent RP, et al. Demographic and behavioral predictors of *Trichomonas vaginalis* infection among pregnant women. Obstet Gynecol 1991;78:1087–92.
[55] Cotch MF, Pastorek JG II, Nugent RP, et al. *Trichomonas vaginalis* associated with low birth weight and preterm delivery. The Vaginal Infections and Prematurity Study Group. Sex Transm Dis 1997;24:353–60.
[56] Read J, Klebanoff M. Sexual intercourse during pregnancy and preterm delivery: effects of vaginal microorganisms. The Vaginal Infections and Prematurity Study Group. Am J Obstet Gynecol 1993;168:514–9.
[57] Moodley P, Wilkinson D, Connolly C, et al. *Trichomonas vaginalis* is associated with pelvic inflammatory disease in women infected with human immunodeficiency virus. Clin Infect Dis 2002;34:519–22.
[58] Hoosen AA, Quinlan DJ, Moodley J, et al. Sexually transmitted pathogens in acute pelvic inflammatory disease. S Afr Med J 1989;76:251–4.
[59] Hobbs MM, Kazembe P, Reed AW, et al. *Trichomonas vaginalis* as a cause of urethritis in Malawian men. Sex Transm Dis 1999;26:381–7.
[60] Levine WC, Pope V, Bhoomaker A, et al. Increase in endocervical CD4 lymphocytes among women with nonulceratvie sexually transmitted diseases. J Infect Dis 1998;177:167–74.
[61] Miller WC, Swygard H, Hobbs MM, et al. The prevalence of trichomoniasis in young adults in the United States. Sex Transm Dis 2005, in press.
[62] Crosby R, DiClemente RJ, Wingood GM, et al. Predictors of infection with *Trichomonas vaginalis*: a prospective study of low income African-American adolescent females. Sex Transm Infect 2002;78:360–4.

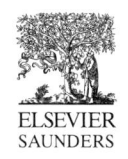

Modern Day Influences on Sexual Behavior

Sevgi O. Aral, PhD, MSc, MA[a,*], Helen Ward, MB ChB, FFPHM, MSc[b]

[a]*Division of STD Prevention, National Centers for HIV, STD and TB Prevention, Centers for Disease Control and Prevention, 1600 Clifton Road, Mailstop E-02, Atlanta, GA 30333, USA*
[b]*School of Medicine, Imperial College of Science Technology and Medicine, London W2 1PG, UK*

Understanding sexual behavior is key to the effective prevention planning of sexually transmitted diseases (STDs) and developing effective intervention programs. As a social activity, sex and the activities that surround it, are linked intimately to the society and the context in which they occur. Sexual partnerships, and the factors that are related to their creation and dissolution, have received particular interest as a key determinant of STD risk. Sexual risk and partnership development patterns respond to societal economic, sociologic, political and technologic change. This article explores these patterns and relationships.

Recent years have brought unprecedented changes to human life and its physical, social, and economic context. Given the increased interconnectedness of populations, people all over the world are impacted, at least in part, by events that take place in a local area. Over the past few decades, globally, societal evolution has included several interrelated processes of change. Among these processes are increasing levels of inequality within countries; growing inequality between countries; increased levels of globalization; increased proportions (and numbers) of people who live in cultures in which they were not born; an increased proportion of the world population living in postconflict/postwar societies; and a declining demand for low skilled labor which has a major impact on the life conditions of the lower classes in all countries [1]. Technologic changes and related changes in public health and medicine have resulted in the interconnected and parallel

---

* Corresponding author.
E-mail address: saral@cdc.gov (S.O. Aral).

changes that are known as the "demographic transition" and the "epidemiologic transition" [1]. In predicting the impact of these changes on the pattern of disease, Mosley and colleagues [2] considered the effects of the demographic transition, the epidemiologic transition, changing risk environments, and the widening gap in health problems and health needs across social and economic classes; together, these changes were termed the "health transition." In this model, the demographic transition leads to declining infectious disease mortality, declining fertility, and an aging population; the epidemiologic transition leads to the emergence and increase of chronic and noncommunicable diseases; and the protracted-polarized epidemiologic transition leads to the persistence or re-emergence of communicable diseases as a result of economic recession and increasing inequality (Fig. 1). The health transition model was adopted to address the evolution of STD epidemics [1]. The STD health transition model suggests that future decades may witness increases in viral STDs and the persistence and re-emergence of viral STDs.

These earlier analyses of the potential impact of social, economic, political, and demographic changes on the incidence and prevalence of sexually transmitted infections largely have been based locally, and particular attention was not paid to wide scale changes in sexual behavior and its determinants. This article briefly reviews what is known about "globalization" and "the second demographic transition," and explores their effects on the structure of marriage and the family and values,

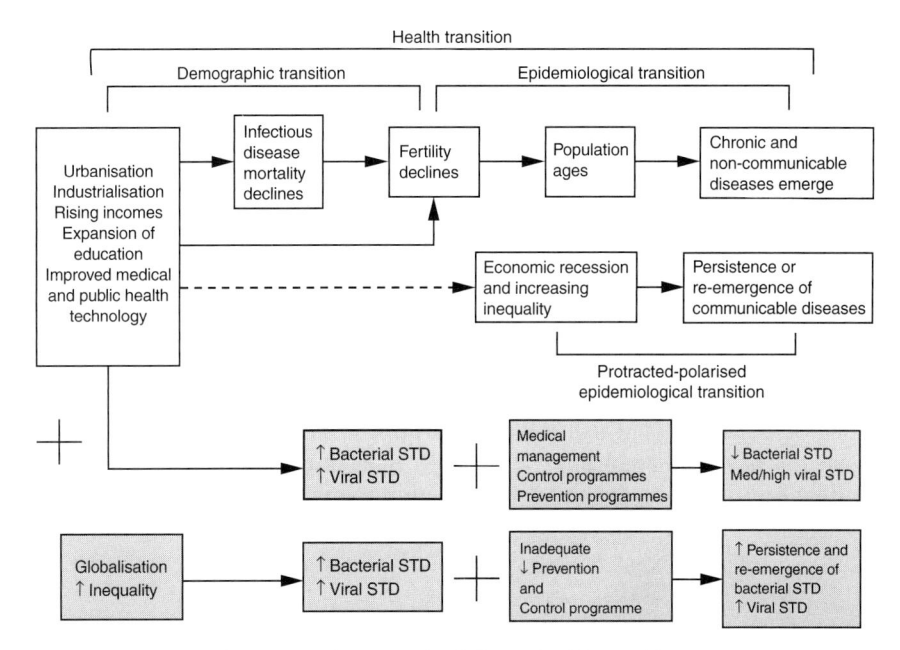

Fig. 1. Sexually transmitted disease health transition.

attitudes, and expectations. The recent data on changes in technologies that are relevant to sexual behavior, mental health, and childhood sexual abuse (CSA) are described as they relate to sexual behaviors and some recent findings on changes in sexual behavior. The discussion refers predominantly to the changes that have observed in the United States and the United Kingdom, but similar trends are observable in other Western industrialized countries.

The global socio-political and economic structure

The past few decades have witnessed major political, technologic, and economic shifts, all of which have the potential to impact on sexual behavior, sexual risk taking, and partner mixing. Included among these are the breakdowns of the Berlin wall, the opening of China to the rest of the world, the establishment of democracy in South Africa, the information revolution, and the emergence of the global economy (or the globalization of capitalism) [1,3]. In Europe, a related dramatic change involved the demise of the former state socialist economics through a combination of internal collapse, popular unrest, and external pressure [4]. The old regimes were marked by no democracy, heavy repression, and limited opportunities; however, there were jobs and incomes for most people, and extensive, if poor quality, social provision of schools, childcare, and health services [4]. These factors combined to mitigate STD risk, albeit at a cost that was unacceptable to democratic societies. In these countries, secure employment has disappeared and women particularly have been affected by unemployment.

Globalization has been a particularly controversial issue. Globalization may be defined as a change in the nature of human interaction across economic, social, political, technologic, and environmental spheres [1,5]. The change often is defined in three dimensions: spatial, temporal, and cognitive. In the spatial dimension, globalization encompasses vast increases in communication and transportation and the resulting shared experiences. In the temporal dimension, globalization refers to decreases in the actual and perceived time that is required or allowed for human activity to occur. In the cognitive dimension, globalization includes the globalized production of knowledge, ideas, beliefs, and values. In everyday experience, the contraction in the spatial dimension often is experienced as "the small world"; the contraction in the temporal dimension, as an accelerated time frame; and the changes in cognitive processes reflect themselves in homogenizing cognitive processes.

More recently, Stiglitz [3] defined globalization as the "closer integration of the countries and peoples of the world which has been brought about by the reduction of costs of transportation and communication, and the breaking down of artificial barriers to the flows of goods, services, capital, knowledge, and to a lesser extent, people across borders." This process is driven by international corporations that move capital, goods, and technology across borders and has renewed attention to intergovernmental institutions, such as the United Nations and the World Health Organization. Although many aspects of globalization have been welcomed throughout the world, economic aspects of globalization have created concern and controversy. Economic globalization involved the collapse of national regulatory frameworks and an increase in international trade and investment. Policies of the World Bank and International Monetary Fund in developing countries ensured production for export and a decrease in public spending in many, and especially, the poorest countries. Consequently, agriculture and factories that produce commodities for export expanded, whereas subsistence production disappeared. In this current system, capital can be—and is—moved anywhere in the world to find the cheapest production costs. For example, textile production has declined significantly in Europe and North America as production shifted to Latin America and Asia [3]. Recently, communication jobs have been exported from the United States and United Kingdom as massive telephone service centers have been created in India. Increasing mobility among workers mirrors the mobility of capital; however, in general, population mobility brings with it potential for social, cultural, political, and behavioral problems inequities, that, in turn, can increase sexual risk-taking behavior.

In Western Europe, large-scale manufacturing has declined together with the secure, long-term employment that characterized the decades after the Second World War. Job security is reduced markedly, more people work part-time and on temporary contracts, and social welfare entitlements have been cut. Economic inequalities have increased and the structure of employment has changed. Similar changes have been observed in the United States. For example, in early 2005, there have been multiple pension system defaults, especially in the airline and steel industries, and major structural and funding changes have been proposed for the social security system. Macrolevel changes in economic and social patterns can have a major impact on structure of sexual partnerships; on the formation, maintenance, and dissolution of marriages; on the family institution, and consequently, sexual behaviors. These, in turn, affect disease risk and transmission patterns.

Demography and its impact

The demographic transitions

The Industrial Revolution and ascent of science and technology, two centuries ago, dramatically reduced disease and famine in Europe and North America, led to reduced mortality, and triggered a sustained and unprecedented growth in population. This was followed by declines in fertility. This change in mortality, fertility, and population growth is termed "the first demographic transition" (Fig. 2). According to United Nations' projections, the global demographic transition will end by 2050. Current estimates suggest that demographic growth rates are declining nearly everywhere, even more rapidly than was projected earlier [6]. Regional growth rates differ, but international migration redistributes a considerable portion of the continuing natural increase [7]. According to United Nations' estimates, even regions that were late in joining the world demographic transition will undergo declines from high mortality and high fertility to low mortality and low fertility by the middle of the twenty-first century. Ultimately, as the age distribution stabilizes, "zero population growth" will follow the global demographic transition.

During the first demographic transition, as societies moved from the preindustrial stage through the transitional and industrial stages, they experienced rapid, slow, and zero growth, respectively. The United States and the United Kingdom (and most of Europe) currently are in the postindustrial stage, which is marked by below replacement fertility levels, aging populations, and decreasing population size. By 1991, 18 European countries had reached or were close to zero population growth; Germany and Hungary were experiencing population declines [8]. Without external factors, STD rates would decrease.

The postindustrial stage in the demographic transition has been called "the second demographic transition" [8]. It is defined by an unexpected low level of fertility; below replacement, which results in disequilibrium between mortality and fertility rates and declining population size; and a compensatory trend in migration patterns (Fig. 3; Table 1). The demographic mechanisms of action that are involved in the second demographic transition are multiple and multidimensional. They include, in addition to

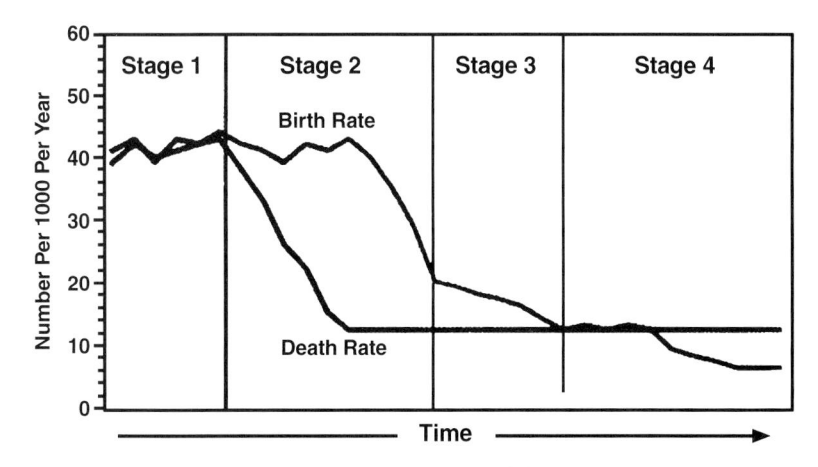

Fig. 2. Demographic transition.

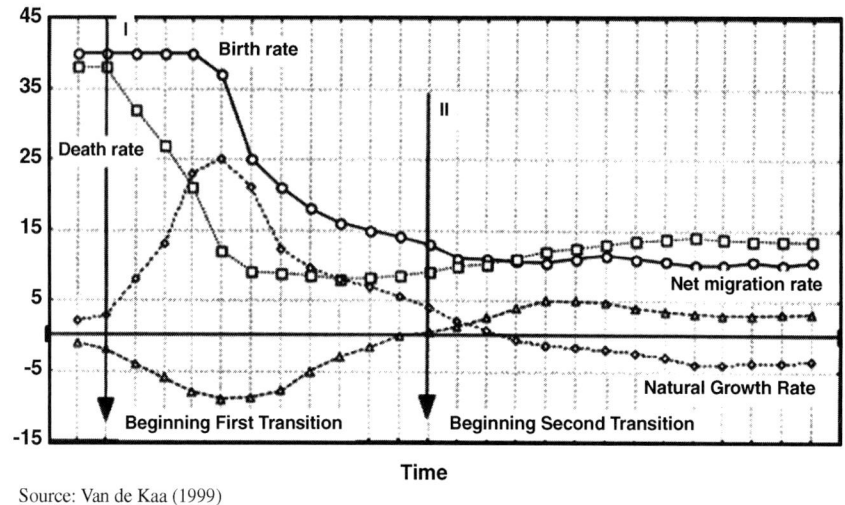

Fig. 3. Second demographic transition. (*From* Van de Kaa DJ. Europe and its populations: the long view. In: Van de Kaa DJ, Leridon H, Gesano G, et al, editors. European populations: unity in diversity. Dordrecht, Netherlands: Kluwer Academic Publishers. p. 1–194.

large decreases in period and cohort fertility, decreases in the total first marriage rate; strong and large increases in mean age at marriage and childbearing; divorce and union dissolution; cohabitation; proportion of extramarital births; and maternal employment [9–13]. Empiric patterns in these demographic parameters are explored (see later discussion).

Table 1
Evidence for the second demographic transition. Industrialized countries by date below replacement fertility was first experienced

On/before 1965	Idem 1970	Idem 1975	Idem 1980	Idem 1985	Idem 1990	Idem 1995
Japan	Germany	Austria	Italy	Iceland	Macedonia	Ireland
Hungary	Denmark	Belgium	Bosnia-II	Spain	Yugoslavia	Moldova
Latvia	Finland	France	Bulgaria	Greece	Poland	
	Luxembourg	Norway	Lithuania	Portugal	Romania	
	Sweden	Netherlands	Belarus	Slovenia	Slovak R.	
	Czech R.	United Kingdom	Australia			
	Croatia	Switzerland	New-Zealand			
	Russia	Estonia	Canada			
	Ukraine	United States				

Data from Frejka T, Ross J. Paths to subreplacement fertility: the empirical evidence. In: Bulatao RA, Casterline JB, editors. Global fertility transition, supplement to PDR, vol. 27. New York: Population Council; 2001. p. 213–55; and Council of Europe. Recent demographic developments in Europe 2000. Strasbourg: Council of Europe Publishing; 2000.

International migration plays an important role in redistributing population from low-income countries with high population growth to high-income countries with low or negative population growth. During the past 2 decades, economic, social, and demographic changes promoted migration into and within Western Europe. In the early 1990s, there was considerable migration from Eastern to Western Europe; however, in the mid-1990s, restrictions on movement were introduced and the migrations slowed considerably [14]. During the 1990s, migration from Asia, sub-Saharan Africa, and Central and Latin America to Western Europe also increased. In the early 1990s, there was a net in migration of people at the rate of 3.1 per 1000 population for the European Economic Area; this decreased to 1.7 per 1000 in 1995–1999, and increased to 2.5 per 1000 in 2000. These official data exclude those who enter as visitors or students [4].

Toward the end of the 1990s and in the early 2000s there has been a sharp increase in employment-related migration into Western Europe. This trend is due to growing skills shortages in many European countries. An increasing proportion of the migrants who are entering Western Europe is women. These migration patterns may be related to the increasing proportion of foreigners among sex workers. Many people enter Western Europe with the right to study and work; others enter as tourists or illegally. Economic survival can be difficult for all of these groups, especially during downturns in the economic cycle when they would be the first to be laid off. Consequently, some choose sex work; others may be coerced into the sex industry [4]. Openings are restricted for migrants with the right to work because of a host of social and other barriers. Official statistics show that legal migrants have higher rates of unemployment than nationals, and migrant women are more likely to be unemployed than men [14]. For example, in Belgium, 16.5% of migrant women are unemployed compared with 7.0% of nationals; these proportions are 13.0% versus 4.6% and 21.3% versus 13.9% in Sweden and Italy, respectively. People without the right to work have even fewer options. Lack of legal papers forces them into the informal economy. Some of these people enter the sex industry; others work in low-level manufacturing and service occupations, such as entry level jobs in catering, hotels, and domestic service.

Migration into the United States also has increased over the past 2 decades. Although the United States is the recipient of migration streams from a large and increasing number of countries, illegal migration from Mexico apparently constitutes the largest stream of persons who enter the informal economy in large numbers.

Moreover, in 1999, the rate of immigration for most countries that were experiencing the second demographic transition was positive and between 0.2% and 0.5% or more [8]. An interesting feature of the second demographic transition is that there often are large demographic mismatches by gender. For example, early immigration from developing to developed countries often involves predominantly younger men who are seeking jobs with the objective of sending wages home to their spouse, family, or community of origin. This situation can lead to an inequality between the number of available and female partners, which, in turn, leads to development of a commercial sex industry to service the unpartnered male population. STD transmission within these networks can be extremely efficient.

Changes in the structure of marriage and the family

According to Frejka and Calot [9], the structure of marriage and the family has been undergoing major change in industrialized countries since the beginning of the 1970s. Mean age at marriage and mean age at childbearing have been increasing—by an average of 2 years in some places. Similar increases have been observed in the United States. The total divorce rate is approximately or greater than 30 per 100 marriages in most industrialized countries and has increased between 1980 and 1999 [9].

In Europe, many women choose not to marry, and their average age at the time of first marriage is increasing. Marriage is increasingly less popular; the marriage rate decreased by 40% from 1960 to 1995 [15]. Among those who do get married, 1 in 3 now divorce, compared with 1 in 15 during the 1960s. The number of children born to a woman has declined and stabilized at 1.42, and more of these children are born later in a woman's life [15]. With a decline in marriage and an increase in divorce, household structures have changed. From 1981 to 1996 in urban centers in Europe, the size of the average household declined from 2.8 persons to 2.3 persons; the number of people living alone increased from 27% to 38%; and the proportion of lone parent households increased from 6.5% to 7.5% [16]. More people now live in a variety of household arrangements: single people with friends or children, gay couples and friends, and stepfamilies.

Similar trends are observed in the United States; the percentage of men and women ages 15 and older who were married declined from 69.3% and 65.9% in 1960 to 57.1% and 54% in 2003, respectively [17], Conversely, over the same time period, the percentage of men and women aged 15 and older who were divorced increased from 1.8% and 2.6% to 8.3% and 10.9%, respectively [17]. Traditionally, family households had predominated in the United States—81% of all households in 1970 were family households; however, this proportion dropped to 68% by 2003 [18].

Changes in values, attitudes, and expectations

The demographic shifts of the second demographic transition were accompanied by large-scale changes in values and attitudes. Emphasis on values, such as individual autonomy, self-fulfillment, tolerance, democratic decision-making, individual freedoms, and individual rights increased [19]. Minimally acceptable standards for partnership quality were raised and consumerism and market orientation expanded. These shifts in values and attitudes coincided with the changing role of women in society, and perhaps more importantly, with women's changing expectations. Women now are less likely to stay in abusive or unhappy marriages; they assume that they have equal rights to education and work outside of the home, and expect an enjoyable sex life with control over their fertility [4].

The second demographic transition also was accompanied by major ideational and cultural shifts that occurred since the mid-1960s. These include the shift from the golden age of marriage to the dawn of cohabitation, and that from the "king-child" with parents to the "king-pair" with or without child, which underscores the disinvestment in children. There was the move from the nuclear family to pluralistic family and households and a shift in contraceptive practices to where contraception is the norm, and conception is the exception [19].

The impact of hierarchy

Hardly any phenomenon is experienced similarly by all socioeconomic strata in stratified societies; the second demographic transition is no exception. A recent analysis of the transition in the United States showed that it is not homogeneous across social strata [20]. It seems that increases in mother's age at childbirth have been greater among high and middle education groups than among low education groups. Similarly, increases in mothers' employment were greater among those with more education. Conversely, single motherhood was more prevalent among groups with low levels of education and has not increased much among those with high levels of education. Finally, divorce also was more prevalent and increasing among those without a college degree and was less prevalent and decreasing among those with a college degree.

Patterns similar to those described above are observed in many other countries that are going through the second demographic transition. These socio-demographic patterns suggest that existing inequalities may be reproducing and leading to even greater disparities between the upper and lower strata in industrialized populations.

Technology and its consequences

Rapid technologic developments, such as the Internet and cell phone communication, have significant impact on the ways in which people relate to each other—as acquaintances, friends, colleagues, family members, or sex partners. Both technologies have functioned to collapse time and space by making it possible for people to "hook up" with each other, independent of time and space. Cell phones have made it possible for adolescents to communicate with friends without parents' knowledge.

The effect of the Internet on sexual behavior is still evolving. The extent of its use by distinct groups of people, for specific purposes, is not known.

An increasing number of people apparently use the Internet to find dates and potential marriage partners, and an increasing number of people use it to identify one-time partners. Internet-based sex partner recruitment facilitates purposive, conscious sexual mixing. Some websites, such as the "Right Stuff" or "Latin Singles," are open only to members of particular subgroups and facilitate assortative mixing (ie, partnering individuals from similar backgrounds). Other websites, for example,www.interracialmatch.com, selectively serve people who are interested in disassortative mixing. Whether the impact of increased purposive mixing will change the sexual mixing patterns of Americans significantly remains to be seen.

It is not known whether Internet use for sex partner recruitment is gender selective. Based on reports in the popular media, women account for more than a quarter of all visitors to websites with adult content; more than 10 million women logged on to such sites during the month of December 2003. Online purchases of sex toys by women apparently soared in the past 4 years, perhaps as a result of changing expectations about sex and the privacy this is provided by the Internet.

Mental health and childhood sexual abuse

In recent years, mental disorders and CSA have emerged as important factors that may influence sexual behavior [21]. By now, it is clear that CSA and mental disorders have remarkably high prevalence levels. A recent study found that the prevalence of various mental disorders are twofold to fivefold higher in populations that are seen at STD clinics than in the community [22]. It is important to explore the evolutionary dynamics of this association which may be causal, or it may be an artifact of the demographic composition of the study population. Mental disorders, often socially constructed themselves, tend to be more prevalent among racial ethnic minorities and among subpopulations with lower socioeconomic status [21].

A recent review suggests that the estimated prevalence of CSA (ever) among American women ranges from 8% to 62% in convenience samples and from 8% to 27% in representative samples [23]. Even after estimates are adjusted for response errors, prevalence ranges between 12% and 17%. Girls were up to five times more likely to report sexual abuse than boys. There were no major differences in reports of sexual abuse by race or ethnicity.

The prevalence of CSA is considerably higher among HIV-infected women [23]. Nine studies explored this association; they found that 31% to 53% of HIV-infected women reported CSA. Prevalence of CSA also is high among matched controls to HIV-infected women; this supports the importance of the relationship between CSA and HIV risk characteristics.

The exact nature of the associations between sexual behavior, mental disorders, and CSA are not yet understood, and neither are the mechanisms of action through which these parameters may influence sexual behavior. It is clear that mental health disorders and CSA figure importantly in sexual behaviors. Whether the socio-political context in which we live—marked by terrorism, war, and economic and political upheaval—will have further negative effects on mental disorders and CSA remains to be seen.

Impact on sexual behaviors: demographics, changes, mobility, and technology

Data collected between 1995 and 1997 in Chicago showed that in the mid-1990s, Americans ages 18 to 59 spent 50% of their lives as singles, longer than ever before; were in the market for a sex partner for longer periods and at older ages; cohabited on the average of 4 years; were married for an average of 18 years; and dated or searched for a partner for an average of 19 years [24]. These data also showed that sexual activity was no longer coupled with marriage and that weak institutional controls, moral heterogeneity, and atomization surrounded sexual behaviors. Sex partner markets were embedded in networks and social space and the structure of opportunities in sex markets varied over the life course.

Technology-based sex partner recruitment continues to change sexual behavior patterns. In the late 1980s and early 1990s, cell phones began to transform the social organization of sex work in London; in big cities in Russia, and elsewhere, the remarkable growth of cyber brothels changed the way in which sexual services are provided [25–27]; and chat rooms have provided a powerful mechanism for connecting men who have sex with men with each other, in contracted time and space [28].

Thus, the impact of the second demographic transition in the United States involves an increase in the number of persons who are at risk for nonmutually monogamous sex partnerships; a lengthening of the duration of time that the average person spends at risk for nonmutually monogamous sex partnerships—before, after, during marriage and in between marriages; and an increase in heterogeneity of sexual expression.

Data from the United Kingdom suggest that there and elsewhere in Europe, similar changes in sexual behavior are taking place. A large survey in the United Kingdom found that 43.7% of all men were single or previously married [29]. This group accounted for 81% of new sex partnerships that were formed by men. Similar proportions—77.8% of new partnerships—were formed by 37.6% of women. Two surveys found an increase from 1990 to 2000 in the numbers of heterosexual partners, the proportion who reported homosexual partnerships, and the numbers of concurrent partnerships; young people were having their first sexual experiences at an earlier age than 10 years previously [29].

Other changes reported from the United Kingdom involve the sex industry and lesbian, gay, bisexual, and transgender people. Over the recent decades, the size of the sex industry apparently increased. The numbers of men who reported having paid women for sex in the previous 5 years doubled from 2.1% in 1990 to 4.3% in 2000. Because of greater numbers of workers and clients the sex industry also diversified, and the services it provides became more specialized [4]. The use of mobile phones and personal websites slowly modify the organization of the industry. Lesbian, gay, bisexual, and transgender people are more open about their sexuality and demand respect and an end to repression.

Summary

To better understand temporal trends in sexual behavior and their determinants, it is important to look at the demographic and technologic context in which we live; both affect sexual behaviors. Mental disorders and CSA emerge as important correlates of high-risk sexual behaviors. The changing role and expectations of women—the result of major economic and social transformation—transform society further through changes to family and community structures. These changes occur alongside increasing inequality and upheavals in the world, all of which are more visible through increased mobility and communication in the "global village." Changes in sexual norms, relationships, abuse, and mental health are better understood in the context of this broad political background.

Acknowledgments

The authors thank Patricia Jackson and Melanie Ross for their outstanding support in the preparation of this article.

References

[1] Aral SO. Determinants of STD epidemics: implications for phase appropriate intervention strategies. Sex Transm Infect 2002;78(Suppl 1):i3–13.
[2] Mosley WH, Bobadilla JL, Jamison DT. The health transition: implications for health policy in developing countries. In: Jamison DT, Mosley WH, Meashem AR, et al, editors. Disease control priorities in developing countries. Oxford (UK): Oxford University Press; 1993. p. 673–99.
[3] Stiglitz JE. Globalization and its discontents. New York: WW Norton and Company Inc.; 2002.
[4] Ward H, Day S. Sex work in context. Sex work, mobility and health in Europe. London: Kegan Paul; 2004.
[5] Jolly R. Global inequalities prospects and challenges for the 21st century. Presented at the 9th Annual Public Health Forum, London School of Hygiene and Tropical Medicine, London, April 1999.
[6] United Nations 2001 World Population Prospects: The 2000 revision. Volume 1: comprehensive tables. New York: United Nations Department of Economic and Social Affairs; 2001.
[7] Harbison SF, Robinson WC. Policy implications of the next world demographic transition. Stud Fam Plann 2002;33(1):37–48.

[8] van de Kaa D. Europe's second demographic transition. Popul Bull 1987;42(1):1–59.
[9] Frejka T, Calot G. Cohort reproductive patterns in low-fertility countries. Popul Dev Rev 2001;27(1):103–32.
[10] UNECE. Fertility decline in the transition economics, 1989–1998: economic and social factors revisited. Economic Survey of Europe 2000;1:189–207.
[11] Halman L. The European values study—a third wave. Tilburg, Germany: WORC Tilburg University; 2001.
[12] Dalla Zuana G, Atoh M, Castiglioni M, et al. Late marriage among young people: the case of Italy and Japan. Genus 1997;53(3–4):187–232.
[13] Pena JA, Alfonso-Sanchez MA, Calderon R. Inbreeding and demographic transition in the Orozco Valley (Basque Country, Spain). Am J Human Biol 2002;14:713–20.
[14] Organisation for Economic Co-operation and Development. Trends in international migration annual report. 2002 edition. Paris: OECD Publications; 2003.
[15] MISSOC. Family benefits and family policies in Europe. Missoc-Info 01/2002, European Commission Directorate-General for Employment and Social Affairs. Available at: http://europa.eu.int/comm/employment_social/missoc. Accessed April 2004.
[16] European Commission. The Urban Audit. Towards the benchmarking of quality of life in 58 European cities. Luxembourg: Office for Official Publications of the European Communities; 2000.
[17] America's families and living arrangements: 2003. U.S. Census Bureau, Annual Social and Economic Supplement: 2003 Current Population Survey, Current Population Reports, Series. p. 20–553.
[18] U.S. Census Bureau America's Families and Living Arrangements: 2003. Washington, DC: U.S. Department of Commerce Economics and Statistics Administration; 2004.
[19] Lesthaeghe R, Moors G. Life course transitions and value orientations: selection and adaptation. In: Lesthaeghe R, editor. Meaning and choice—value orientations and life course decisions, NIDI-CBGS Monograph No. 37. The Hague (Netherlands): Netherlands Interdisciplinary Demographic Institute; 2002. p. 1–44.
[20] Marcia C, McLanahan S. Poverty and gender in highly industrialized nations. In: McLanahan SS, Carlson MJ, editors. International encyclopedia of the social and behavioral sciences. Oxford (UK): Elsevier Science Limited; 2001.
[21] Aral SO. Editorial response: mental health: a powerful predictor of sexual health? Sex Transm Dis 2004;31(1):13–4.
[22] Erbelding EJ, Hutton HE, Zenilman JM, et al. The prevalence of psychiatric disorders in STD clinic patients and their association with STD risk. Sex Transm Dis 2003;31:8–12.
[23] Koenig LJ, Doll LS, O'Leary A, et al, editors. From child sexual abuse to adult sexual risk: trauma, revictimization, and intervention. Washington, DC: American Psychological Association; 2004.
[24] Laumann EO, Ellingson S, Mahay J, et al. The sexual organization of the city. Chicago: University of Chicago Press; 2004.
[25] Aral SO, St. Lawrence JS, Tikhonova L, et al. The social organization of commercial sex work in Moscow, Russia. Sex Transm Dis 2003;30(1):39–45.
[26] Aral SO, St. Lawrence JS. The ecology of sex work and drug use in Saratov Oblast, Russia. Sex Transm Dis 2002;29(12):798–805.
[27] Aral SO, St. Lawrence JS, Dyatlov R, et al. Commercial sex work, drug use, and sexually transmitted infections in St. Petersburg, Russia. Soc Sci Med 2005;60:2181–90.
[28] Bull S, McFarlane M. HIV and sexually transmitted infection risk behaviors among men who have sex with men on-line. Am J Public Health 2001;91:988–9.
[29] Johnson AM, Mercer CH, Erens B, et al. Sexual behaviour in Britain: partnerships, practices, and HIV risk behaviours. Lancet 2001;358:1835–69.

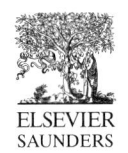

Increasing Rates of Sexually Transmitted Diseases in Homosexual Men in Western Europe and the United States: Why?

Kevin A. Fenton, MD, PhD[a,b,]*, John Imrie, PhD[c]

[a]*Division of STD Prevention, National Centers for HIV, STD and TB Prevention, Centers for Disease Control and Prevention (CDC), 1600 Clifton Road, Mailstop E02, Atlanta, GA 30333, USA*
[b]*HIV/STI Department, Health Protection Agency Centre for Infections, 61 Colindale Avenue, London NW9 5EQ, UK*
[c]*Centre for Sexual Health and HIV Research, Royal Free & University College Medical School, University College London, Mortimer Market Centre, Off Capper Street, London WC1E 6AU, UK*

For over a decade following the identification of HIV/AIDS, marked declines in numbers and rates of bacterial sexually transmitted diseases (STDs) were reported in many western industrialized countries [1,2]. These declines occurred across a range of demographic and social groups, including men who have sex with men (MSM). The belief is that these declines resulted from an interaction between the widespread adoption and implementation of safer-sex behavior (including use of condoms and reductions in rate of partner acquisition); selective mortality of individuals who had high-risk sexual lifestyles; and the effectiveness of generalized and targeted public education and health promotion strategies [3,4].

By the mid-1990s, rates of syphilis and gonorrhea approached their lowest point since recording began in the United States and many Western European countries, and the possibility of eliminating specific STDs appeared achievable. In the United States, a national plan to eliminate syphilis was developed [5] as a result of the highly concentrated nature of the disease and its vulnerability to concerted, targeted intervention. Several European countries developed sexual health strategies to capitalize on the gains being made with STD control, and to regalvanize HIV prevention and

---

* Corresponding author. Division of STD Prevention, National Centers for HIV, STD and TB Prevention, Centers for Disease Control and Prevention (CDC), 1600 Clifton Road, Mailstop E02, Atlanta, GA 30333.

E-mail address: kif2@cdc.gov (K.A. Fenton).

control efforts that had lost some impetus and urgency in the era of effective treatment [6–8]. However, initial indications of a reversal in these declining trends were first recorded in the late 1990s. Since then, many countries have been struggling against a resurgence of STDs among MSM, and in some areas, disease rates have reached or even surpassed pre-1980 levels [9,10].

This article examines the research and surveillance evidence regarding the changing epidemiology of acute STDs (excluding HIV infection) among homosexually active men in industrialized settings and explores possible explanations for this phenomenon. Published reports of STD surveillance data from the United States and Western Europe and published research reports are examined. In general, some of the most comprehensive STD surveillance data on infections acquired through sex between men come from the United Kingdom, Netherlands, and Scandinavian countries [11]. In the United States, sentinel surveillance or STD prevalence–monitoring studies have greatly added to our understanding of the disease burden among MSM [12]. However, variations in the structure of STD surveillance systems and inconsistencies in the collection and reporting of data on sexual orientation limit direct wider cross-country comparisons.

Changing disease epidemiology

Western Europe

In England, Wales, and Northern Ireland, MSM continue to bear a disproportionate burden of newly diagnosed acute STDs, accounting for 55% of HIV infections, 19% of gonorrhea diagnoses, and 58% of syphilis diagnoses [9,13]. Rates of gonorrhea among MSM in England and Wales doubled between 1999 and 2001, from 553 per 100,000 population to 1140 per 100,000 population, and, although a slight decrease was observed in 2002, rates increased in all age groups in 2003. Large increases in infectious syphilis rates among MSM have been observed between 1999 and 2003 (616%) as a result of ongoing outbreaks in Manchester, Brighton, London, and elsewhere in the United Kingdom. Increases (183%) in genital chlamydial infections in MSM have also been observed since 1999.

These overall trends mask substantial heterogeneity within the United Kingdom MSM population by age-group, ethnicity, HIV status, and geographic area of residence. Recent increases have been most marked in areas of England outside of London, in particular the northwest, midland, and southeast regions that contain expanding metropolitan areas with large MSM communities [9]. MSM who have diagnosed HIV infection account for a disproportionate burden of new bacterial STD infections. Data from the London Enhanced Syphilis Surveillance collected between April 2001 and September 2004 indicate that 53% (558 per 1048 population) of MSM diagnosed with syphilis in London were known to have coinfection with

HIV [14]. This reflects the large prevalent pool of diagnosed HIV infection in London and the concentration of the syphilis epidemic in this group.

In the rest of Western Europe, increases in gonorrhea among MSM were first observed in the mid-1990s [15,16]. Herida and colleagues [17] analyzed data from RENAGO, a voluntary-based laboratory surveillance system, including private and public laboratories in France. The average number of *Neisseria Gonorrhoea* isolates per laboratory per year decreased steadily from 10.6 in 1986 to 0.6 in 1997, but then increased each year and reached 1.9 in 2000. Increasing gonorrhea was observed mostly in men in the Paris region. The proportion of rectal strains increased significantly from 0.9% in 1986 to 9.2% in 2000. In Denmark [18], a trend toward an increase in the annual incidence of gonorrhea has been observed annually since 1997, with an increase of 35% from 1997 to 1998 and a further increase of 41% from 1998 to 1999. The increase appears mainly because of rises in the number and proportion of cases among MSM. Among MSM, the estimated mean annual reported incidence of gonorrhea was six times greater in MSM known to be HIV-positive than among other MSM ($P < .001$).

The recent resurgence in syphilis in MSM was first recorded toward the end of the last decade and has been well described [19–24]. Initially characterized by focal outbreaks occurring in major conurbations in Western Europe and the United States, the epidemics have been characterized by high male-to-female ratios, with a high proportion of male cases being MSM, and the proportion of MSM who are HIV positive ranging between 20% in Ireland [23] to nearly 60% in Belgium [20]. Data from enhanced surveillance studies confirm the strong association between the incidence of infectious syphilis and high rates of sex partner change and social and commercial venues that facilitate this behavior (eg, saunas, "sex on premises" clubs) [23–28].

Other disease outbreaks among MSM have been reported more recently. In 2004, hepatitis A outbreaks were reported in several European countries, including Denmark, Norway, Sweden, and the United Kingdom [25–27], with some cases being linked through viral genotyping of the outbreak strain. Investigation of the Danish outbreak revealed that sex in saunas and with casual partners was associated with an increased risk for infection [28]. Lymphogranuloma venereum (LGV) outbreaks were initially reported among HIV-positive MSM in Rotterdam, the Netherlands in early 2004. Within a year, confirmed cases were identified in other parts of the Netherlands [29], Antwerp, Belgium [30], Paris [31], Stockholm [32], Hamburg [33], and the United States [29]. Most cases of LGV have been identified among HIV-positive MSM of white ethnicity who present with proctitis. High levels of concurrent STDs (gonorrhoea, syphilis, hepatitis B virus, and genital herpes) are also common among LGV cases. Contact tracing has been of limited use in addressing these outbreaks as most LGV cases report multiple sexual contacts, mostly anonymous.

United States

Examination of United States national STD surveillance data indicates that trends in the male-to-female syphilis rate ratio have been increasing in recent years (Fig. 1). In 2003, the rate of reported primary and secondary (ie, infectious) syphilis among men (4.2 cases per 100,000 men) was 5.2 times greater than the rate among women (0.8 cases per 100,000 women) [34]. The overall male-to-female syphilis rate ratio has risen steadily since 1996 when it was 1.2. The increase in the male-to-female rate ratio occurred among all racial and ethnic groups between 2002 and 2003.

Between 1999 and 2003, nine United States cities participating in the MSM Prevalence Monitoring Project submitted results of 67,588 syphilis, gonorrhea, chlamydia, and HIV culture and nonculture tests collected from MSM visits to STD clinics and in routine care to the Centers for Disease Control and Prevention (CDC) [34]. These results suggest that increases have occurred in median syphilis seroreactivity among MSM (from 4.1% to 10.5% in 2003) and median gonorrhea positivity (13.7% to 15.3%) between 1999 and 2003. During 2003, particularly high prevalence of gonorrhea positivity was recorded among MSM, ranging from median 13.3% urethral gonorrhea positivity; 6.0% median rectal gonorrhea positivity; and 2.8% median pharyngeal gonorrhea positivity. Marked geographic and ethnic variations in disease prevalence were also found. Urethral gonorrhea positivity was 11.5% (range, 6.3%–17.2%) in whites, 18.8% (range, 10.5%–30.3%) in African-Americans, and 12.4% (range, 5.3%–21.9%) in Hispanics. Gonorrhea positivity was higher in HIV-positive MSM

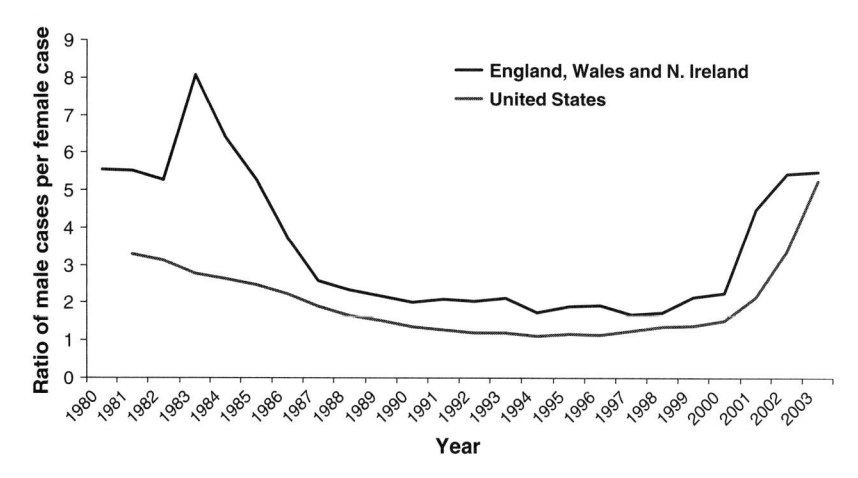

Fig. 1. Trends in the male-to-female ratio of early syphilis in United States and England, Wales, and Northern Ireland 1980–2003. Note: United States data includes primary and secondary syphilis only and England and Wales data includes primary, secondary, and early latent syphilis.

compared with MSM who were HIV-negative or of unknown HIV status: 17.8% (range, 10.3%–25.8%) versus 12.1% (range, 5.4%–16.9%).

Why are we seeing these increases?

STD transmission is influenced by numerous interconnected factors that each operate at different levels. For example, an individual's STD transmission and acquisition risk is influenced by biologic and behavioral factors. The individual's risk is further influenced by their sexual partnerships and the sexual networks within which these partnerships occur. In turn, individuals, their partners, and the sexual networks from which partners are drawn are all embedded within various MSM subcommunities that together constitute the affected population. Each level is also influenced by social, behavioral, and biomedical factors, such as the response of public health services and interventions (Fig. 2) [35].

Biologic factors

The presence of immunity has important effects on the dynamics of infectious diseases. When the period of infectiousness is short compared

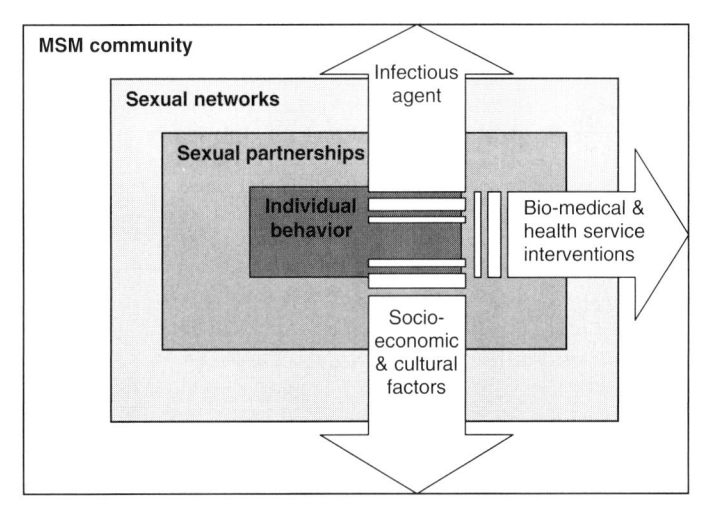

Fig. 2. A multilevel approach to understanding the interaction between the infectious agent, behaviors, populations, and biomedical interventions. Note: the factors that influence STD transmission among MSM will operate at different levels ranging from the individual, their sexual partnerships, and the sexual networks in which they are found. However, sexual networks are in turn embedded in subpopulations that constitute a population. Each of these levels is in turn influenced by social, behavioral, and biomedical factors, including the response of public health services and interventions. (*Adapted from* Aral SO, Padian NS, Holmes KK. Advances in multilevel approaches to understanding the epidemiology and prevention of sexually transmitted infections and HIV: an overview. J Infect Dis 2005;191(Suppl 1):S1–6; with permission.)

with immunity, fluctuations in incidence may occur over a period determined by the supply of susceptible individuals. Although there is no such evidence for gonorrhea, the recent publication by Grassly and colleagues [36] postulated that national trends of syphilis in the United States demonstrate a rare example of unforced, endogenous oscillations in disease incidence, with an 8- to 11-year period that is predicted by the natural dynamics of syphilis infection. Their hypothesis was based on limited evidence that partial immunity to reinfection may occur in treated and untreated syphilis, either because of acquired immune memory or continued presence of antigens. Although their analysis did not control for infections acquired though sex between men, the findings hinted at the possible role of partial immunity in the disease cycles for syphilis.

Phenotypic and genotypic changes in STDs may facilitate rapid disease spread of a particular strain. Much has been made of the recent reports of transmission of the HIV superbug among HIV-positive MSM in New York that may have implications for onward transmission of highly resistant viral strain and for rapid progression of drug-resistant HIV infection [37]. Emerging evidence of *Treponema pallidum* resistance to azithromycin [38,39] has limited its recommendation for disease management, whereas ciprofloxacin-resistant gonorrhea among MSM in Europe and parts of the United States [40,41] have also necessitated changes in first-line treatment recommendations for these infections.

Epidemiologic synergy, which is the biologic interaction between STDs [42], may be of importance in understanding the recent evolution of syphilis and other acute STDs among MSM. Chesson and colleagues [43] found that increases in AIDS-associated mortality in the early 1990s may have accounted for one third to one half of the decline in syphilis rates among men. By using a fixed-effects regression analysis of state-level AIDS mortality rates and primary and secondary syphilis incidence rates for men, the investigators showed a significant association between higher AIDS mortality and lower rates of syphilis incidence after controlling for confounding factors. They estimated that every 20 AIDS deaths per 100,000 adult men were associated with a decline of about 7% to 12% in syphilis incidence rates. More recent expansions in the prevalent pool of high-risk HIV-infected individuals may be contributing to STD increases through behavioral and biologic means. Evidence from the recent syphilis outbreak sites in Europe and the United States suggests that HIV may impact on clinical presentation and progression and the efficacy of treatment [42,44,45]. However, a recent United States study [46] suggests that rising HIV incidence in the presence of increases in gonorrhea and syphilis among MSM may not be as dramatic as initially feared. Similar stable HIV incidence in an environment of increasing STDs has been observed in the United Kingdom [47,48] and the Netherlands [49]. The reasons for this remain to be elucidated; however, one possibility is that seroconcordant high-risk sexual mixing among HIV-infected individuals may be increasing

STD transmission risk while limiting concomitant increases in HIV incidence.

Demographic trends

Increases in the proportion of men reporting homosexual experience and in the sexual activity of MSM have been recorded in several industrialized countries. Based on data from the 2000 National Surveys of Sexual Attitudes and Lifestyles (Natsal) in Britain, Mercer and colleagues [50] found that 2.8% of British men reported sex with men in the past 5 years, 46% of MSM reported five or more partners in the past 5 years, and 59.8% of MSM reported unprotected anal intercourse (UAI) in the past year. Compared with the 1990 Natsal, there were significant increases in the overall proportion of MSM in the population in 2000, and among these men, in the proportion reporting receptive anal intercourse in the past year. The increased reporting of these behaviors may partly reflect more socially tolerant attitudes toward homosexual behavior and a reduction in social desirability biases that impeded honest reporting in the previous survey [51]. However, genuine increases in the male homosexual population may also have occurred [50,52]. Understanding the impact of such demographic change is important because expansions in the base population of homosexual men may result in increases in total numbers of reported STDs, despite disease rates remaining constant within this group. This point underscores the importance of probability sample surveys that provide appropriate prevalence estimates of male homosexual behavior and aid in the interpretation of STD surveillance trends.

Expansions in the homosexually active male population in industrialized countries may also have occurred through improved survival of HIV-positive MSM as a result of widespread use of highly active antiretroviral therapies (HAART), thus reducing the selective mortality from HIV seen in the 1980s and 1990s [53]. Boily and colleagues [54] examined this hypothesis and its impact on STD incidence, using a mathematical model of bacterial STDs and treated/untreated HIV/AIDS infection for an open homosexual population. They found that over 10 years, 0% to 55% of new bacterial STDs could be attributed to the wide-scale use of HAART as a result of more modest increases (0%–25%) in risky sex occurring at the population level rather than at the individual level.

High-risk sexual behavior

At the individual level, sexual behavior remains the strongest determinant of an individual's risk for acquiring an acute STD; a relationship that appears to be independent of social or demographic factors [55]. Key behavioral determinants of STD transmission include numbers of partnerships, rate of new partner acquisition, and partner concurrency, all of which increase the probability of contact with someone who is infected with an STD, thereby facilitating STD transmission between individuals and across networks. Changes in high-risk behavior among MSM have now been widely reported in behavioral surveillance surveys, repeat panel surveys, and prospective cohort studies [50,51,56,57].

In London, Dodds and colleagues [58] estimated changes in sexual behavior among 8052 MSM attending commercial gay venues between 1996 and 2000. The proportion of men having UAI increased significantly each year from 30% in 1996 to 42% in 2000 ($P < .001$). Approximately half of HIV-positive and HIV-negative and untested men reported UAI in the past year. HIV antibody positivity was associated with increasing numbers of UAI partners and having a sexually transmitted infection (STI) in the past year (odds ratio, 2.15). Elford and colleagues [59], examining sexual behavior change among MSM in London gyms, found that the percentage of men reporting high-risk behavior with a casual partner increased from 6.7% to 16.1% between 1998 and 2003. They also found that the percentage of HIV-positive men reporting UAI with a casual partner who was also HIV-positive increased from 6.8% to 10.3% over the same period.

Similar increasing sexual risk behaviors have been reported from nearly all major European centers, with anal penetration (regardless of the nature of the relationship), UAI, and ejaculation in the mouth—in particular with casual partners—all being reported more frequently. In Switzerland [60], where ongoing behavioral surveillance surveys among MSM have been undertaken since 1987, the median number of partners in the latest 12 months was two to five until 1990 and six to ten since 1992. By 2000, three quarters of respondents had more than one partner in the last 12 months, and over one third had more than ten. In these surveys, the proportion who reported anal penetration with casual partners in the past 12 months increased from 60% in 1992 and 1994 to 69% in 1997 and 2000.

In Amsterdam [61], a cohort study of MSM followed since 1984 indicated that among HIV-positive and HIV-negative MSM, anal sex was practiced more often in the period after the introduction of HAART. Among HIV-negative homosexual men who reported practicing anal sex, the frequency of unsafe sex with steady partners increased from 70% (in 1996) to 78% (in 1999), and with casual partners from 28% to 33% for the same time periods. In Barcelona [62], repeated cross-sectional surveys performed since 1993 in gay community settings and through community organization mailing lists have shown anal intercourse to be practiced by 87% with a steady partner and 83% with casual partners, and orogenital sex by 98% and 96%, respectively. UAI with a steady partner was reported by 59%, and with casual partners by 25%; in both cases the proportions showed a slight increasing trend, but this was not statistically significant.

In the United States, although no national MSM behavioral surveillance surveys exist, data from major cities confirm that similar behavioral trends are taking place [63,64], although caution may be required when interpreting STD clinic–based studies that will tend to overestimate risk. In San Francisco [65], community surveys of MSM showed that the use of HAART among MSM living with AIDS increased from 4% in 1995 to 54% in 1999. The percentage of MSM who reported UAI and multiple sexual partners increased from 24% in 1994 to 45% in 1999. McFarland and colleagues [66] identified significant increases in UAI with multiple partners, UAI with multiple partners of unknown HIV serostatus, the incidence of male rectal gonorrhea, and the incidence of early syphilis among Asian Pacific Islander MSM between 1999 and 2002. Chen and colleagues [67] conducted 10,579 interviews with MSM at gay-oriented venues in San Francisco and the surrounding area between 1999 and 2001. They found that potentially serodiscordant UAI with at least two anal sex partners was reported by 12.7% of all men sampled between 1999 and 2001 and increased from 11% in 1999 to 16.2% in 2001. In this sample, 20.8% of HIV-positive respondents, 12.1% of HIV-negative respondents, and 13.4% of MSM who did not know or report their HIV serostatus reported potentially serodiscordant UAI. Among those who had unknown HIV serostatus, MSM of color were the more likely to engage in potentially serodiscordant UAI.

Risk behavior of HIV-positive MSM, including their more frequent reporting of the practice of "barebacking," or intentional unprotected anal sex, has gained considerable attention especially because of the higher STD burden borne by this group. Between May 2000 and December 2002, 2491 HIV-positive MSM were interviewed at 16 surveillance sites in the United States [68]. Of 77% who had HIV diagnosed for more than 12 months, 61% reported sex with a male partner during the preceding 12 months. Overall, 40% of sexually active HIV-positive MSM reported insertive anal intercourse at last sexual encounter; of these, 25% did not use a condom. No significant differences were observed by partner type (steady versus nonsteady) for insertive anal intercourse at last sexual encounter (43% versus 38%, respectively). Insertive anal intercourse at last sexual encounter was significantly less likely with an HIV-negative partner or partner of unknown serostatus than with known HIV-positive partners.

Halkitis and colleagues [69] studied the prevalence of barebacking among 518 MSM who completed a brief intercept survey in New York City. Of the 448 men who were familiar with the term barebacking, 45.5% reported engaging in bareback sex in the past 3 months. HIV-positive men were significantly more likely than HIV-negative men to report barebacking and also reported significantly more sexual partners with whom they had engaged in bareback sex. Participants reported significantly more acts of seroconcordant bareback sex than serodiscordant bareback sex. The Internet, availability of sexually oriented chat rooms, HIV treatment advances, emotional fatigue regarding HIV, and the increased popularity of "club" drugs were all cited by the respondents as reasons for the growing barebacking phenomenon.

The sexual marketplace

Dramatic changes to the social and sexual environments of MSM include the substantial expansion of sexual and social networks that facilitate the rapid acquisition of new sexual partners, and in turn, the onward transmission of STDs. The Internet is undoubtedly a central feature of this expanding sexual marketplace, with a growing proportion of MSM reporting Internet access and acquisition of sexual partners through this route [70,71]. In addition to providing mainstream MSM with another vehicle for locating potential sexual partners, the Internet allows non–gay identified and bisexual men greater access to wider online networks of MSM seeking sexual partners. It also facilitates the almost instantaneous worldwide dissemination of ideas and new behavioral norms and ultimately links sexual networks that may traverse vast physical distances. The addition of increased international travel, sexual partner acquisition while overseas, "sex tourism," globalization of traditional gay community events (eg, Pride Festivals, "circuit parties"), and rapid diffusion of novel sexual practices or new behavioral norms creates the potential for rapid global spread of localized STD outbreaks among MSM.

Emerging evidence suggests that "circuit parties," which are scheduled weekend-long dance parties in different cities across the United States, Canada, Europe, Brazil, and South Africa, are frequently characterized by high levels of recreational drug use and high-risk sexual behavior, especially among HIV-positive men. Lee and colleagues [72] examined the characteristics of men attending United States circuit parties and their drug use. The role of methylenediomethamphetamine (MDMA, "ecstasy") in particular was considered in relation to other drug use and sexual behavior. The investigators surveyed 173 men, of whom most were gay-identified, Caucasian, employed, and well-educated MSM. Of these men, 25% were self-identified as HIV-positive and 86% reported using at least one substance on the day of the party, with polydrug use also being frequently reported. The most common substances reported and used in combination were MDMA, ketamine, and methamphetamine. MDMA use was highly associated with ketamine, methamphetamine, and cocaine use. MDMA use was also associated with significantly more receptive anal intercourse.

The study by Mansergh and colleagues [73] considered the characteristics of MSM who attend circuit parties by examining drug use and sexual behavior during circuit party weekends in a cross-sectional survey of 295 MSM from the San Francisco Bay Area who had attended a circuit party in the previous year. Nearly all respondents reported use of drugs during circuit party weekends, including ecstasy (75%), ketamine (58%), crystal methamphetamine (36%), gamma hydroxybutyrate or gamma butyrolactone (25%), and sildenafil citrate (12%). A quarter of the men reported a drug overuse incident in the previous year. Two thirds of the men reported having sex (oral or anal), 49% reported anal sex, and 28% reported unprotected anal sex during the 3-day period. An association was found between use of drugs and sexual risk behavior. A better understanding of the role played by recreational drug use in the lives of MSM is needed before appropriate interventions can be developed that aim to reduce the drug use/sexual risk-taking combinations evident among MSM who attend circuit parties.

The increased international leisure travel of MSM; visits to localities that attempt to cultivate an image of "gay holiday destinations"; and a rise in the proportion of MSM who report sex with a casual partner while aboard also influence potential rapid STD diffusion. Over the past 15 years, cheaper travel, promotion of weekend breaks, and the emergence several Eastern European, Latin American, and South African cities as gay holiday hot spots have all increased opportunities for MSM to extend the numbers and range of possible sexual partners. For example, in the 2000 Natsal survey, among all British men who reported travel outside the United Kingdom in the last 5 years, MSM were significantly more likely to report a new sexual partner while abroad and to report sex with a new partner from overseas while abroad compared with non-MSM (Catherine Mercer, PhD, personal communication, 2005). The effect of these expanded opportunities to find new sexual partners may be less important for American and Western European men than it is for MSM who live in the countries being visited, where safer-sex norms, HIV prevalence, and access to appropriate or targeted sexual health services may be substantially poorer than in industrialized countries.

Expansion of the sexual marketplace is not only characterized by quantitative changes in the number, nature, and forms of outlets but also qualitative changes that may favor STD transmission. For example, increased Internet use for meeting sexual partners has been accompanied by reductions in the use of cruising grounds and cottages in the United Kingdom [74]. These sorts of changes at a population level may increase STD transmission risk if the new outlets facilitate higher-risk sexual practices than those associated with more traditional public sex environments. Binson and colleagues [75] investigated differences in risk behaviors among MSM who went to gay bathhouses, public cruising areas, or both in a probability sample survey of 2881 MSM residing in four United States cities. They found that men who used party drugs and had UAI with non–primary partners were more likely to go to any sex venue than men who did not. Men who only went to public cruising areas were least likely to report risky sex, whereas those who went to public cruising areas and bathhouses were the most likely to report high-risk practices. The investigators concluded that distinguishing between different types of sex venues may reveal significant associations between patterns of venue use and sexual risk.

However, to avoid a knee-jerk reaction, it needs to be borne in mind that high-risk venues such as saunas also provide important prevention and sexual health promotion opportunities [76]. Evidence is now emerging about other types of interventions that aim to reduce sexual risk-taking within "sex on premises" venues (eg, more lighting, open booths, use of safer-sex monitors, on-site STD screening and referral services, and regulated opening times) [77,78]. Similarly, Internet-based interventions (eg, online partner notification, safer-sex interactive banners) developed in partnership with Webmasters are an operational way to increase safer Web-based environments [79,80].

Psychosocial contexts

Although much has been made about the potential role of HIV optimism on risk behavior of MSM, several studies [81–84] have now demonstrated that even when a causal association exists, the contribution of HIV treatment optimism to the overall increase in high-risk sexual behavior remains extremely modest at a population level. The reality is that few gay men are optimistic in the light of HAART, and that at a population level, HIV optimism is unlikely to explain the recent increase in high-risk sexual behavior among gay men. Crepaz and colleagues [85] reviewed 25 papers published between 1996 and 2003 and conducted three meta-analyses to determine whether being treated with HAART, having an undetectable viral load, or holding specific beliefs about HAART and viral load were associated with an increased likelihood of engaging in unprotected sex. They found that HIV-positive people who had an undetectable viral load were no more likely to engage in unprotected sex than those whose viral load was detectable. This absence of an association did not vary by risk group, by country of study, or whether viral load was self-reported or taken from medical records. They also found no significant overall association between taking HAART and unprotected sex (odds ratio, 0.92; 95% CI, 0.65–1.31). Speculation that taking HAART or having an undetectable viral load might trigger risky sexual behavior among people who have HIV was not supported by these meta-analyses.

Changes in the legal position of MSM, such as the greater recognition of partnership rights, are indicative of the increased social acceptability of homosexuality in some countries [86,87]. However, although greater tolerance in the general population may reduce the social stigma attached to homosexuality, it may also contribute to increased tolerance within MSM communities for alternative ideas and higher-risk sexual lifestyles. For example, during the late 1990s much was made of the rising incidence of self-reported bareback sex and the practice's rapid diffusion among geographically disparate MSM communities [88–90]. The emerging discourse and proliferation of Internet sites and chat rooms that allow MSM to advertise as seeking this type of sex is an example of how the diffusion of ideas may contribute to changing sexual behavior norms.

The role of recreational drug use in the lives of MSM and its association with high-risk behavior is an area in need of further study [91,92]. In 2000, Stueve and colleagues [93] assessed the extent to which urban young MSM report being high on drugs or alcohol during sex and the association between being high and UAI. In their study, 3075 MSM aged 15 to 25 years completed a 20-minute interview for the Community Intervention Trial for Youth Project. Overall, 18.6% of MSM who had a main partner reported being high during their last sexual encounter and 25.0% reported UAI. Among men who reported sex with a non–main partner, 29.3% reported being high and 12.3% reported UAI. The investigators found that being high was significantly associated with receptive UAI with non–main partners (odds ratio, 1.66, $P = .02$). Klitzman and colleagues [94] assessed patterns of MDMA use in a sample of 733 MSM in New York City. They found that 13.7% reported using MDMA in the past 6 months, with a mean frequency of use of 6.24 times for the period. MDMA users were younger, less educated, had more male partners, had more one night stands, had more visits to bars or clubs and sex clubs or bathhouses, had more unprotected anal sex with a man, were more likely to have been the victim of physical domestic violence, and were more likely to have higher levels of gay community participation and affiliation than nonusers. The investigators concluded that MDMA use is associated with being more "out," which may be advantageous in helping gay men deal with harmful psychologic effects of stigma but may place them in situations that have greater sexual health risks.

Researchers have also studied the role of depression and sexual risk behaviors of MSM. In two Seattle studies [95], 1228 IDUs and 429 young MSM completed the Center for Epidemiologic Studies Depression Scale (CES-D). Of the injecting drug users (IDUs), 47% had CES-D scores of 23 or less. High scores were significantly related to injection with a syringe used by another IDU (adjusted odds ratio, 1.4) but no other injection risk behavior. Among MSM, CES-D scores of 16 or less corresponded to reporting three or more sex partners in the last 6 months, but not to other sexual risk behavior. This analysis suggests that psychologic depression may influence certain HIV risk behavior in young MSM and IDUs and that interventions addressing depression may be needed. Similar emerging evidence has highlighted the association between childhood sexual abuse, mental health problems, and high-risk sexual behavior in MSM. Kalichman and colleagues [96] studied the psychologic and behavioral correlates of HIV risk behavior associated with childhood sexual abuse in a sample of 647 MSM attending a large gay Pride event. They found that MSM who had a history of childhood sexual abuse were more likely to engage in high-risk sexual behavior (ie, unprotected receptive anal intercourse), trade sex for money or drugs, report being HIV positive, and experience nonsexual relationship violence.

Box 1. A conceptual framework for understanding reasons for recent increases in sexually transmitted diseases among men who have sex with men

Individual level
Demographic changes
- Increases in the proportion of men reporting same sex experiences and intercourse
- Increased survival of MSM because of HAART
- Increases in HIV-positive MSM population

Sexual risk behaviors
- Increases in unsafe sex
- Increased sex partner change rates
- Increased sex partner concurrency
- Increased HIV seroconcordant sexual mixing (serosorting)
- Increases in payment for sex

Proximal determinants of sexual risk behavior
- Recreational drug use
- Drug abuse
- Mental ill health (depression)

Infectious Agents
Resistance and the interaction between STDs
- Antimicrobial and antiretroviral resistance
- Interaction between HIV and bacterial STDs
- Epidemiologic synergy

Sociocultural environment
Growth of the sexual marketplace
- Internet
- Sex on premises venues (eg, bathhouses, bookstores)
- Circuit parties, sex parties
- Sex tourism

Socioeconomic status
- Lower socioeconomic status
- Lower educational attainment

Changing cultural environments that facilitate high-risk behavior
- Barebacking
- Discrimination (increasing or decreasing)
- Homophobia
- HAART optimism

Biomedical environment
Inability of health services to effectively intervene
- MSM seek care within private sector, which may be less amenable or accessible to STD prevention interventions
- Public health department staff less used to dealing with MSM issues or clients
- Lack of effectiveness of traditional disease control interventions (eg, partner notification) with MSM because of changing social and behavioral contexts

Among MSM, there is little evidence regarding the relationship between education, occupation, and social stratification and STD risk and morbidity [97–99]; this remains an area for further work. In England, the annual Gay Men's Sex Survey (GMSS) [100] uses educational qualifications as an indicator of socioeconomic status. GMSS data indicate that men who have less formal education (usually leaving school at the age of 16) have a higher prevalence of diagnosed HIV infection than men educated to A-level or above. GMSS data also indicate that men who have less formal educational qualifications have more UAI with regular partners than better-educated men and, despite being less likely to have casual sex, are more likely to have casual and serodiscordant UAI.

Finally, recent interest has surrounded the role of stigma, discrimination, and internalized homophobia on MSM sexuality and sexual risk behavior [101–103]. Diaz and colleagues [104] used data from a probability sample of 912 Latino gay men in three United States cities to test a multivariate model of sexual risk, including experiences of homophobia, racism, and poverty as predictors. Participants reported multiple instances of verbal and physical abuse, rude mistreatment, and discrimination on account of their sexual orientation and their race or ethnicity. Many reported experiences of poverty, such as inability to pay for basic necessities of food or shelter. Men who reported more instances of social discrimination and financial hardship were more psychologically distressed and more likely to participate in "difficult" sexual situations. Participation in difficult sexual situations mediates the effects of social oppression and psychologic distress on sexual risk behavior.

Box 1 lists a conceptual framework for understanding the reasons for the recent increases in STDs among MSM.

Summary

The recent increases in acute STDs among MSM must be viewed in the context of a post-AIDS era that is characterized by demographic shifts, changing sexual attitudes, and rapidly changing social contexts. A key driver seems to be the growing prevalent pool of HIV-positive MSM for whom the crucial motivator for safer sex (primary HIV prevention) no longer exists and where, given the prevalence of seroconcordant sexual mixing, considerable uncertainty and conflicting advice regarding the rationale and benefits for continued safer-sex practice are unclear [105,106]. Although it is tempting to ascribe these changes to increases in risk behavior, it is essential that the contexts in which the changes are occurring are also considered. It may also be appropriate to contemplate whether further changes to the social environment (eg, structural interventions) are a suitable adjunct to our traditional prevention activities that operate largely in isolation from each other. It seems natural to advocate that interventions that adopt holistic approaches to the sexual health of MSM and that address upstream factors such as mental health, drug use, discrimination, and internalized homophobia should be included in the efforts to create more healthy environments for MSM. However, there is still some way to go in identifying which of these upstream interventions are effective, how they may be implemented within or alongside existing health care systems, and what impact, if any, they are likely to have on STD transmission. Such interventions are also likely to be long on implementation time, require consider political will, and be extremely hard to evaluate, and the benefits may not be seen within the same generation in which they are implemented. Therefore, there must be confidence that this is the appropriate route of travel.

The consistency of findings from across industrialized countries confirms an increasing connectivity within the global MSM community; a community that is decreasingly defined by geographic boundaries and, in the era of the Internet and easier foreign travel, increasingly linked by shared interests and social and sexual networks. This is powerfully demonstrated in the near-simultaneous syphilis and LGV outbreaks among MSM in Europe and the United States [29]. In this regard, greater collaboration between researchers and providers working with MSM in different countries is now required. More specifically, consideration should be given to creating closer partnerships between sentinel cities, such as London, New York, San Francisco, Berlin, Paris, and Amsterdam, that have large MSM populations and are likely to be emerging, or rapid diffusion sites for new social and sexual trends that may impact on disease transmission. There are many benefits to such cross-national working, including earlier recognition and improved response to emerging threats, sharing innovative practice, avoiding duplication of effort, and creating a united front for dealing with what must be considered a cause for concern domestically and globally.

References

[1] Fox KK, del Rio C, Holmes KK, et al. Gonorrhea in the HIV era: a reversal in trends among men who have sex with men. Am J Public Health 2001;91(6):959–64.

[2] Fenton KA, Lowndes CM. Recent trends in the epidemiology of sexually transmitted infections in the European Union. Sex Transm Infect 2004;80(4):255–63.

[3] Nicoll A, Hamers FF. Are trends in HIV, gonorrhoea, and syphilis worsening in western Europe? BMJ 2002;324(7349):1324–7.

[4] Boily MC, Bastos FI, Desai K, et al. Increasing prevalence of male homosexual partnerships and practices in Britain 1990–2000: but why? AIDS 2005;19(3):352–4.

[5] Division of STD Prevention, National Center for HIV, STD, and TB Prevention, Centers for Disease Control and Prevention. The National Plan to Eliminate Syphilis from the United States. Atlanta (GA): Centers for Disease Control and Prevention; 1999.

[6] Department of Health. The national strategy for sexual health and HIV implementation action plan. London: Department of Health; 2002.

[7] Scottish Executive. Enhancing sexual wellbeing in Scotland: a sexual health & relationship strategy. Edinburgh: Scottish Executive; 2003.

[8] World Health Organization. WHO regional strategy on sexual and reproductive health. Reproductive Health/Pregnancy Programme. Copenhagen: World Health Organization; 2001.
[9] Macdonald N, Dougan S, McGarrigle CA, et al. Recent trends in diagnoses of HIV and other sexually transmitted infections in England and Wales among men who have sex with men. Sex Transm Infect 2004;80(6):492–7.
[10] Resurgent bacterial sexually transmitted disease among men who have sex with men–King County, Washington, 1997–1999. MMWR Morb Mortal Wkly Rep 1999;48(35): 773–7.
[11] Lowndes CM, Fenton KA. European Surveillance of STI's Network. Surveillance systems for STIs in the European Union: facing a changing epidemiology. Sex Transm Infect 2004; 80(4):264–71.
[12] Centers for Disease Control and Prevention. Sexually transmitted disease surveillance 2003. Atlanta (GA): US Department of Health and Human Services; 2003.
[13] The UK Collaborative Group for HIV and STI Surveillance. Focus on prevention. HIV and other sexually transmitted infections in the United Kingdom in 2003. London: Health Protection Agency Centre for Infections; 2004.
[14] Righarts AA, Simms I, Wallace L, et al. Syphilis surveillance and epidemiology in the United Kingdom. Euro Surveill 2004;9(12):15–6.
[15] Nicoll A, Hamers FF. Are trends in HIV, gonorrhoea, and syphilis worsening in western Europe? BMJ 2002;324(7349):1324–7.
[16] Berglund T, Fredlund H, Giesecke J. Epidemiology of the reemergence of gonorrhea in Sweden. Sex Transm Dis 2001;28(2):111–4.
[17] Herida M, Sednaoui P, Goulet V. Gonorrhoea surveillance system in France: 1986–2000. Sex Transm Dis 2004;31(4):209–14.
[18] Johansen JD, Smith E. Gonorrhoea in Denmark: high incidence among HIV-infected men who have sex with men. Acta Derm Venereol 2002;82(5):365–8.
[19] Fenton KA. A multilevel approach to understanding the resurgence and evolution of infectious syphilis in Western Europe. Euro Surveill 2004;9:2–4.
[20] Sasse A, Defraye A, Ducoffre G. Recent syphilis trends in Belgium and enhancement of STI surveillance systems. Euro Surveill 2004;9(12):5–6.
[21] Couturier E, Michel A, Janier M, et al. Syphilis surveillance in France 2000–2003. Euro Surveill 2004;9(12):7–8.
[22] Cowan S. Syphilis in Denmark–Outbreak among MSM in Copenhagen 2003–2004. Euro Surveill 2004;9(12):17–8.
[23] Cronin M, Domegan L, Thornton L, et al. The epidemiology of infectious syphilis in the Republic of Ireland. Euro Surveill 2004;9(12):11–2.
[24] Marcus U, Bremer V, Hamouda O. Syphilis surveillance and trends of the syphilis epidemic in Germany since the mid-90s. Euro Surveill 2004;9(12):9–10.
[25] Mølbak K. Increase in hepatitis A in MSM in Denmark. Available at: http://www.eurosurveillance.org/ew2004/040527/.asp. Accessed May 10, 2005.
[26] HPA. Outbreak of hepatitis A in men who have sex with men in south east London. Available at: http://www.hpa.org.uk/cdr/index.html. Accessed May 10, 2005.
[27] De Jager C, Heijne J. Increase in hepatitis A in MSM in the Netherlands. Available at: http://www.eurosurveillance.org/ew2004/040527.asp#. Accessed May 10, 2005.
[28] EPi News. Available at: http://www.ssi.dk/sw23055.asp. Accessed May 10, 2005.
[29] Laar MJ van de, Götz HM, Zwart O, et al. Lymphogranuloma venereum among men have sex with men–Netherlands, 2003–2004. MMWR Morb Mortal Wkly Rep 2004;53(42): 985–8.
[30] Vandenbruaene M. Uitbraak van lymphogranuloma venereum in Antwerpen en Rotterdam. Available at: http://www.wvc.vlaanderen.be/epibul/47/lymphogranuloma.htm. Accessed May 10, 2005.

[31] Institut de Vieille Sanitaire. Emergence de la Lymphogranulomatose vénérienne rectale en France: cas estimés au 31 mars 2004. Synthèse réalisée le 1er Juin 2004. Available at: http://www.invs.sante.fr/presse/2004/le_point_sur/lgv_160604/. Accessed May 10, 2005.

[32] Berglund T, Herrmann B. Utbrott av Lymfogranuloma venereum (LGV) i Europa. Available at: http://www.smittskyddsinstitutet.se/SMItemplates/BigArticle____3942.aspx#LGV. Accessed May 10, 2005.

[33] Plettenberg A, von Krosigk A, Stoehr A, et al. Four cases of lymphogranuloma venereum in Hamburg, 2003. Available at: http://www.eurosurveillance.org/ew/2004/040722.asp#4. Accessed May 10, 2005.

[34] Centers for Disease Control and Prevention. Sexually transmitted disease surveillance 2003. Atlanta (GA): US Department of Health and Human Services; 2003.

[35] Aral SO, Padian NS, Holmes KK. Advances in multilevel approaches to understanding the epidemiology and prevention of sexually transmitted infections and HIV: an overview. J Infect Dis 2005;191(Suppl 1):S1–6.

[36] Grassly NC, Fraser C, Garnett GP. Host immunity and synchronized epidemics of syphilis across the United States. Nature 2005;433:417–21.

[37] Smith SM. New York City HIV superbug: fear or fear not? Available at http://www.retrovirology.com/content/2/1/14. Accessed March 9, 2005.

[38] Lukehart SA, Godornes C, Molini BJ, et al. Macrolide resistance in Treponema pallidum in the United States and Ireland. N Engl J Med 2004;351(2):154–8.

[39] Chen JC. Update on emerging infections: news from the Centers for Disease Control and Prevention. Brief report: azithromycin treatment failures in syphilis infections–San Francisco, California, 2002–2003. Ann Emerg Med 2004;44(3):232–4.

[40] Centers for Disease Control and Prevention (CDC). Increases in fluoroquinolone-resistant Neisseria gonorrhoeae among men who have sex with men–United States, 2003, and revised recommendations for gonorrhea treatment, 2004. MMWR Morb Mortal Wkly Rep 2004;53(16):335–8.

[41] Fenton KA, Ison C, Johnson AP, et al. GRASP collaboration. Ciprofloxacin resistance in *Neisseria gonorrhoeae* in England and Wales in 2002. Lancet 2003;361(9372):1867–9.

[42] Rottingen JA, Cameron DW, Garnett GP. A systematic review of the epidemiologic interactions between classic sexually transmitted diseases and HIV: how much really is known? Sex Transm Dis 2001;28(10):579–97.

[43] Chesson HW, Dee TS, Aral SO. AIDS mortality may have contributed to the decline in syphilis rates in the United States in the 1990s. Sex Transm Dis 2003;30(5):419–24.

[44] Fenton KA, Nicoll A, Kinghorn G. Resurgence of syphilis in England: time for more radical and nationally coordinated approaches. Sex Transm Infect 2001;77(5):309–10.

[45] Paz-Bailey G, Meyers A, Blank S, et al. A case-control study of syphilis among men who have sex with men in New York City: association With HIV infection. Sex Transm Dis 2004;31(10):581–7.

[46] Centers for Disease Control and Prevention (CDC). Trends in primary and secondary syphilis and HIV infections in men who have sex with men–San Francisco and Los Angeles, California, 1998–2002. MMWR Morb Mortal Wkly Rep 2004;53(26):575–8.

[47] Murphy G, Charlett A, Jordan LF, et al. HIV incidence appears constant in men who have sex with men despite widespread use of effective antiretroviral therapy. AIDS 2004;18(2):265–72.

[48] Murphy G, Parry JV, Gupta SB, et al. Test of HIV incidence shows continuing HIV transmission in homosexual/bisexual men in England and Wales. Commun Dis Public Health 2001;4(1):33–7.

[49] van der Bij AK, Stolte IG, Coutinho RA, et al. Increase of sexually transmitted infections, but not HIV, among young homosexual men in Amsterdam: are STIs still reliable markers for HIV transmission? Sex Transm Infect 2005;81(1):34–7.

[50] Mercer CH, Fenton KA, Copas AJ, et al. Increasing prevalence of male homosexual partnerships and practices in Britain 1990–2000: evidence from national probability surveys. AIDS 2004;18(10):1453–8.
[51] Mercer C, Johnson A, Copas A, et al. Possible explanations for the increase in the prevalence of male homosexual partnerships and practices in Britain 1990–2000. A response to Boily et al. AIDS 2005;19(3):354–5.
[52] Johnson AM, Mercer CH, Erens B, et al. Sexual behaviour in Britain: partnerships, practices, and HIV risk behaviours. Lancet 2001;358(9296):1835–42.
[53] Boily MC, Bastos FI, Desai K, et al. Increasing prevalence of male homosexual partnerships and practices in Britain 1990–2000: but why? AIDS 2005;19(3):352–4.
[54] Boily MC, Bastos FI, Desai K, et al. Changes in the transmission dynamics of the HIV epidemic after the wide-scale use of antiretroviral therapy could explain increases in sexually transmitted infections: results from mathematical models. Sex Transm Dis 2004;31(2):100–13.
[55] Fenton KA, Mercer CH, Johnson AM, et al. Reported sexually transmitted disease clinic attendance and sexually transmitted infections in Britain: prevalence, risk factors, and proportionate population burden. J Infect Dis 2005;191(Suppl 1):S127–38.
[56] Valleroy LA, MacKellar DA, Karon JM, et al. HIV prevalence and associated risks in young men who have sex with men. Young Men's Survey Study Group. JAMA 2000;284(2):198–204.
[57] Laporte A. A new decline in preventive behaviours among homosexual men: the role of highly active antiretroviral therapy? Euro Surveill 2002;7(2):15–6.
[58] Dodds JP, Mercey DE, Parry JV, et al. Increasing risk behaviour and high levels of undiagnosed HIV infection in a community sample of homosexual men. Sex Transm Infect 2004;80(3):236–40.
[59] Elford J, Bolding G, Davis M, et al. Trends in sexual behaviour among London homosexual men 1998–2003: implications for HIV prevention and sexual health promotion. Sex Transm Infect 2004;80(6):451–4.
[60] Dubois-Arber F, Moreau-Gruet F, Jeannin A. Men having sex with men and HIV/AIDS prevention in Switzerland: 1987–2000. Euro Surveill 2002;7(2):16–8.
[61] Stolte G, Dukers NH, de Wit JB, et al. A summary report from Amsterdam: increase in sexually transmitted diseases and risky sexual behaviour among homosexual men in relation to the introduction of new anti-HIV drugs. Euro Surveill 2002;7(2):19–22.
[62] Perez K, Rodes A, Casabona J. Monitoring HIV prevalence and behaviour of men who have sex with men in Barcelona, Spain. Euro Surveill 2002;7(2):19–22.
[63] Rietmeijer CA, Patnaik JL, Judson FN, et al. Increases in gonorrhea and sexual risk behaviors among men who have sex with men: a 12-year trend analysis at the Denver Metro Health Clinic. Sex Transm Dis 2003;30(7):562–7.
[64] Chen SY, Gibson S, Katz MH, et al. Continuing increases in sexual risk behavior and sexually transmitted diseases among men who have sex with men: San Francisco, Calif, 1999–2001, USA. Am J Public Health 2002;92(9):1387–8.
[65] Katz MH, Schwarcz SK, Kellogg TA, et al. Impact of highly active antiretroviral treatment on HIV seroincidence among men who have sex with men: San Francisco. Am J Public Health 2002;92(3):388–94.
[66] McFarland W, Chen S, Weide D, et al. Gay Asian men in San Francisco follow the international trend: increases in rates of unprotected anal intercourse and sexually transmitted diseases, 1999–2002. AIDS Educ Prev 2004;16(1):13–8.
[67] Chen SY, Gibson S, Weide D, et al. Unprotected anal intercourse between potentially HIV-serodiscordant men who have sex with men, San Francisco. J Acquir Immune Defic Syndr 2003;33(2):166–70.
[68] Centers for Disease Control and Prevention (CDC). High-risk sexual behavior by HIV-positive men who have sex with men–16 sites, United States, 2000–2002. MMWR Morb Mortal Wkly Rep 2004;53(38):891–4.

[69] Halkitis PN, Parsons JT, Wilton L. Barebacking among gay and bisexual men in New York City: explanations for the emergence of intentional unsafe behavior. Arch Sex Behav 2003; 32(4):351–7.
[70] Bolding G, Davis M, Sherr L, et al. Use of gay Internet sites and views about online health promotion among men who have sex with men. AIDS Care 2004;16(8):993–1001.
[71] McFarlane M, Ross MW, Elford J. The Internet and HIV/STD prevention. AIDS Care 2004;16(8):929–30.
[72] Lee SJ, Galanter M, Dermatis H, et al. Circuit parties and patterns of drug use in a subset of gay men. J Addict Dis 2003;22(4):47–60.
[73] Mansergh G, Colfax GN, Marks G, et al. The Circuit Party Men's Health Survey: findings and implications for gay and bisexual men. Am J Public Health 2001;91(6):953–8.
[74] Hickson F, Weatherburn P, Reid D, et al. Out and about: findings from the United Kingdom gay men's sex survey 2002. London: Sigma Research; 2003.
[75] Binson D, Woods WJ, Pollack L, et al. Differential HIV risk in bathhouses and public cruising areas. Am J Public Health 2001;91(9):1482–6.
[76] Lambert N, Fisher M, Imrie J, et al. Community-based syphilis screening: feasibility, acceptability and effectiveness in case finding. Sex Transm Infect, in press.
[77] Binson D, Woods WJ. A theoretical approach to bathhouse environments. J Homosex 2003;44(3–4):23–31.
[78] Mutchler MG, Bingham T, Chion M, et al. Comparing sexual behavioral patterns between two bathhouses: implications for HIV prevention intervention policy. J Homosex 2003; 44(3–4):221–42.
[79] Klausner JD, Levine DK, Kent CK. Internet-based site-specific interventions for syphilis prevention among gay and bisexual men. AIDS Care 2004;16(8):964–70.
[80] Levine DK, Scott KC, Klausner JD. Online syphilis testing–confidential and convenient. Sex Transm Dis 2005;32(2):139–41.
[81] Stolte I, Dukers N, Geskus R, et al. Homosexual men change to risky sex when perceiving less threat of HIV/AIDS since availability of highly active antiretroviral therapy: a longitudinal study. AIDS 2004;18:303–9.
[82] International Collaboration on HIV Optimism. HIV treatments optimism among gay men: an international perspective. J Acquir Immune Defic Syndr 2003;32:545–50.
[83] Vanable P, Ostrow D, McKirnan D, et al. Impact of combination therapies on HIV risk perceptions and sexual risk among HIV-positive and HIV-negative gay and bisexual men. Health Psychol 2000;8:241–8.
[84] Elford J, Bolding G, Maguire M, et al. Combination therapies for HIV and sexual risk behavior among gay men. J Acquir Immune Defic Syndr 2000;23:266–71.
[85] Crepaz N, Hart T, Marks G. Highly active antiretroviral therapy and sexual risk behaviour. JAMA 2004;292:224–36.
[86] Rotello G. Sexual ecology - AIDS and the destiny of gay men. London: Penguin/Plume; 1998.
[87] Schumm WR. Differential risk theory as a subset of social exchange theory: implications for making gay marriage culturally normative and for understanding stigma against homosexuals. Psychol Rep 2004;94(1):208–10.
[88] Mansergh G, Marks G, Colfax GN, et al. "Barebacking" in a diverse sample of men who have sex with men. AIDS 2002;16(4):653–9.
[89] Halkitis PN, Parsons JT. Intentional unsafe sex (barebacking) among HIV-positive gay men who seek sexual partners on the internet. AIDS Care 2003;15(3):367–78.
[90] Halkitis PN, Parsons JT, Wilton L. Barebacking among gay and bisexual men in New York City: explanations for the emergence of intentional unsafe behavior. Arch Sex Behav 2003; 32(4):351–7.
[91] Semple SJ, Patterson TL, Grant I. Binge use of methamphetamine among HIV-positive men who have sex with men: pilot data and HIV prevention implications. AIDS Educ Prev 2003;15(2):133–47.

[92] Romanelli F, Smith KM, Pomeroy C. Use of club drugs by HIV-seropositive and HIV-seronegative gay and bisexual men. Top HIV Med 2003;11(1):25–32.
[93] Stueve A, O'Donnell L, Duran R, et al. Community Intervention Trial for Youth Study Team. Being high and taking sexual risks: findings from a multisite survey of urban young men who have sex with men. AIDS Educ Prev 2002;14(6):482–95.
[94] Klitzman RL, Greenberg JD, Pollack LM, et al. MDMA ('ecstasy') use, and its association with high risk behaviors, mental health, and other factors among gay/bisexual men in New York City. Drug Alcohol Depend 2002;66(2):115–25.
[95] Perdue T, Hagan H, Thiede H, et al. Depression and HIV risk behavior among Seattle-area injection drug users and young men who have sex with men. AIDS Educ Prev 2003;15(1):81–92.
[96] Kalichman SC, Gore-Felton C, Benotsch E, et al. Trauma symptoms, sexual behaviors, and substance abuse: correlates of childhood sexual abuse and HIV risks among men who have sex with men. J Child Sex Abus 2004;13(1):1–15.
[97] Hope VD, MacArthur C. Safer sex and social class: findings from a study of men using the 'gay scene' in the West Midlands region of the United Kingdom. AIDS Care 1998;10(1):81–8.
[98] Strathdee SA, Hogg RS, Martindale SL, et al. Determinants of sexual risk-taking among young HIV-negative gay and bisexual men. J Acquir Immune Defic Syndr Hum Retrovirol 1998;19(1):61–6.
[99] Hart GJ, Flowers P, Der GJ, et al. Homosexual men's HIV related sexual risk behaviour in Scotland. Sex Transm Infect 1999;75(4):242–6.
[100] Hickson F, Weatherburn P, Reid D, et al. Out and about: findings from the United Kingdom Gay Men's Sex Survey, 2002. London: Sigma Research. Available at: www.sigmaresearch.org.uk/downloads/report03f.pdf. Accessed May 10, 2005.
[101] Dudley MG, Rostosky SS, Korfhage BA, et al. Correlates of high-risk sexual behavior among young men who have sex with men. AIDS Educ Prev 2004;16(4):328–40.
[102] Moss D. Internalized homophobia in men: wanting in the first person singular, hating in the first person plural. Psychoanal Q 2002;71(1):21–50.
[103] Rowen CJ, Malcolm JP. Correlates of internalized homophobia and homosexual identity formation in a sample of gay men. J Homosex 2002;43(2):77–92.
[104] Diaz RM, Ayala G, Bein E. Sexual risk as an outcome of social oppression: data from a probability sample of Latino gay men in three US cities. Cultur Divers Ethnic Minor Psychol 2004;10(3):255–67.
[105] Colfax GN, Guzman R, Wheeler S, et al. Beliefs about HIV reinfection (superinfection) and sexual behavior among a diverse sample of HIV-positive men who have sex with men. J Acquir Immune Defic Syndr 2004;36(4):990–2.
[106] Guzman R, Colfax GN, Wheeler S, et al. Negotiated safety relationships and sexual behavior among a diverse sample of HIV-negative men who have sex with men. J Acquir Immune Defic Syndr 2005;38(1):82–6.

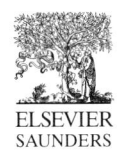

Mucopurulent Cervicitis: No Longer Ignored, but Still Misunderstood

Jeanne M. Marrazzo, MD, MPH[a,b,*]

[a]Division of Allergy and Infectious Diseases, University of Washington, Seattle, WA, USA
[b]Seattle STD/HIV Prevention Training Center, Seattle, WA, USA

Mucopurulent cervicitis (MPC) is an inflammatory condition of the cervix that has been viewed primarily as the consequence of infection with sexually acquired pathogens, typically *Chlamydia trachomatis* or *Neisseria gonorrhoeae*, and occasionally, *Trichomonas vaginalis* or herpes simplex virus (HSV) [1]. In practice, MPC is a clinical diagnosis made when mucopurulent discharge or easily induced bleeding (friability) is present at the endocervical os; more subtle signs include edema of the cervical ectropion (edematous ectopy) and the presence of an elevated number of polymorphonuclear (PMN) white blood cells as detected by Gram stain of a smear of endocervical secretions. Superficially, at least, the clinical syndrome of MPC seems to be a fairly simple female version of male urethritis—what a landmark study published in 1984 termed "the ignored counterpart in women of urethritis in men" [2]. As with many syndromes, however, appearances can be deceptive, and MPC is an area that is ripe for discussion, research, and controversy.

Anatomy and physiology

The cervix consists of an underlying connective tissue matrix that is overlaid by two types of distinct epithelium (Fig. 1). The endocervical canal and ectropion, if present, are lined by columnar epithelial cells. These cells provide targets of entry for the pathogens that are associated most commonly with endocervicitis, namely, *C trachomatis* and *N gonorrhoeae*. In contrast, the ectocervix is lined by squamous epithelium that is

---

* Harborview Medical Center, Division of Infectious Diseases, 325 Ninth Avenue, Mailbox #359931, Seattle, WA 98104.
  E-mail address: jmm2@u.washington.edu

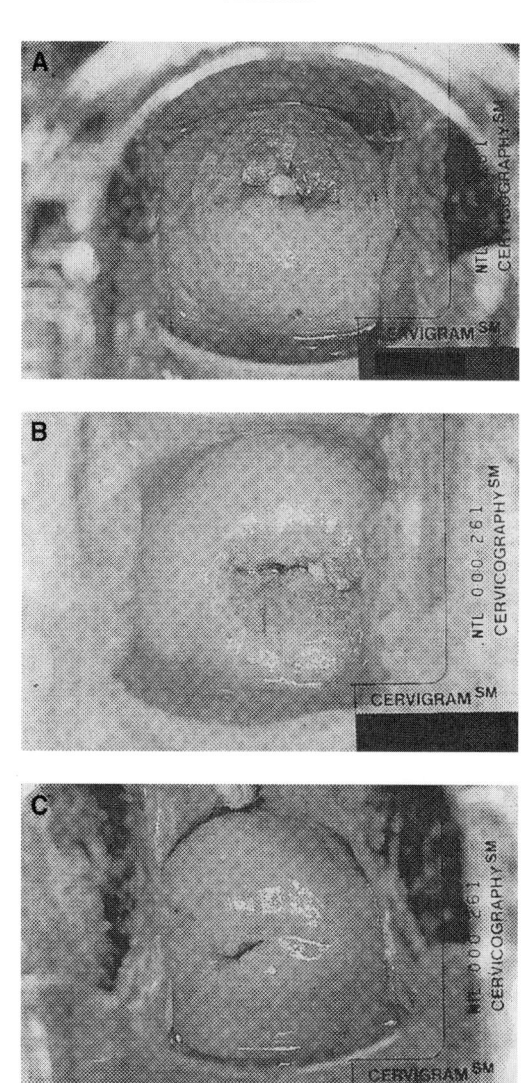

Fig. 1. The cervix at different stages of transformation, seen by colposcopy after application of acetic acid. (*A*) Cervical ectopy, consisting of columnar epithelium, appears as the darker area adjacent to the external os. (*B*) Squamous metaplasia, with columnar and squamous epithelium adjacent to the external os. (*C*) Mature squamous epithelium surrounding the external os, except for small transformational zone which appears light. (*From* Jacobson DL, Peralta L, Graham NM, et al. Histologic development of cervical ectopy: relationship to reproductive hormones. Sex Transm Dis 2000;27:253; with permission.)

contiguous with the vaginal mucosa, and thus, is susceptible to pathogenesis associated with vaginitis, including trichomoniasis and vulvovaginal candidiasis. Both types of epithelium are responsive to sustained hormonal changes [3]. Estrogen, either endogenous or exogenous, has numerous effects at cervicovaginal mucosa (see later discussion), but two are important to mention here. First, estrogen promotes formation and maintenance of cervical ectopy, which is present in adolescents, pregnancy, and in women who take estrogen-containing contraceptives. Second, estrogen is critical for maintaining adequate thickness of the squamous cervicovaginal epithelium (≥ 20 cell layers). Progesterone, in contrast, can cause relative thinning of this epithelium. The quality of endocervical mucus also is impacted by these hormones. High levels of estrogen during the follicular phase leading up to ovulation, for example, work to thin the endocervical mucus plug and facilitate the passage of spermatozoa through the endocervical canal. Progesterone, conversely, dominates the luteal phase of the cycle and acts to increase the viscosity and reduce the volume of endocervical mucus; this makes this material more tenacious, and, potentially, more resistant to passage by sperm and possibly by pathogens. More recently, some investigators proposed a direct role for these hormones in modulating the balance of cell-mediated (Th1) and humoral (Th2) immune responses, with estrogen predominance promoting Th2 responses and progesterone augmenting Th1 responses [4].

Physiologically, endocervical mucus evidences considerable intrinsic antimicrobial activity effected by lactic acid, low pH, and antimicrobial peptides [5–7].

Definition and epidemiology

The presence of easily induced bleeding and mucopurulent discharge from the endocervical canal are the most straightforward signs of the endocervical inflammation that defines MPC. These signs, along with the more subtle presence of edematous ectopy, do confer a considerably higher likelihood of detecting the sexually transmitted infections (STIs) that classically are associated with MPC, including *N gonorrhoeae* and *C trachomatis* [2,8–11]. It is worth noting, however, that some important perceptions about these signs have changed over the last several years. First, the use of nucleic acid amplified tests (NAATs) for both of these STIs, in particular *C trachomatis*, have enhanced sensitivity markedly relative to earlier generations of diagnostic tests, while maintaining excellent specificity [12–14]. This has resulted in an increasing proportion of cervical chlamydial and gonococcal infections that are not associated with signs that are typical of MPC. The quantity of organisms in endocervical and urethral chlamydial infections correlates directly with the presence of mucosal inflammatory signs [15,16] and with the ability of any diagnostic test to detect infection

[17]. NAATs detect more infections in women who do not have signs of MPC than in those who do have signs of MPC [18]. Thus, the proportion of women who have no endocervical signs whose cervical chlamydial infection is detected by NAAT is likely to be greater than for women whose infection is detected by less sensitive tests. This finding has resulted in a decrease in the estimated proportion of cervical chlamydial infections that are believed to cause cervical signs, which is likely 10% to 20%. Second, even seemingly obvious signs of endocervical inflammation may have variable precision for these STIs because the predictive value of individual cervical findings that are suggestive of MPC may vary with patients' age and other STI-related risk factors [19].

Two tests that are used to assess endocervical inflammation are cited in much of the literature on MPC, and deserve comment. The independent value of inflammation as detected by Gram stain of a smear of endocervical secretions or by Papanicolaou smear as a criterion for MPC, especially in predicting chlamydial infection, has been variable [2,20–26]. The Centers for Disease Control and Prevention's (CDC) Sexually Transmitted Disease Treatment Guidelines stopped including inflammation on endocervical Gram stain as presumptive evidence and indication for empiric treatment of chlamydial infection in 1993 [27]; the sensitivity of endocervical Gram stain for detection of *N gonorrhoeae* at the cervix is only 50% [28,29]. Gram stain of endocervical secretions continues to be used in many settings, particularly those that provide focused STI care (sexually transmitted disease [STD] clinics), and is still recommended by some investigators [25]. Most clinic practice guidelines recommend a threshold level of 10 to 30 PMN leukocytes per high-power (1000×, oil immersion) field; PMN counts above this level support a diagnosis of MPC. As expected, the sensitivity of this test increases and the specificity decreases as the threshold cutoff is decreased [22]. Although inflammatory changes on Papanicolaou smear are associated with an increased likelihood of detection of several STIs [30,31], including *C trachomatis, N gonorrhoeae*, trichomoniasis, and human papillomavirus, this test is neither specific enough to direct empiric therapy for these pathogens nor practical in delineating immediate etiologies of MPC for empiric therapy to recommend its unqualified use for this purpose [32–35].

Finally, it is worth emphasizing that no consensus definition for MPC as a research outcome exists. This has led to a literature that is difficult to interpret and to findings that may be less than generalizable. At the most basic level, many studies have not distinguished between the presence of signs at the endocervix—lined by the columnar epithelial cells that are the target for chlamydial and gonococcal infection—or the ectocervix—made up of the squamous epithelium that also lines the vagina. These epithelia differ in the target organisms that they host, endogenous defense mechanisms, secretory capacity, and vulnerability to infection with HIV-1. Some studies have required the presence of inflammation detected by Gram stain of endocervical secretions to substantiate the clinical diagnosis of MPC, whereas others have not collected information on endocervical induced bleeding. These inconsistencies make generalizing across studies difficult, and point out the need for consistent definitions and protocols in clinical research.

What causes mucopurulent cervicitis? Some old and new culprits

C trachomatis and *N gonorrhoeae* are well-described causes of MPC (Table 1). Other common STIs also can cause clinically evident cervical inflammation. *T vaginalis* may cause an erosive inflammation of the ectocervical epithelium which classically is manifest as "strawberry cervix" or colpitis macularis. This process may cause a range of epithelial disruption, from small isolated petechiae to large punctuate hemorrhages with surrounding areas of pale mucosa. The pathogenesis of these lesions probably arises, in part, from the variety of cytotoxic factors that *T vaginalis* can elaborate, including cystine proteases, which degrade endogenous factors that protect the integrity of the cervicovaginal epithelium, most notably secretory leukocyte protease inhibitor (SLPI) [36]. Again, why some women develop evident cervical changes with trichomoniasis is not clear. Possible reasons include a direct relationship between quantitative burden of *T vaginalis*, strain of organism involved, or host factors that might increase susceptibility to cervical inflammation [37–39].

Genital infection with HSV types 1 and 2 also can cause MPC. The most striking example occurs in women who experience severe clinical manifestations of primary infection with HSV-2. Although most primary HSV-2 infections are asymptomatic, some women experience a severe primary infection that may include MPC. Typically, MPC in this setting is characterized by diffuse erosive and hemorrhagic lesions, usually in the ectocervical epithelium, and often accompanied by frank ulceration. MPC is believed to occur in approximately 15% to 20% of women who experience clinically evident primary HSV-2 genital infection [40]. When MPC occurs in this setting, other manifestations of primary HSV-2 genital infection usually are evident, including external herpetic lesions, neurologic manifestations (including aseptic meningitis, urinary retention, and lumbosacral radiculitis), fever, and inguinal lymphadenopathy. Any of these symptoms and signs, including MPC, may reoccur with clinical recurrences of genital HSV-2; however, typically, they are less severe during recurrences. Subclinical shedding of HSV-2 does not seem to be related directly to MPC [41]. HSV-1 also may cause MPC similar to those described for HSV-2; however, the manifestations typically are less severe, and usually occur only during the primary genital infection with HSV-1 [40].

Mycoplasma genitalium recently was implicated as a sexually transmissible cause of MPC [42,43]. Manhart and colleagues [42] studied archived endocervical fluid samples that were collected from 779 women who attended an STD clinic from 1984 to 1986. Of the 719 samples that

Table 1
Etiologies of mucopurulent cervicitis and suggested management

Etiology	Management	Comments
Chlamydia trachomatis	Azithromycin, 1 g po (single dose); or doxycycline, 100 mg po twice daily for 7 days	Minority of infected women have signs of MPC Urine NAAT highly sensitive for diagnosis of endocervical chlamydial infection
Neisseria gonorrhoeae	A single dose of any of following: Cefixime, 400 mg po Ciprofloxacin, 500 mg po Levofloxacin, 250 mg po Ceftriaxone, 125 mg IM	Availability of oral cefixime has been precarious, leading many experts to advocate use of cefpodoxime, 400 mg po; formal efficacy studies underway Fluoroquinolone resistance increasing rapidly in *N gonorrhoeae*; may not be appropriate empiric therapy in some areas [96,97] Minority of infected women have signs of MPC Urine NAAT highly sensitive for diagnosis of endocervical chlamydial infection
Trichomonas vaginalis	Metronidazole, 2 g po (single dose); or Tinidazole, 2 g po (single dose); or Metronidazole, 500 mg po twice daily for 7 days	
HSV	Any of the following given orally for 7–10 days: Acyclovir, 400 mg three times daily Famciclovir, 250 mg three times daily Valacyclovir, 1 g twice daily	Primary infection with HSV-2 may cause an especially erosive, hemorrhagic cervicitis
Empiric therapy	Most women should be treated for chlamydial infection Consider therapy for gonococcal infection based on age, risk, local or patient subgroup prevalence [88,89] Treat concomitant causes of any vaginitis present appropriately	All women should have diagnostic tests for *C trachomatis* and *N gonorrhoeae* using most sensitive assays available (ideally, NAAT) Evaluate for history suggestive of genital herpes, vaginitis, use of irritative intravaginal preparations (spermicides, deodorants, chemical douches) Evaluate and treat sex partners appropriately

Abbreviations: IM, intramuscularly; NAAT, nucleic acid amplified test; po, by month. Include PCR, transcription-mediated amplification, strand displacement assay.

contained material that was polymerase chain reaction (PCR)-amplifiable, women with *M genitalium* isolated were 3.3 times more likely to have MPC as defined by the presence of endocervical mucopurulent discharge, easily induced bleeding, and Gram stain with at least 30 PMN cells/high-power field. Detection of *M genitalium* also was associated with each of these individual findings. This association persisted even when multiple cofactors were accounted for, including chlamydial and gonococcal coinfection, proliferative phase of the menstrual cycle, and age. The investigators concluded that *M genitalium* was associated independently with MPC in this population, may cause cervical inflammation, and should be considered among potential etiologies of MPC. More recent studies seem to confirm this preliminary finding [43]; efforts to examine the response of this organism to standard antibiotics that are used to treat MPC are underway. Establishing a definitive role for *M genitalium* in the causation of MPC and other inflammatory genital syndromes will require prospective studies that examine the response of associated clinical syndromes to appropriate antibiotics, concurrent infection of sex partners, and the true predilection of the anatomic site for this intriguing organism. Like *M pneumoniae*, *M genitalium* seems to be sensitive to macrolides and tetracyclines, but further study is required to confirm the efficacy of these antibiotics in curing lower genital tract infection with this organism. *M genitalium* is difficult to culture; to date, clinical studies have relied on PCR to detect it. The implication of this for determining microbiologic cure in such studies is not yet clear.

Other infectious agents have been invoked as causes of MPC. Cytomegalovirus (CMV), a herpesvirus that is known to be sexually transmitted, has been isolated in some of the few studies of MPC that have looked for it [44]. Given the small number of studies and subjects involved, as well as the limited descriptions of study design and subject selection, it is difficult to generalize about how much nonchlamydial, nongonococcal MPC that CMV might cause. CMV is shed in secretions at several mucosal sites, and its detection in the setting of MPC may represent an "epiphenomenon" of endocervical inflammation. Recently, cervical shedding of human T-cell lymphotrophic virus (HTLV)-1 was associated with the presence of MPC as defined by Gram stain of endocervical secretions or by visible endocervical secretions in a cohort of commercial sex workers in Peru [45]. Whether HTLV-1 plays an etiologic role in cervical inflammation, or is simply shed in greater quantity during episodes of MPC, is not known. Various case reports have attributed the presence of MPC in individual women to infection with certain *Streptococcus* species [46–48]—most notably, *S agalactiae* (group B streptococcus) and *S pyogenes*—but reliable estimates of how commonly this might occur, if a causal relationship does exist, are not available.

Apart from the infections that were noted above, a variety of noninfectious and infectious systemic inflammatory processes and local insults can induce endocervical inflammation which can result in clinically evident MPC. Among the former are Behcet's disease, sarcoidosis, ligneous conjunctivitis [49], and tuberculosis. In the latter group are substances that erode cervicovaginal mucosa or cause an irritant mucositis, usually through frequent use of high concentrations. These substances include chemical douches [8,50], some spermicides (specifically those with surfactant properties; nonoxynol-9 [N-9] is the prototype), and chemical deodorants. In one large study in which commercial sex workers were randomized to use vaginal sponges that were impregnated with 1 g of N-9, cervical erosions as assessed by colposcopy were seen more commonly among N-9 users, who also were more likely to acquire HIV infection during the course of the study than were nonusers. The mucosal erosion was believed to be the means by which N-9 conferred an increased risk of HIV-1 acquisition in this cohort of women [51]. Because at least one other study has demonstrated harm from the use of N-9 [52], and none showed clear benefit, this preparation cannot be recommended for the purpose of preventing STIs [53,54].

Nongonococcal, nonchlamydial mucopurulent cervicitis: further considerations

A vexing clinical problem is that in many cases of MPC, neither of the two major associated STIs (*C trachomatis* and *N gonorrhoeae*) are detected, even when highly sensitive diagnostic tests are used [2,10,19,55]. For example, among 520 women who had chlamydial or gonococcal endocervical infection as detected by culture at a Seattle STD clinic from 1995–1999, only 58% had any sign that was consistent with MPC [19]. Nonetheless, MPC that occurs in the absence of detectable gonococcal or chlamydial infection may confer an increased risk of poor pregnancy outcome [26] and predict upper genital tract disease [56–58]. The etiology of the large proportion of MPC in which neither gonorrhea nor chlamydia is detected is not clear. Endocervical inflammation may be mediated through several different pathways. One possible categorization for how MPC might occur apart from a direct effect of a known pathogen is presented in Table 2. An undefined local inflammatory process might be induced or maintained through several pathways, including the effects of a persistent undefined pathogen, persistently abnormal vaginal flora, or an inappropriately exuberant primary host immune response. Such processes probably are modulated further by the effect of endogenous and exogenous hormones, including those that are experienced throughout the menstrual cycle and with the use of contraceptive formulations.

A possible association between bacterial vaginosis (BV) and MPC, independent of concomitant chlamydial and gonococcal infection, emerged in several recent studies [59–61]. BV is the most common cause of vaginitis in diverse clinical settings, and is characterized by overgrowth of commensal anaerobic flora relative to the hydrogen peroxide (H_2O_2)-producing *Lactobacillus* species that predominate in the healthy vagina [62]. The observation that BV is associated with acquisition of *C trachomatis* and *N gonorrhoeae* [63,64] poses a challenge to demonstrating a definitive, independent relationship between BV and MPC. BV is associated strongly with adverse outcomes that are related to the upper genital tract [65], and the vaginal bacteria that characterize BV must cross the endocervical

Table 2
Factors that may play a role in mucopurulent cervicitis in which typical sexually transmitted pathogens are not detected

Process	Comments	References
Persistent disruptions of vaginal flora	Mechanism unclear, but may involve effect of glycosidases produced by bacteria associated with BV Treatment of BV associated with enhanced resolution of MPC in one small study	[67,76]
Persistent infection with an undefined pathogen	No direct research in MPC yet, but use of cultivation-independent molecular techniques is rapidly expanding the spectrum of bacteria associated with BV, including *Atopobium vaginalis*	[98]
Sustained primary host immune response	Genital mucosa affected in many diseases with immune basis, including psoriasis, Behcet's syndrome May be augmented further by effect of endogenous or exogenous sex hormones	[77]
Sustained use of commercial products that disrupt or irritate cervicovaginal mucosa	Many over-the-counter products contain surfactants or other potentially irritating substances (betadine, corn starch, topical anesthestics)	[53,54,99]

mucous barrier where they may elicit a local inflammatory response as a result. More persuasively, including intravaginal antibiotic therapy for BV in the treatment regimen for women who had MPC was associated with enhanced cure of MPC in two small studies [66,67]. Finally, cervical shedding of HIV is increased in the setting of BV; this suggests that BV itself may have direct effects at the endocervical mucosa [68,69].

Emerging data suggest that the risk profile of women who develop MPC in the setting of BV is different from that of women who are at risk for chlamydial or gonococcal infection. In a study of 424 women who had BV, MPC was common and occurred in 15%; most cases (87%) were not associated with chlamydial or gonococcal infection of the cervix [70]. Increasing age, fewer years of formal education, report of a new male sex partner or of a current female sex partner, more recent receptive oral sex, and absence of H_2O_2-producing *Lactobacillus* species were associated independently with an increased likelihood of MPC among women who had BV. Vaginal colonization with H_2O_2-producing *Lactobacillus* species was associated with a 60% reduction in the likelihood of MPC.

Although few studies have addressed the issue of BV and MPC, the available data suggest a potential role for multiple factors, especially vaginal cytokines. Cytokines that help to regulate the normal function of mucosal defense systems include SLPI, which helps to maintain healthy vaginal mucosa and is decreased in the presence of several STIs [36]; interleukin (IL)-10, which may increase susceptibility of macrophages to HIV-1 infection [71]; and IL-1β, which has been associated with a higher number of vaginal neutrophils among women who have BV [72]. Even when vaginal flora is normal, the balance of pro- and anti-inflammatory cervical cytokines may play a key role in modulating evident cervical inflammation and in permitting ascension of STIs or other potential pathogens to the upper genital tract. One recent study demonstrated that decreased cervical proinflammatory cytokines—IL-1β, IL-6, and IL-8—were associated with an increased likelihood of clinical chorioamnionitis [73]. A role for proinflammatory vaginal cytokines, such as IL-1β, IL-6, and IL-8, is suggested by the observation that these cytokines decline after successful treatment of BV [74].

Other players that are important in a potential connection between MPC and BV include lactobacilli that produce H_2O_2. H_2O_2 may exert a direct effect against pathogens that are known to cause MPC and against potentially pathogenic anaerobes that are associated with BV itself [75]. Finally, glycosidases and proteinases that are produced in abundance by BV-associated flora may degrade cervicovaginal mucus, along with its protective physical and immunologic components [76].

It is increasingly clear that endogenous hormones have a role in maintaining the integrity of cervicovaginal mucosa. Estrogen likely upregulates, and progesterone down-regulates, the local immune response to some pathogens [77]. Women who have relative estrogen deficiency (eg, those who are postmenopausal, post partum, have very low body fat, or take drugs with androgenic effects) are known to have an increased risk of atrophic vaginitis; however, more subtle effects of their inability to maintain a normal vaginal pH (<4.5) may include gradual erosion of the endocervical mucous layer. Progesterone, which can promote thinning of the vaginal mucosa and in animal models enhances susceptibility to infection with simian immunodeficiency virus [78], also may increase a woman's risk for MPC for reasons that are not clear. In one large recent study, women who used depot progesterone as their primary source of contraception were more likely to be diagnosed with endocervical chlamydial and gonococcal infection, as well as clinically diagnosed MPC [79]; this association also was noted in earlier studies [80]. Although this particular study has several limitations that preclude a definite assignation of MPC or STI risk to progesterone use [81], the reported association concords with our limited knowledge of the mucosal effect of this hormone, and supports the need for more careful prospective study of larger numbers of women.

Guidelines for management

Clinical definition of MPC is syndromic. Most clinicians do not have access to endocervical Gram stain, and even when this test is performed, its predictive value is highly variable. Because the association between MPC and cervical infection with *C trachomatis* and *N gonorrhoeae* is well-established, the CDC recommends testing for both of these organisms if MPC is present [82]. It is important that one of the most sensitive diagnostic tests, NAAT, be used if at all possible, particularly for chlamydial infections, because the sensitivity of NAAT (including PCR, transcription mediated amplification, and strand displacement amplification) for *C trachomatis* is at least 20% higher than that of unamplified DNA probes [13]. Examination of vaginal fluid should be performed to look for the presence of BV because treatment of concurrent BV might enhance the resolution of MPC. Three of four Amsel criteria are sufficient to establish the diagnosis of BV, including presence of homogeneous vaginal discharge, vaginal fluid pH greater than 4.5, clue cells greater than 20% of total vaginal epithelial cells seen on 100× magnification on saline microscopy, and amine (fishy) odor on addition of potassium hydroxide [83]. Saline microscopy also offers the opportunity to look for motile trichomonads (although newer diagnostic tests may enhance clinicians' ability to make this diagnosis more readily and accurately [84]), and for an elevated number of PMN cells, which may indicate a higher likelihood of cervical infection with *C trachomatis* or *N gonorrhoeae* [85].

The 2002 CDC STD Treatment Guidelines also recommend that empiric treatment of MPC that is directed at *C trachomatis* and *N gonorrhoeae* should be provided if the local prevalence of these infections is high, or if the likelihood of a woman's return for treatment based on a diagnostic test that turns out to be positive is judged to be low. No specific prevalence parameters are provided to help guide providers' approach regarding empiric treatment. Consensus establishment of a threshold prevalence of these infections above which empiric therapy should be provided would be useful. Other considerations that should weigh toward empiric therapy for these infections include report of STI-related risk behavior (especially new or multiple sex partners in the past 60 days) and recent history of STI (especially chlamydial or gonococcal infection in the past year). Recurrent infection with *C trachomatis* is common among women (8%–25% in several studies) [86,87], and probably relates predominantly to resumption of unprotected sex with untreated partners. Although treatment for *C trachomatis* should be a mainstay of empiric therapy regimens, the approach that involves possible infection with *N gonorrhoeae* is less clear. Certainly, women who have MPC and fall into subgroups with high previous likelihood of gonococcal infection should be treated empirically; these subgroups include adolescents in inner-city areas in many parts of the United States [88,89]. Treating MPC—especially if it is caused by *C trachomatis* or *N gonorrhoeae*—is especially important among HIV-infected women, because MPC undoubtedly increases the amount of HIV-1 that is shed from the cervix [90,91]. At least one small study demonstrated a decline in the amount of HIV-1 that was shed from the cervical mucosa after empiric treatment of MPC that was aimed at chlamydial and gonococcal infection [92]; this likely reduces these women's risk of transmitting HIV-1 to sex partners.

The limited available data suggest that antibiotics that are aimed at *C trachomatis* and *N gonorrhoeae* do not treat nonchlamydial, nongonococcal MPC adequately. This contrasts with the parallel syndrome in men—nonchlamydial, nongonococcal urethritis—in which single-dose therapy with azithromycin resolved the condition in most men [93]. Although the combination of doxycycline and amoxicillin initially was effective in treating MPC among STD clinic clients in one study, high rates (30%) of persistent or recurrent MPC (23% and 33%, respectively) were observed 3 months after treatment, usually in the absence of detectable infection with *C trachomatis*, *N gonorrhoeae*, genital mycoplasma, or *T vaginalis* (a surrogate measure for BV) [94]. In another study, treatment with ofloxacin yielded similar improvement in MPC, regardless of whether *C trachomatis* was detected [95]. Finally, among 51 women who had MPC and BV who were randomized to receive doxycycline and ofloxacin plus intravaginal metronidazole or placebo, those who received metronidazole had a higher rate of resolution of MPC at 2 and 4 weeks posttreatment; women whose BV resolved were more likely to have resolution of MPC at 2 weeks, regardless of which regimen they received [67]. Further management of MPC for which neither identifiable STI nor BV plays a role is empiric, and is substantiated by little rigorous evidence; approaches include more extended courses of broad-spectrum antibiotics or ablative therapy [55].

Areas of controversy and challenges for future efforts

Although our understanding of MPC and its pathogenesis has advanced considerably in the last 2 decades, many areas of uncertainty remain. What should constitute appropriate empiric management of MPC in women who are at low risk for chlamydial or gonococcal infection, or in settings in which gonococcal disease is uncommon? Does BV really cause clinical MPC and if so, what is the mechanism for this? Are "new" pathogens that elude identification by traditional culture methods playing a role in MPC? If the association between adequate levels of vaginal H_2O_2-producing lactobacilli and the absence of MPC is confirmed, how do these organisms help to maintain a healthy cervicovaginal environment? Because MPC increases the risk of poor pregnancy outcome, predicts upper genital tract disease, and is associated with increased shedding of HIV-1 from the cervix, defining alternate etiologies and effective treatment for this condition should be a priority. Future research should focus on these issues, including clarification of the cervix's immune response to disruptions in the normal vaginal flora and to varying levels of sex hormones. For this purpose, a consensus definition of MPC needs to be established, and clear guidance on the approach to empiric therapy defined.

References

[1] Holmes KK, Stamm WE. Lower genital tract infection syndromes in women. In: Holmes KK, Sparling F, Mardh P-A, et al, editors. Sexually transmitted diseases. 3rd edition. New York: McGraw-Hill; 1999. p. 761–81.
[2] Brunham RC, Paavonen J, Stevens CE, et al. Mucopurulent cervicitis—the ignored counterpart in women of urethritis in men. N Engl J Med 1984;311:1–6.
[3] Jacobson DL, Peralta L, Graham NM, et al. Histologic development of cervical ectopy: relationship to reproductive hormones. Sex Transm Dis 2000;27:252–8.
[4] Whitacre CA, Reingold SC, O'Looney PA. A gender gap in autoimmunity. Science 1999; 283:1277–8.
[5] Eggert-Krause W, Botz I, Pohl S, et al. Antimicrobial activity of human cervical mucus. Hum Reprod 2000;15:778–84.
[6] Hein M, Valore EV, Helmig RB, et al. Antimicrobial factors in the cervical mucus plug. Am J Obstet Gynecol 2002;187:137–44.
[7] Valore EV, Park CH, Igreti SL, et al. Antimicrobial components of vaginal fluid. Am J Obstet Gynecol 2002;187:561–8.
[8] Critchlow CW, Wolner-Hanssen P, Eschenbach DA, et al. Determinants of cervical ectopia and of cervicitis: age, oral contraception, specific cervical infection, smoking, and douching. Am J Obstet Gynecol 1995;173:534–43.
[9] Lindner LE, Geerling S, Nettum JA, et al. Clinical characteristics of women with chlamydial cervicitis. J Reprod Med 1988;33:684–90.
[10] Paavonen J, Critchlow CW, DeRouen T, et al. Etiology of cervical inflammation. Am J Obstet Gynecol 1986;154:556–64.
[11] Paavonen J, Vesterinen E. Chlamydia trachomatis in cervicitis and urethritis in women. Scand J Infect Dis Suppl 1982;32:45–54.
[12] Koumans EH, Johnson RE, Knapp JS, et al. Laboratory testing for *Neisseria gonorrhoeae* by recently introduced nonculture tests: a performance review with clinical and public health considerations. Clin Infect Dis 1998;27:1171–80.
[13] Black CM, Marrazzo J, Johnson RE, et al. Head-to-head multicenter comparison of DNA probe and nucleic acid amplification tests for *Chlamydia trachomatis* infection in women performed with an improved reference standard. J Clin Microbiol 2002;40: 3757–63.
[14] Cosentino LA, Landers DV, Hillier SL. Detection of *Chlamydia trachomatis* and *Neisseria gonorrhoeae* by strand displacement amplification and relevance of the amplification control for use with vaginal swab specimens. J Clin Microbiol 2003;41: 3592–6.
[15] Geisler W, Suchland RJ, Whittington WLH, et al. Quantitative culture of *Chlamydia trachomatis*: relationship of inclusion-forming units produced in culture to clinical manifestations and acute inflammation in urogenital disease. J Infect Dis 2001;184:879–84.
[16] Marrazzo JM, Whittington WL, Celum CL, et al. Urine-based screening for *Chlamydia trachomatis* in men attending sexually transmitted disease clinics. Sex Transm Dis 2001;28: 219–25.
[17] Black CM. Current methods of laboratory diagnosis of *Chlamydia trachomatis* infections. Clin Microbiol Rev 1997;10:160–84.
[18] Marrazzo JM, Johnson RE, Green TA, et al. Impact of patient characteristics on performance of nucleic acid amplification tests and DNA probe for Chlamydia trachomatis genital infection in women. J Clin Microbiol 2005;43:577–84.
[19] Marrazzo JM, Handsfield HH, Whittington WL. Predicting chlamydial and gonococcal cervical infection: implications for management of cervicitis. Obstet Gynecol 2002;100: 579–84.
[20] Katz BP, Caine VA, Jones RB. Diagnosis of mucopurulent cervicitis among women at risk for *Chlamydia trachomatis* infection. Sex Transm Dis 1989;16:103–6.

[21] Knud-Hansen CR, Dallabetta GA, Reichart C, et al. Surrogate methods to diagnose gonococcal and chlamydial cervicitis: comparison of leukocyte esterase dipstick, endocervical Gram stain, and culture. Sex Transm Dis 1991;18:211–6.
[22] Manavi K, Conlan R, Barrie G. The performance of microscopic cervicitis for the detection of chlamydial infection. Sex Transm Infect 2004;80:415.
[23] Moore SG, Miller WC, Hoffman IF, et al. Clinical utility of measuring white blood cells on vaginal wet mount and endocervical gram stain for the prediction of chlamydial and gonococcal infections. Sex Transm Dis 2000;27:530–8.
[24] Moscicki B, Shafer MA, Millstein SG, et al. The use and limitations of endocervical Gram stains and mucopurulent cervicitis as predictors for *Chlamydia trachomatis* in female adolescents. Am J Obstet Gynecol 1987;157:65–71.
[25] Myziuk L, Romanowski B, Brown M. Endocervical Gram stain smears and their usefulness in the diagnosis of *Chlamydia trachomatis*. Sex Transm Infect 2001;77:103–6.
[26] Nugent RP, Hillier SL. Mucopurulent cervicitis as a predictor of chlamydial infection and adverse pregnancy outcome. The Investigators of the Johns Hopkins Study of Cervicitis and Adverse Pregnancy Outcome. Sex Transm Dis 1992;19:198–202.
[27] Centers for Disease Control and Prevention. 1993 sexually transmitted diseases treatment guidelines. MMWR Morb Mortal Wkly Rep 1993;42:1–102.
[28] Hook EW III, Handsfield HH. Gonococcal infections in the adult. In: Holmes KK SP, Mardh P-A, Lemon SM, et al, editors. Sexually transmitted diseases. 3rd edition. New York: McGraw-Hill; 1999. p. 451–66.
[29] Manavi K, Young H, Clutterbuck D. Sensitivity of microscopy for the rapid diagnosis of gonorrhoea in men and women and the role of gonorrhoea serovars. Int J STD AIDS 2003; 14:390–4.
[30] Kiviat NB, Paavonen JA, Wolner-Hanssen P, et al. Histopathology of endocervical infection caused by Chlamydia trachomatis, herpes simplex virus, *Trichomonas vaginalis*, and *Neisseria gonorrhoeae*. Hum Pathol 1990;21:831–7.
[31] Kiviat NB, Wolner-Hanssen P, Eschenbach DA, et al. Endometrial histopathology in patients with culture-proved upper genital tract infection and laparoscopically diagnosed acute salpingitis. Am J Surg Pathol 1990;14:167–75.
[32] Addiss DG, Vaughn ML, Golubjatnikov R, et al. *Chlamydia trachomatis* infection in women attending urban midwestern family planning and community health clinics: risk factors, selective screening, and evaluation of non-culture techniques. Sex Transm Dis 1990;17: 138–46.
[33] Bertolino JG, Rangel JE, Blake RL Jr, et al. Inflammation on the cervical Papanicolaou smear: the predictive value for infection in asymptomatic women. Fam Med 1992;24: 447–52.
[34] Edelman M, Fox A, Alderman E, et al. Cervical Papanicolaou smear abnormalities and *Chlamydia trachomatis* in sexually active adolescent females. J Pediatr Adolesc Gynecol 2000;13:65–9.
[35] Garozzo G, Lomeo E, La Greca M, et al. *Chlamydia trachomatis* diagnosis: a correlative study of pap smear and direct immunofluorescence. Clin Exp Obstet Gynecol 1993;20: 259–63.
[36] Draper D, Landers D, Krohn M, et al. Levels of vaginal secretory leukocyte protease inhibitor are decreased in women with lower reproductive tract infections. Am J Obstet Gynecol 2000;183:1243–8.
[37] Fiori PL, Rappelli P, Addis MF. The flagellated parasite *Trichomonas vaginalis*: new insights into cytopathogenicity mechanisms. Microbes Infect 1999;1:149–56.
[38] Petrin D, Delgaty K, Bhatt R, et al. Clinical and microbiological aspects of *Trichomonas vaginalis*. Clin Microbiol Rev 1998;11:300–17.
[39] Schwebke JR. Update of trichomoniasis. Sex Transm Infect 2002;78:378–9.
[40] Corey L, Wald A. Genital herpes. In: Holmes KK SP, Mardh P-A, Lemon SM, et al, editors. Sexually transmitted diseases. 3rd edition. New York: McGraw-Hill, 1999. p. 285–312.

[41] Koelle DM, Benedetti J, Langenberg A, et al. Asymptomatic reactivation of herpes simplex virus in women after the first episode of genital herpes. Ann Intern Med 1992;116:433–7.
[42] Manhart LE, Critchlow CW, Holmes KK, et al. Mucopurulent cervicitis and *Mycoplasma genitalium*. J Infect Dis 2003;187:650–7.
[43] Schlicht MJ, Lovrich SD, Sartin JS, et al. High prevalence of genital mycoplasmas among sexually active young adults with urethritis or cervicitis symptoms in La Crosse, Wisconsin. J Clin Microbiol 2004;42:4636–40.
[44] McGalie CE, McBride HA, McCluggage WG. Cytomegalovirus infection of the cervix: morphological observations in five cases of a possibly under-recognised condition. J Clin Pathol 2004;57:691–4.
[45] Zunt JR, Dezzutti CS, Montano SM, et al. Cervical shedding of human T cell lymphotropic virus type I is associated with cervicitis. J Infect Dis 2002;186:1669–72.
[46] Buttigieg G. Cervicitis and urethritis caused by group B streptococcus: case report. Genitourin Med 1985;61:343–4.
[47] Paavonen J, Kiviat N, Brunham RC, et al. Prevalence and manifestations of endometritis among women with cervicitis. Am J Obstet Gynecol 1985;152:280–6.
[48] Paraskevaides EC, Wilson MC. Fatal disseminated intravascular coagulation secondary to streptococcal cervicitis. Eur J Obstet Gynecol Reprod Biol 1988;29:39–40.
[49] Chakravarti S, Pickrell MD, Dunn PJ, et al. Ligneous conjunctivitis and the cervix. BJOG 2003;110:1032–3.
[50] Scholes D, Stergachis A, Ichikawa LE, et al. Vaginal douching as a risk factor for cervical *Chlamydia trachomatis* infection. Obstet Gynecol 1998;91:993–7.
[51] Kreiss J, Ngugi E, Holmes K, et al. Efficacy of nonoxynol 9 contraceptive sponge use in preventing heterosexual acquisition of HIV in Nairobi prostitutes. JAMA 1992;268:477–82.
[52] Richardson BA, Lavreys L, Martin HL. Evaluation of a low-dose nonoxynol-9 gel for the prevention of sexually transmitted diseases. Sex Transm Dis 2001;28:394–400.
[53] Richardson BA. Nonoxynol-9 as a vaginal microbicide for prevention of sexually transmitted infections: it's time to move on. JAMA 2002;287:1171–2.
[54] Wilkinson D, Tholandi M, Ramjee G, et al. Nonoxynol-9 spermicide for prevention of vaginally acquired HIV and other sexually transmitted infections: systematic review and meta-analysis of randomised controlled trials including more than 5000 women. Lancet Infect Dis 2002;2:613–7.
[55] Nyirjesy P. Nongonococcal and nonchlamydial cervicitis. Curr Infect Dis Rep 2001;3:540–5.
[56] Peipert JF, Ness RB, Soper DE, et al. Association of lower genital tract inflammation with objective evidence of endometritis. Infect Dis Obstet Gynecol 2000;8:83–7.
[57] Paavonen J, Kiviat N, Holmes KK. Prevalence and manifestations of endometritis among women with cervicitis. Am J Obstet Gynecol 1985;173:534–43.
[58] Wiesenfeld HC, Hillier SL, Krohn MA, et al. Lower genital tract infection and endometritis: insight into subclinical pelvic inflammatory disease. Obstet Gynecol 2002;100:456–63.
[59] Keshavarz H, Duffy SW, Sadeghi-Hassanabadi A, et al. Risk factors for and relationship between bacterial vaginosis and cervicitis in a high risk population for cervicitis in Southern Iran. Eur J Epidemiol 2001;17:89–95.
[60] Peipert JF, Montagno AB, Cooper AS, et al. Bacterial vaginosis as a risk factor for upper genital tract infection. Am J Obstet Gynecol 1997;177:1184–7.
[61] Willmott FE. Mucopurulent cervicitis: a clinical entity? Genitourin Med 1988;64:169–71.
[62] Hillier S, Holmes KK. Bacterial vaginosis. In: Holmes KK SP, Mardh P-A, Lemon SM, et al, editors. Sexually transmitted diseases. 3rd edition. New York: McGraw-Hill, 1999. p. 563–86.
[63] Martin HL, Richardson BA, Nyange PM, et al. Vaginal lactobacilli, microbial flora, and risk of human immunodeficiency virus type 1 and sexually transmitted disease acquisition. J Infect Dis 1999;180:1863–8.

[64] Wiesenfeld HC, Hillier SL, Krohn MA, et al. Bacterial vaginosis is a strong predictor of *Neisseria gonorrhoeae* and *Chlamydia trachomatis* infection. Clin Infect Dis 2003;36:663–8.
[65] Sweet RL. Gynecologic conditions and bacterial vaginosis: implications for the non-pregnant patient. Infect Dis Obstet Gynecol 2000;8:184–90.
[66] Schwebke JR, Schulien MB, Zajackowski M. Pilot study to evaluate the appropriate management of patients with coexistent bacterial vaginosis and cervicitis. Infect Dis Obstet Gynecol 1995;3:199–202.
[67] Schwebke JR, Weiss HL. Interrelationships of bacterial vaginosis and cervical inflammation. Sex Transm Dis 2002;29:59–64.
[68] Cu-Uvin S, Hogan JW, Caliendo AM, et al. Association between bacterial vaginosis and expression of human immunodeficiency virus type 1 RNA in the female genital tract. Clin Infect Dis 2001;33:894–6.
[69] Seck K, Samb N, Tempesta S, et al. Prevalence and risk factors of cervicovaginal HIV shedding among HIV-1 and HIV-2 infected women in Dakar, Senegal. Sex Transm Inf 2001; 77:190–3.
[70] Marrazzo JM, Wiesenfeld HC, Murray P, et al. Risk factors for mucopurulent cervicitis among women with bacterial vaginosis. Presented at the International Society for Sexually Transmitted Diseases Research Congress. Ottawa, Canada. August 27–30, 2003.
[71] Cohen CR, Plummer FA, Mugo N, et al. Increased interleukin-10 in the endocervical secretions of women with non-ulcerative sexually transmitted diseases: a mechanism for enhanced HIV-1 transmission? AIDS 1999;13:327–32.
[72] Cauci S, Guaschino S, De Aloysio D, et al. Interrelationships of interleukin-8 with interleukin-1beta and neutrophils in vaginal fluid of healthy and bacterial vaginosis positive women. Mol Hum Reprod 2003;9:53–8.
[73] Simhan HN, Caritis SN, Krohn MA, et al. Decreased cervical proinflammatory cytokines permit subsequent upper genital tract infection during pregnancy. Am J Obstet Gynecol 2003;189:560–7.
[74] Yudin MH, Landers DV, Meyn L, et al. Clinical and cervical cytokine response to treatment with oral or vaginal metronidazole for bacterial vaginosis during pregnancy: a randomized trial. Obstet Gynecol 2003;102:527–34.
[75] Hashemi FB, Ghassemi M, Faro S, et al. Induction of human immunodeficiency virus type 1 expression by anaerobes associated with bacterial vaginosis. J Infect Dis 2000;181:1574–80.
[76] Olmsted SS, Meyn LA, Rohan LC, et al. Glycosidase and proteinase activity of anaerobic gram-negative bacteria isolated from women with bacterial vaginosis. Sex Transm Dis 2003;30:257–61.
[77] Brabin L. Interactions of the female hormonal environment, susceptibility to viral infections, and disease progression. AIDS Patient Care STDS 2002;15:211–21.
[78] Smith SM, Baskin GB, Marx PA. Estrogen protects against vaginal transmission of simian immunodeficiency virus. J Infect Dis 2000;182:708–15.
[79] Morrison CS, Bright P, Wong EL, et al. Hormonal contraceptive use, cervical ectopy, and the acquisition of cervical infections. Sex Transm Dis 2004;31:561–7.
[80] Jacobson DL, Peralta L, Farmer M, et al. Relationship of hormonal contraception and cervical ectopy as measured by computerized planimetry to chlamydial infection in adolescents. Sex Transm Dis 2000;27:313–9.
[81] Dayan L, Donovan B. Chlamydia, gonorrhoea, and injectable progesterone. Lancet 2004; 364:1387–8.
[82] Centers for Disease Control and Prevention. Sexually transmitted disease treatment guidelines. MMWR Morb Mortal Wkly Rep 2002;51:32–42.
[83] Amsel R, Totten PA, Spiegel CA, et al. Nonspecific vaginitis. Diagnostic criteria and microbial and epidemiologic associations. Am J Med 1983;74:14–22.
[84] Kurth A, Whittington WL, Golden MR, et al. Performance of a new, rapid assay for detection of *Trichomonas vaginalis*. J Clin Microbiol 2004;42:2940–3.

[85] Geisler WM, Yu S, Venglarik M, et al. Vaginal leucocyte counts in women with bacterial vaginosis: relation to vaginal and cervical infections. Sex Transm Infect 2004;80:401–5.
[86] Burstein GR, Zenilman JM, Gaydos CA, et al. Predictors of repeat *Chlamydia trachomatis* infections diagnosed by DNA amplification testing among inner city females. Sex Transm Infect 2001;77:26–32.
[87] Whittington WL, Kent C, Kissinger P, et al. Determinants of persistent and recurrent *Chlamydia trachomatis* infection in young women: results of a multicenter cohort study. Sex Transm Dis 2001;28:117–23.
[88] Sexually Transmitted Disease Surveillance, 2003. Atlanta (GA): Centers for Disease Control and Prevention; 2004.
[89] Miller WC, Ford CA, Morris M, et al. Prevalence of chlamydial and gonococcal infections among young adults in the United States. JAMA 2004;291:2229–36.
[90] Gadkari DA, Quinn TC, Gangakhedkar RR, et al. HIV-1 DNA shedding in genital ulcers and its associated risk factors in Pune, India. J Acquir Immune Defic Syndr Hum Retrovirol 1998;18:277–81.
[91] Mostad SB, Overbaugh J, DeVange DM, et al. Hormonal contraception, vitamin A deficiency, and other risk factors for shedding of HIV-1 infected cells from the cervix and vagina. Lancet 1997;350:922–7.
[92] McClelland RS, Wang CC, Mandaliya K, et al. Treatment of cervicitis is associated with decreased cervical shedding of HIV-1. AIDS 2001;15:105–10.
[93] Stamm WE, Hicks CB, Martin DH, et al. Azithromycin for empirical treatment of the nongonococcal urethritis syndrome in men. A randomized double-blind study. JAMA 1995;274:545–9.
[94] Paavonen J, Roberts PL, Stevens CE, et al. Randomized treatment of mucopurulent cervicitis with doxycycline or amoxicillin. Am J Obstet Gynecol 1989;161:128–35.
[95] Chandeying V, Sutthijumroon S, Tungphaisal S. Evaluation of ofloxacin in the treatment of mucopurulent cervicitis: a response of chlamydia-positive and chlamydia-negative forms. J Med Assoc Thai 1989;72:331–7.
[96] Berman SM, Moran JS, Wang SA, Workowski KA. Fluoroquinolones, gonorrhea, and the CDC STD treatment guidelines. Sex Transm Dis 2003;30:528–9; author reply 530.
[97] Centers for Disease Control and Prevention. Increases in fluoroquinolone-resistant Neisseria gonorrhoeae among men who have sex with men–United States, 2003, and revised recommendations for gonorrhea treatment, 2004. MMWR Morb Mortal Wkly Rep 2004;53:335–8.
[98] Ferris MJ, Masztal A, Aldridge KE, et al. Association of *Atopobium vaginae*, a recently described metronidazole resistant anaerobe, with bacterial vaginosis. BMC Infect Dis 2004;4:5.
[99] Sobel J. Current concepts: vaginitis. N Engl J Med 1997;337:1896–903.

Fluoroquinolone-resistant *Neisseria gonorrhoeae*: the Inevitable Epidemic

Khalil G. Ghanem, MD*, Julie A. Giles, MS, Jonathan M. Zenilman, MD

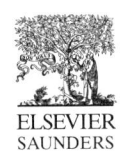

Division of Infectious Diseases, Johns Hopkins University, Bayview Medical Center, 4940 Eastern Avenue, B3 North, Suite 352, Baltimore, MD 21224, USA

The World Health Organization has estimated that over 60 million incident cases of gonorrhea occur worldwide every year [1]. In the United States 335,104 gonorrhea cases were reported to health departments in 2003 for an annual estimated rate of 116.2 cases per 100,000 persons—one of the highest rates among industrialized countries [2]. As with most other sexually transmitted infections (STIs), these numbers underestimate the true burden of this disease. Many cases of gonorrhea diagnosed by primary care physicians are never reported to local health departments, and others are asymptomatic and are never diagnosed. For example, in a probability sample of adults living in Baltimore, the estimated number of subclinical gonococcal infections was 1.3-fold higher than the number of infections diagnosed and treated in a given year [3]. The sequelae of not treating gonococcal infections can be devastating. These include infertility [4], ectopic pregnancy [5], chronic pelvic pain [6], and increased HIV-1 transmission and acquisition [7].

Diagnostic methods for *Neisseria gonorrhoeae* have changed dramatically. The Gram stain is still widely used because of its low cost and overall simplicity. In symptomatic men, it is up to 90% sensitive [8]. However, the sensitivity decreases significantly in women and asymptomatic men. The test must also be performed in a laboratory certified according to the Clinical Laboratory Improvement Amendments, which often reduces the cost advantage. Culture remains the gold standard for diagnosing *N gonorrhoeae* infections, with a reported sensitivity of more than 90% and a specificity of nearly 100% when obtained from the urethra or cervix [9]. Anorectal and

---

* Corresponding author.
E-mail address: kghanem@jhmi.edu (K.G. Ghanem).

oropharyngeal specimens may be less sensitive, unless more selective media are used to prevent commensal bacterial overgrowth. Despite the low cost and the good performance measures of culture, a recent survey of public and private laboratories reported that over 60% of tests to diagnose gonococcal infections were nucleic acid-based [10]. Nonamplified (eg, probes, enzyme immunoassays) and amplified (eg, polymerase chain reaction, transcription-mediated amplification, strand displacement assays) tests are readily available. These tests have revolutionized the field of STI diagnostic testing and have several advantages over culture: they need no special handling, such as special temperature and CO_2 conditions, because they do not require live organisms; and most can be performed on urine and self-collected vaginal swabs in addition to urethral and endocervical specimens, which facilitates specimen collection in a variety of field settings. In addition, several commercial test formulations allow for the concomitant detection of more than one STI from a single sample (eg, multiplex polymerase chain reaction assays) [11]. The main disadvantage of these tests is that antimicrobial susceptibility testing cannot be performed on the infecting strain [9].

In the United States, the Gonococcal Isolate Surveillance Project (GISP) was established by the Centers for Disease Control and Prevention (CDC) in 1986 to monitor the trends in *N gonorrhoeae* antimicrobial resistance [12]. GISP consists of a number of sexually transmitted diseases clinics (27 clinics in 2002) around the country that submit the first 25 male *N gonorrhoeae* isolates each month to a regional reference laboratory. A similar program, the Gonococcal Antimicrobial Surveillance Program (GASP), was established by the World Health Organization to monitor trends worldwide [13]. The antimicrobial susceptibility testing of strains by GISP in the United States provides data that inform national treatment guidelines for treating *N gonorrhoeae* infections. However, GISP collects data in a limited number of sites that may not reflect the distribution of resistant strains in other areas of the country. With the increasing use of non–culture-based testing to diagnose *N gonorrhoeae* infections, this has made epidemiologic studies of *N gonorrhoeae* resistance more difficult and less reliable at the local level, increasing the risk of suboptimal therapy in some patients who have *N gonorrhoeae* infections and also posing a challenge for *N gonorrhoeae* surveillance.

The increasing prevalence of different types of *N gonorrhoeae* resistance has had an impact on *N gonorrhoeae* treatment options. For 40 years, penicillin was the drug of choice. The organism was also sensitive to tetracycline. By the early 1960s, reports of penicillin [14] and tetracycline resistance began to surface [15], and by the mid-1980s, penicillin was no longer a recommended therapy for *N gonorrhoeae* infections. In the United States, resistance to penicillin and tetracycline peaked in 1992 (33.6% of strains were resistant to one or both classes). Over ten years later, and despite the lack of use of these drugs to treat *N gonorrhoeae* infections, 18%

of strains are still resistant [2]. Subsequently, resistance to spectinomycin [16], macrolides [17], aminoglycosides [18], trimethoprim-sulfamethoxazole [19], and most recently, fluoroquinolones [20] has been reported. Currently, resistance to spectinomycin and cephalosporins is exceedingly low among isolates in the United States [2]. In 2002, the drugs most frequently used to treat N gonorrhoeae infections among GISP participants were fluoroquinolones (~40%), and cephalosporins (~60%) [21].

One of the leading principles that has guided N gonorrhoeae treatment guidelines is the use of oral antimicrobials that eradicate the infection after a single dose. Table 1 lists the current CDC recommendations for treating gonococcal infections in the United States. Oral options are limited to the fluoroquinolones and the cephalosporin cefixime. Although the 2-g dose of azithromycin is approved by the US Food and Drug Administration (FDA) to treat N gonorrhoeae infections, it is no longer recommended because of the high rates of gastrointestinal adverse effects and increasing resistance [22]. In 2002, the maker of the orally administered cephalosporin cefixime discontinued manufacturing the drug, leaving fluoroquinolones as the only oral alternative [23]. Some authorities have suggested using cefpodoxime as an alternate orally administered cephalosporin, but there are no clinical trials to demonstrate efficacy. As a result, pregnant women, patients who have a history of penicillin allergy, and individuals residing in areas with increased fluoroquinolone resistance (FQR) were left with no oral options.

Table 1
Antimicrobial recommendations in the 2002 Centers for Disease Control and Prevention guidelines for treating uncomplicated gonococcal infections

Antimicrobial	Dosage and route of administration
Cefixime[a,d]	400 mg po (1 dose)
Ceftriaxone[d]	125 mg IM (1 dose)
Ciprofloxacin[b,d]	500 mg po (1 dose)
Ofloxacin[b,d]	400 mg po (1 dose)
Levofloxacin[b,d]	250 mg po (1 dose)
Spectinomycin[c]	2 g IM (1 dose)

All patients treated for gonorrhea should be concomitantly treated for *Chlamydia trachomatis* infection with either doxycycline or azithromycin.

Abbreviation: IM, intramuscular administration.

[a] Manufacturing was halted from 2002 until mid-2004 when a new company assumed production.

[b] Not recommended for treating infections acquired in the Far East, Pacific Islands, California, other areas with a high prevalence of fluoroquinolone-resistant strains, or for men who have sex with men.

[c] Oropharyngeal cultures should be performed on individuals treated with spectinomycin. If positive, a test of cure should be performed to ensure eradication of infection.

[d] Alternate cephalosporins include ceftizoxime, cefoxitin, and cefotaxime all administered IM. Alternate fluoroquinolones include gatifloxacin, norfloxacin, and lomefloxacin administered orally.

In February, 2004, another drug maker, Lupin, received FDA approval to begin manufacturing cefixime. However, as of this writing cefixime is still not widely available. Thus, for a patient who is allergic to penicillin and who resides in an area with high FQR, spectinomycin is the only CDC-recommended option that can be used to treat the infection. Spectinomycin, which is delivered intramuscularly, has suboptimal activity against rectal and oropharyngeal *N gonorrhoeae* infections [24]. The CDC recommends that oropharyngeal *N gonorrhoeae* cultures be obtained on all patients treated with spectinomycin, and if positive, the recommendation is to perform a test of cure following spectinomycin therapy [21]. This simple example makes it clear that the loss of fluoroquinolones as a mainstay of therapy in *N gonorrhoeae* infections will make what has been considered an easy infection to treat much more challenging.

Fluoroquinolones: mechanisms of action and resistance determinants in *N gonorrhoeae*

Fluoroquinolones act by disrupting bacterial DNA synthesis through binding and subsequent inhibition of specific members of the topoisomerase family of enzymes, DNA gyrase, and DNA topoisomerase IV [25]. Although the enzymes exhibit similar functions, their distinct structures afford functional specificity under certain conditions. DNA gyrase and topoisomerase IV untangle DNA by forming DNA–enzyme complexes during bacterial replication; DNA gyrase releases the supercoiling at the front of the replication fork, and topoisomerase IV decatenates the DNA sister strands at the end of replication [26,27]. To perform these functions, the enzymes catalyze full breaks in the double-stranded DNA. Quinolones bind the DNA–enzyme complex while the DNA is broken, forming DNA–enzyme–quinolone complexes that block the progression of the replication fork (halting DNA replication) and prevent sister strands from dissociating (halting bacterial reproduction). As in other gram-negative bacteria, DNA gyrase is the primary target for fluoroquinolones in *N gonorrhoeae*, whereas topoisomerase IV is the drugs' secondary target. Mutations in DNA encoding these enzymes have been correlated with decreased susceptibility to fluoroquinolones [28]. Secondary resistance mechanisms to fluoroquinolones also include overexpression of efflux pumps and reduced membrane permeability to antimicrobials [29]. A mobile element, *qnr*, has been implicated in FQR by insulating DNA gyrase from quinolone attack, but has not yet been described in *N gonorrhoeae* [30].

There has been substantial work on the molecular genetics of FQR. Primary mechanisms of resistance in *N gonorrhoeae* are associated with point mutations within the *gyrA* and *parC* genes, which code for the DNA gyrase and topoisomerase IV proteins respectively (Table 2). The *gyrA* and *parC* genes contain sequences that are referred to as *'quinolone resistance*

Table 2
Common mutations associated with fluoroquinolone resistance in *Neisseria gonorrhoeae*

	GyrA					ParC				
	91	92	95	85	86	87	88	91	92	100	116
Amino acid changes associated with FQR	Ser→Tyr Ser→Phe Ser→Leu	Ala→Pro	Asp→Tyr Asp→Asn Asp→Gly Asp→Ala	Gly→Cys	Asp→Asn	Ser→Ile Ser→Asn Ser→Arg	Ser→Pro	Glu→Gln Glu→Lys Glu→Gly Glu→Val	Ala→Gly	Phe→Tyr	Arg→Leu Arg→His

determining regions (QRDR) [28,31]. Single-base or point mutations at specific positions of the *gyrA* gene are the major cause of resistance in *N gonorrhoeae*, whereas point mutations within the *parC* gene contribute to increased resistance. Mutations in the *parC* QRDR alone have not been associated with high-level resistance to fluoroquinolones in *N gonorrhoeae* [28,32]. The *gyrA* and *parC* mutations result in conformational changes in the DNA gyrase and DNA topoisomerase IV proteins, preventing the drugs from binding to their target enzymes. The unbound drug molecules are then removed from the cell [29].

Reduced intracellular drug concentrations mediated by efflux pumps have also been implicated in FQR [33]. When point mutations are present in the *N gonorrhoeae NorM* efflux pump promoter region, more *NorM* pumps are produced. More drug molecules can then be pumped out of the cell, resulting in reduced susceptibility to ciprofloxacin and norfloxacin. Efflux pump overexpression alone is not sufficient to cause high-level resistance, but excess pump expression may be a selective factor at critical drug concentrations close to the strain's minimum inhibitory concentration (MIC). Similarly, a reduction in outer membrane porin protein expression is thought to inhibit the entry of drug molecules, thus affecting a strain's MIC [34].

Generally, as the number of QRDR mutations increases, the quinolone MIC increases [35]. Mutation at *gyrA* Ser91 and Asp95 are considered the most important mutations for resistance, which alone or together can afford a 34- to 100-fold increase in MIC to ciprofloxacin [36–38]. Specific point mutations in the *gyrA* QRDR that cause the largest MIC increases include: (1) Ser91→Phe, (2) Ser91→Ile, and (3) Asp95→Gly. Additional *parC* mutations most often associated with high-level resistance include: (1) Asp86→Gly, (2) Ser87→Arg, and (3) Ser88→Pro [39–41]. Many different mutation patterns have been identified, comprising various combinations of the same point mutations [42].

However, strains that have identical mutations have shown highly variable MICs [40,43]. Secondary resistance mechanisms, such as efflux pump overexpression, may help explain these discrepancies [44,45]. Additionally, the molecular characteristics of different fluoroquinolones vary widely; MIC data for each quinolone must be considered individually. The characteristics of the chosen quinolone, for example, can effect how well efflux pumps remove drug molecules, resulting in MIC differences.

Traditionally, antimicrobial susceptibility is determined by culturing clinical isolates in the presence of increasing antibiotic concentrations. The lowest concentration that inhibits bacterial growth is considered the MIC. The interpretive criteria for MIC determinations vary depending on the type of fluoroquinolone and the method used to determine the MIC (eg, agar dilution, disc diffusion, broth microdilution). The Clinical and Laboratory Standards Institute guidelines have established MIC cutoffs in determining sensitive, intermediate, and resistant *N gonorrhoeae* strains to various fluoroquinolones. For ciprofloxacin at the 500-mg dose, strains with an MIC more than one are considered resistant, and those with an MIC less than 0.06 are considered sensitive [46]. These MIC cutoffs differ depending on the type and dose of fluoroquinolone being used.

Each of the available fluoroquinolones has different activities against *gyrA* and *parC*. For example, trovafloxacin (no longer used clinically) preferentially targets gyrase activity, whereas grepafloxacin and moxifloxacin preferentially target topoisomerase IV [47]. As a result, the types and concentrations of fluoroquinolones determine the rate of single-step resistance mutations that occur [29]. Some fluoroquinolones are less likely to select for resistant mutations [48], and it has even been suggested that some of the newer fluoroquinolones with enhanced overall antimicrobial activity may be effective at treating ciprofloxacin-resistant *N gonorrhoeae* isolates [49–51]. However, the limited clinical data on using newer fluoroquinolones in such situations warrants the use of other recommended drug classes instead.

Fluoroquinolone-resistant *N gonorrhoeae*: epidemiology and clinical significance

In 1993, with the increasing rates of penicillin and tetracycline resistance, the CDC recommended single-dose fluoroquinolones (ciprofloxacin, 500 mg and ofloxacin, 400 mg) as a first-line therapy for the treatment of *N gonorrhoeae* infections [52]. In many parts of the world, especially developing countries, lower single doses were being used to save costs [53]. In the early 1990s, strains of *N gonorrhoeae* with decreased sensitivity to fluoroquinolones were reported [54]. In the United States, the first fluoroquinolone resistant strain was identified by GISP in Hawaii in 1991 [55]. Currently, more than 50% of isolates in many parts of the world are resistant to fluoroquinolones (Fig. 1), 17% of GISP isolates in Hawaii are resistant [56], and 16% of isolates from some areas in California are resistant (Fig. 2) [57]. Although the overall rate of FQR in the United States in 2003 was still low at 4.1% (most cases were diagnosed in Hawaii and California) [2], this was double the number from 2002; the 2002 estimate was triple the number from 2001. Fluoroquinolone-resistant strains of *N gonorrhoeae* are also more prevalent among certain high-risk populations. In 2003, high rates were reported in men who have sex with men (MSM) in Massachusetts, New York City, and 30 other GISP sites around the United States [58]. Because of this epidemiologic pattern, the CDC currently recommends not using fluoroquinolones to treat patients who acquired *N gonorrhoeae* in Asia, the Pacific Islands (including Hawaii), England, Wales, California, and other areas with increased prevalence of FQR [21]. Additionally, in 2004 the CDC recommended against routine use of fluoroquinolones to treat *N gonorrhoeae* infections in MSM. It is advised

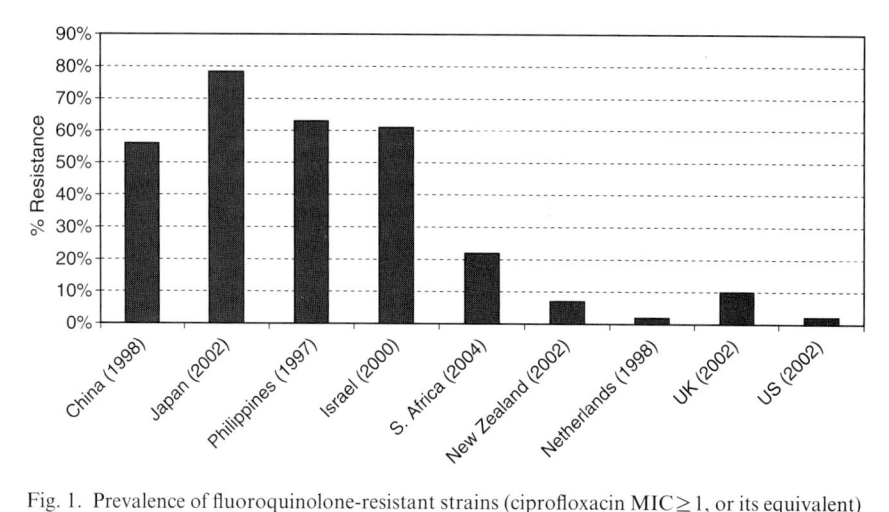

Fig. 1. Prevalence of fluoroquinolone-resistant strains (ciprofloxacin MIC ≥ 1, or its equivalent) of *Neisseria gonorrhoeae* in China [66], Japan [67], Philippines [62], Israel [68], South Africa [69], New Zealand [70], Netherlands [36], United Kingdom [71], and the United States [2]. MIC, minimum inhibitory concentration.

that a detailed travel and behavioral history be obtained in all patients (and their partners) who are currently diagnosed with *N gonorrhoeae* infection.

Incorporating genetic analysis into antimicrobial resistance surveillance prompts a series of molecular and clinical questions. From a treatment standpoint, mutations that confer minimal or no impact on susceptibility would be of little clinical interest. Therefore, the impact of a genetic mutation on the MIC needs to be correlated and the MIC cutoff that predicts clinical treatment failure must be defined. The exact correlation between a strain's MIC and clinical treatment failure with the use of fluoroquinolones is still not well established. In one retrospective study, six out of ten patients who had ciprofloxacin resistant strains (MIC > 1) failed therapy with 500 mg of ciprofloxacin [59]. The individual MICs in the study were not reported, making it difficult to assess whether the treatment failures represented MICs of one or greater. Another retrospective study using ofloxacin demonstrated a positive correlation between increasing failure rates and increasing MICs; for MICs of two, four, eight, and more than eight (where an MIC > 2 was the cutoff used for defining resistance), the failure rates were 18.6%, 18.8%, 36.7%, and 42.9%, respectively [60]. In one prospective study of 217 female sex workers in Bangladesh where the prevalence of fluoroquinolone-resistant *N gonorrhoeae* was 38%, 80 women were found to be infected with *N gonorrhoeae* and were treated with a 500-mg dose of ciprofloxacin; 37.9% failed therapy [61]. All of those who failed had strains with MICs more than 0.5. None of the women who had MIC strains more than 0.5 responded to ciprofloxacin. In that study, however, most women had *N gonorrhoeae* strains with MICs more than four, making

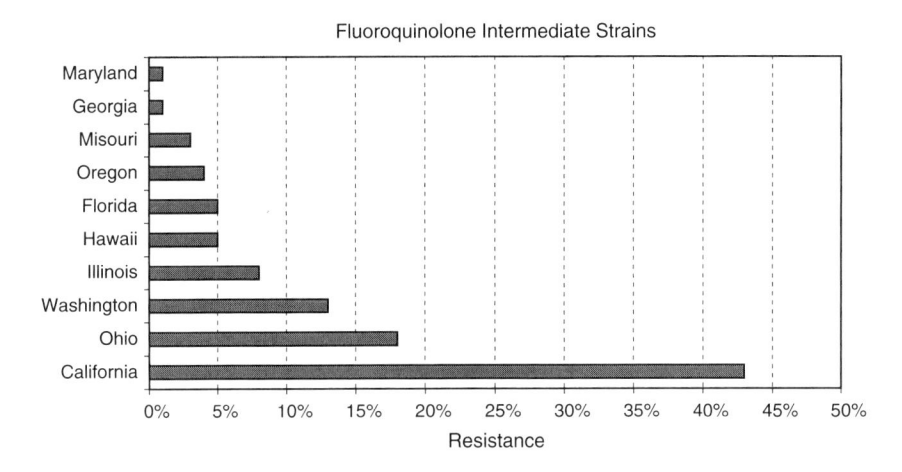

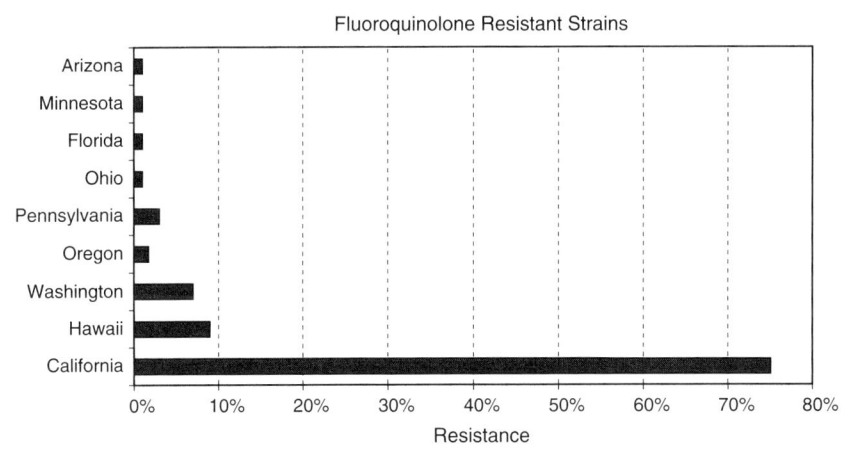

Fig. 2. The percent of fluoroquinolone-intermediate and -resistant strains that each state contributed to the total number of intermediate (80, N = 5367) and resistant (116, N = 5367) strains from the 2002 GISP data. (Note: these numbers do not reflect the prevalence of intermediate and resistant strains in those areas.)

it impossible to extrapolate meaningful estimates of clinical failure at lower MICs. Finally, a randomized study of female sex workers in the Philippines compared 400 mg of cefixime to 500 mg of ciprofloxacin in a population with a 49% prevalence of FQR [62]. Overall, 24 out of 72 women (32.3%) failed ciprofloxacin therapy. Of those women, 14 out of 30 (47%) who were infected with strains whose MIC was more than four failed therapy, compared with one out of 28 (3.6%) whose strains had an MIC less than four. These studies suggest a correlation between increasing MIC and clinical failure, although the exact MIC cutoff to predict treatment failure still needs to be defined. However, based on the available literature, an MIC cutoff of one appears to be adequate for predicting clinical treatment failure.

Once a strain is introduced into the population, the spread of fluoroquinolone-resistant *N gonorrhoeae* can be rapid. In Bangladesh, 9% of *N gonorrhoeae* isolates were resistant to fluoroquinolones in 1997, but the numbers jumped to 41% and 49% in 1998 and 1999, respectively [63]. In other populations, however, there has been a more gradual increase in the numbers of resistant strains [53]. One hypothesis, supported by *N gonorrhoeae* strain typing, is that slower rates are observed when most cases of *N gonorrhoeae* in a community are imported (suggested by many different strain types), but the number of cases rises rapidly once endemic spread (suggested by a decrease in the types of resistant strains) replaces importation [64]. Although few novel mutations have been identified in fluoroquinolone-resistant *N gonorrhoeae* isolates from diverse geographic locales, variability in mutation patterns and typing characteristics demonstrate worldwide strain diversity rather than the spread of a limited number of strains [42].

Future directions

The future of fluoroquinolone-resistant *N gonorrhoeae* is currently being shaped by several forces, including (1) the increasing numbers of resistant strains, (2) the limitations of a national surveillance program such as GISP to reflect local epidemiology, (3) the increasing use of molecular tests to diagnose gonococcal infections at the expense of culture methods, and (4) a paucity of treatment options that are practical and inexpensive in the outpatient setting. Financial and logistical considerations make it unreasonable to assume that the increasing trend in the use of molecular diagnostics will reverse itself even in the face of increasing drug resistance and therapeutic uncertainty. It is therefore imperative that new tools in molecular epidemiology be introduced to take advantage of the increasing reliance on molecular diagnostics to allow for better surveillance.

Where culture is not or cannot be performed, molecular detection of resistance determinants could help increase surveillance and inform treatment guidelines. DNA sequencing [65], nucleic acid hybridization assays [28], rapid genotyping methods [42], and DNA microarrays [65] can successfully detect *N gonorrhoeae* QRDR mutations. These new molecular techniques can be performed on crude cell extracts from samples that are routinely obtained to test for the presence of *N gonorrhoeae* infection, and the requirement for live organisms to perform antimicrobial susceptibility testing is alleviated. The higher costs and complicated logistics of performing these tests will limit their current application to surveillance studies focusing on the molecular epidemiology of drug-resistant *N gonorrhoeae*. In the short term, such studies will more accurately define local trends in *N gonorrhoeae* resistance much more extensively than the GISP program, leading to more accurate clinical decision-making. However, with decreasing costs and improvements in automation techniques, these molecular tests may become a staple that could accompany and supplement the commonly used *N gonorrhoeae* diagnostic tests by providing real-time information about the local epidemiology of *N gonorrhoeae* resistance, and optimizing antimicrobial management of patients presenting for care.

It is only a matter of time before fluoroquinolones can no longer be used as a first-line treatment option in the United States and most other parts of the world. Based on current recommendations, this leaves cefixime as the only approved oral agent. New, orally administered, single-dose alternatives are urgently needed to minimize therapeutic failures and their resulting costly sequelae.

Summary

The worldwide incidence of fluoroquinolone-resistant *Neisseria gonorrhoeae* has increased dramatically in the last few years. Single doses of fluoroquinolones can no longer be used to treat *N gonorrhoeae* infections acquired in the Far East, parts of the Middle East, the Pacific Islands, and parts of Western Europe and the United States. Although California and Hawaii account for most of the current United States cases, the increased incidence of FQR in some high-risk groups independent of geography heralds an imminent spread of drug-resistant strains throughout the rest of the population. The use of molecular tests has revolutionized the diagnostic field in STIs. The main limitation of their application in *N gonorrhoeae* testing has been the loss of culture specimens that allow antimicrobial sensitivity testing. New molecular methods have made it possible to detect antimicrobial resistance without the use of live organisms. These tests hold the promise of improving epidemiologic tracking of *N gonorrhoeae* drug resistance, leading to better patient management at the local level. The loss of fluoroquinolones limits available oral regimens to a single CDC-recommended antibiotic, cefixime. Oral, inexpensive, single-dose alternatives are needed to ensure continued therapeutic success.

References

[1] World Health Organization. Global prevalence and incidence of selected curable sexually transmitted infections overview and estimates. Geneva: World Health Organization; 2001. Report #WHO/CDS/CSR/EDC/2001.10.
[2] Centers for Disease Control and Prevention. Sexually transmitted disease surveillance, 2003. Atlanta (GA): Department of Health and Human Services; 2004.
[3] Turner CF, Rogers SM, Miller HG, et al. Untreated gonococcal and chlamydial infection in a probability sample of adults. JAMA 2002;287(6):726–33.
[4] Westrom L. Effect of acute pelvic inflammatory disease on fertility. Am J Obstet Gynecol 1975;121(5):707–13.

[5] Franklin EW III, Zeiderman AM. Tubal ectopic pregnancy: etiology and obstetric and gynecologic sequelae. Am J Obstet Gynecol 1973;117(2):220–5.
[6] Sweet RL. Pelvic inflammatory disease: etiology, diagnosis, and treatment. Sex Transm Dis 1981;8(Suppl 4):308–15.
[7] Fleming DT, Wasserheit JN. From epidemiological synergy to public health policy and practice: the contribution of other sexually transmitted diseases to sexual transmission of HIV infection. Sex Transm Infect 1999;75(1):3–17.
[8] D'Angelo LJ, Mohla C, Sneed J, et al. Diagnosing gonorrhea. A comparison of standard and rapid techniques. J Adolesc Health Care 1987;8(4):344–8.
[9] Johnson RE, Newhall WJ, Papp JR, et al. Screening tests to detect Chlamydia trachomatis and Neisseria gonorrhoeae infections—2002. MMWR Recomm Rep 2002;51(RR-15):1–38.
[10] Dicker LW, Mosure DJ, Steece R, et al. Laboratory tests used in US public health laboratories for sexually transmitted diseases, 2000. Sex Transm Dis 2004;31(5):259–64.
[11] Mahony JB. Multiplex polymerase chain reaction for the diagnosis of sexually transmitted diseases. Clin Lab Med 1996;16(1):61–71.
[12] Schwarcz SK, Zenilman JM, Schnell D, et al. National surveillance of antimicrobial resistance in Neisseria gonorrhoeae. The Gonococcal Isolate Surveillance Project. JAMA 1990 Sep;19;264(11):1413–7.
[13] Surveillance of antibiotic resistance in Neisseria gonorrhoeae in the WHO Western Pacific Region, 2002. Commun Dis Intell 2003;27(4):488–91.
[14] King AJ. Penicillin resistance in gonorrhoea. Br J Vener Dis 1960;36:34–5.
[15] Tetracycline-resistant Neisseria gonorrhoeae—Georgia, Pennsylvania, New Hampshire. MMWR Morb Mortal Wkly Rep 1985;34(37):563–70.
[16] Reyn A, Schmidt H, Trier M, et al. Spectinomycin hydrochloride (Trobicin) in the treatment of gonorrhoea. Observation of resistant strains of Neisseria gonorrhoeae. Br J Vener Dis 1973;49(1):54–9.
[17] Ehret JM, Nims LJ, Judson FN. A clinical isolate of Neisseria gonorrhoeae with in vitro resistance to erythromycin and decreased susceptibility to azithromycin. Sex Transm Dis 1996;23(4):270–2.
[18] Evans AJ. Relapse of gonorrhoea after treatment with penicillin or streptomycin. Br J Vener Dis 1966;42(4):251–62.
[19] Prior RB, Fass RJ, Perkins RL. A single large dose of trimethoprim-sulfamethoxazole fails to cure gonococcal urethritis in men. Sex Transm Dis 1978;5(2):62–4.
[20] From the Centers for Disease Control and Prevention. Decreased susceptibility of Neisseria gonorrhoeae to fluoroquinolones—Ohio and Hawaii, 1992–1994. JAMA 1994;271(22): 1733–4.
[21] Centers for Disease Control and Prevention. Sexually transmitted diseases treatment guidelines 2002. MMWR Recomm Rep 2002;51(RR-6):1–78.
[22] Fluoroquinolone-resistance in Neisseria gonorrhoeae, Hawaii, 1999, and decreased susceptibility to azithromycin in N. gonorrhoeae, Missouri, 1999. MMWR Morb Mortal Wkly Rep 2000;49(37):833–7.
[23] Discontinuation of cefixime tablets–United States. MMWR Morb Mortal Wkly Rep 2002; 51(46):1052.
[24] Karney WW, Pedersen AH, Nelson M, et al. Spectinomycin versus tetracycline for the treatment of gonorrhea. N Engl J Med 1977;296(16):889–94.
[25] Drlica K, Zhao X. DNA gyrase, topoisomerase IV, and the 4-quinolones. Microbiol Mol Biol Rev 1997;61(3):377–92.
[26] Chen CR, Malik M, Snyder M, et al. DNA gyrase and topoisomerase IV on the bacterial chromosome: quinolone-induced DNA cleavage. J Mol Biol 1996;258(4): 627–37.
[27] Kampranis SC, Maxwell A. The DNA gyrase-quinolone complex. ATP hydrolysis and the mechanism of DNA cleavage. J Biol Chem 1998;273(35):22615–26.

[28] Belland RJ, Morrison SG, Ison C, et al. Neisseria gonorrhoeae acquires mutations in analogous regions of gyrA and parC in fluoroquinolone-resistant isolates. Mol Microbiol 1994;14(2):371–80.
[29] Hooper DC. Emerging mechanisms of fluoroquinolone resistance. Emerg Infect Dis 2001; 7(2):337–41.
[30] Tran JH, Jacoby GA. Mechanism of plasmid-mediated quinolone resistance. Proc Natl Acad Sci USA 2002;99(8):5638–42.
[31] Deguchi T, Saito I, Tanaka M, et al. Fluoroquinolone treatment failure in gonorrhea. Emergence of a Neisseria gonorrhoeae strain with enhanced resistance to fluoroquinolones. Sex Transm Dis 1997;24(5):247–50.
[32] Tanaka M, Takahashi K, Saika T, et al. Development of fluoroquinolone resistance and mutations involving GyrA and ParC proteins among Neisseria gonorrhoeae isolates in Japan. J Urol 1998;159(6):2215–9.
[33] Brenwald NP, Gill MJ, Wise R. The effect of reserpine, an inhibitor of multi-drug efflux pumps, on the in-vitro susceptibilities of fluoroquinolone-resistant strains of Streptococcus pneumoniae to norfloxacin. J Antimicrob Chemother 1997;40(3):458–60.
[34] Yamano Y, Nishikawa T, Komatsu Y. Outer membrane proteins responsible for the penetration of beta-lactams and quinolones in Pseudomonas aeruginosa. J Antimicrob Chemother 1990;26(2):175–84.
[35] Tanaka M, Sakuma S, Takahashi K, et al. Analysis of quinolone resistance mechanisms in Neisseria gonorrhoeae isolates in vitro. Sex Transm Infect 1998;74(1):59–62.
[36] de Neeling AJ, van Santen-Verheuvel M, Spaargaren J, et al. Antimicrobial resistance of Neisseria gonorrhoeae and emerging ciprofloxacin resistance in the Netherlands, 1991 to 1998. Antimicrob Agents Chemother 2000;44(11):3184–5.
[37] Lindback E, Rahman M, Jalal S, et al. Mutations in gyrA, gyrB, parC, and parE in quinolone-resistant strains of Neisseria gonorrhoeae. APMIS 2002;110(9):651–7.
[38] Mavroidi A, Tzouvelekis LS, Tassios PT, et al. Characterization of Neisseria gonorrhoeae strains with decreased susceptibility to fluoroquinolones isolated in Greece from 1996 to 1999. J Clin Microbiol 2000;38(9):3489–91.
[39] Trees DL, Sandul AL, Whittington WL, et al. Identification of novel mutation patterns in the parC gene of ciprofloxacin-resistant isolates of Neisseria gonorrhoeae. Antimicrob Agents Chemother 1998;42(8):2103–5.
[40] Kam KM, Kam SS, Cheung DT, et al. Molecular characterization of quinolone-resistant Neisseria gonorrhoeae in Hong Kong. Antimicrob Agents Chemother 2003;47(1):436–9.
[41] Shigemura K, Shirakawa T, Okada H, et al. Mutations in the gyrA and parC genes and in vitro activities of fluoroquinolones in 91 clinical isolates of Neisseria gonorrhoeae in Japan. Sex Transm Dis 2004;31(3):180–4.
[42] Giles JA, Falconio J, Yuenger JD, et al. Quinolone resistance-determining region mutations and por type of Neisseria gonorrhoeae isolates: resistance surveillance and typing by molecular methodologies. J Infect Dis 2004;189(11):2085–93.
[43] Su X, Lind I. Molecular basis of high-level ciprofloxacin resistance in Neisseria gonorrhoeae strains isolated in Denmark from 1995 to 1998. Antimicrob Agents Chemother 2001;45(1): 117–23.
[44] Tanaka M, Nakayama H, Haraoka M, et al. Analysis of quinolone resistance mechanisms in a sparfloxacin-resistant clinical isolate of Neisseria gonorrhoeae. Sex Transm Dis 1998;25(9): 489–93.
[45] Dewi BE, Akira S, Hayashi H, et al. High occurrence of simultaneous mutations in target enzymes and MtrRCDE efflux system in quinolone-resistant Neisseria gonorrhoeae. Sex Transm Dis 2004;31(6):353–9.
[46] Knapp JS, Hale JA, Neal SW, et al. Proposed criteria for interpretation of susceptibilities of strains of Neisseria gonorrhoeae to ciprofloxacin, ofloxacin, enoxacin, lomefloxacin, and norfloxacin. Antimicrob Agents Chemother 1995;39(11):2442–5.

[47] Saravolatz LD, Leggett J. Gatifloxacin, gemifloxacin, and moxifloxacin: the role of 3 newer fluoroquinolones. Clin Infect Dis 2003;37(9):1210–5.
[48] Ruiz J, Jurado A, Garcia-Mendez E, et al. Frequency of selection of fluoroquinolone-resistant mutants of Neisseria gonorrhoeae exposed to gemifloxacin and four other quinolones. J Antimicrob Chemother 2001;48(4):545–8.
[49] Ruiz J, Marco F, Sierra JM, et al. In vitro activity of gemifloxacin against clinical isolates of Neisseria gonorrhoeae with and without mutations in the gyrA gene. Int J Antimicrob Agents 2003;22(1):73–6.
[50] Deguchi T, Yasuda M, Nakano M, et al. Antimicrobial activity of a new fluoroquinolone, DU-6859a, against quinolone-resistant clinical isolates of Neisseria gonorrhoeae with genetic alterations in the GyrA subunit of DNA gyrase and the ParC subunit of topoisomerase IV. J Antimicrob Chemother 1997;39(2):247–9.
[51] Shultz TR, Tapsall JW, White PA. Correlation of in vitro susceptibilities to newer quinolones of naturally occurring quinolone-resistant Neisseria gonorrhoeae strains with changes in GyrA and ParC. Antimicrob Agents Chemother 2001;45(3):734–8.
[52] Centers for Disease Control and Prevention. 1993 sexually transmitted diseases treatment guidelines. MMWR Recomm Rep 1993;42(RR-14):1–102.
[53] Ison CA, Woodford PJ, Madders H, et al. Drift in susceptibility of Neisseria gonorrhoeae to ciprofloxacin and emergence of therapeutic failure. Antimicrob Agents Chemother 1998; 42(11):2919–22.
[54] Tanaka M, Kumazawa J, Matsumoto T, et al. High prevalence of Neisseria gonorrhoeae strains with reduced susceptibility to fluoroquinolones in Japan. Genitourin Med 1994;70(2): 90–3.
[55] Knapp JS, Ohye R, Neal SW, et al. Emerging in vitro resistance to quinolones in penicillinase-producing Neisseria gonorrhoeae strains in Hawaii. Antimicrob Agents Chemother 1994;38(9):2200–3.
[56] Newman LM, Wang SA, Ohye RG, et al. The epidemiology of fluoroquinolone-resistant Neisseria gonorrhoeae in Hawaii, 2001. Clin Infect Dis 2004;38(5):649–54.
[57] From the Centers for Disease Control and Prevention. Increases in fluoroquinolone-resistant Neisseria gonorrhoeae—Hawaii and California, 2001. JAMA 2002;288(23): 2961–3.
[58] Increases in fluoroquinolone-resistant Neisseria gonorrhoeae among men who have sex with men—United States, 2003, and revised recommendations for gonorrhea treatment, 2004. MMWR Morb Mortal Wkly Rep 2004;53(16):335–8.
[59] Ng PP, Chan RK, Ling AE. Gonorrhoea treatment failure and ciprofloxacin resistance. Int J STD AIDS 1998;9(6):323–5.
[60] Kam KM, Lo KK, Chong LY, et al. Correlation between in vitro quinolone susceptibility of Neisseria gonorrhoeae and outcome of treatment of gonococcal urethritis with single-dose ofloxacin. Clin Infect Dis 1999;28(5):1165–6.
[61] Rahman M, Alam A, Nessa K, et al. Treatment failure with the use of ciprofloxacin for gonorrhea correlates with the prevalence of fluoroquinolone-resistant Neisseria gonorrhoeae strains in Bangladesh. Clin Infect Dis 2001;32(6):884–9.
[62] Aplasca De Los Reyes MR, Pato-Mesola V, Klausner JD, et al. A randomized trial of ciprofloxacin versus cefixime for treatment of gonorrhea after rapid emergence of gonococcal ciprofloxacin resistance in The Philippines. Clin Infect Dis 2001;32(9):1313–8.
[63] Rahman M, Sultan Z, Monira S, et al. Antimicrobial susceptibility of Neisseria gonorrhoeae isolated in Bangladesh (1997 to 1999): rapid shift to fluoroquinolone resistance. J Clin Microbiol 2002;40(6):2037–40.
[64] Knapp JS, Fox KK, Trees DL, et al. Fluoroquinolone resistance in Neisseria gonorrhoeae. Emerg Infect Dis 1997;3(1):33–9.
[65] Ng LK, Sawatzky P, Martin IE, et al. Characterization of ciprofloxacin resistance in Neisseria gonorrhoeae isolates in Canada. Sex Transm Dis 2002;29(12):780–8.

[66] Ye S, Su X, Wang Q, et al. Surveillance of antibiotic resistance of Neisseria gonorrhoeae isolates in China, 1993–1998. Sex Transm Dis 2002;29(4):242–5.
[67] Ito M, Yasuda M, Yokoi S, et al. Remarkable increase in central Japan in 2001–2002 of Neisseria gonorrhoeae isolates with decreased susceptibility to penicillin, tetracycline, oral cephalosporins, and fluoroquinolones. Antimicrob Agents Chemother 2004;48(8):3185–7.
[68] Dan M, Poch F, Sheinberg B. High prevalence of high-level ciprofloxacin resistance in Neisseria gonorrhoeae in Tel Aviv, Israel: correlation with response to therapy. Antimicrob Agents Chemother 2002;46(6):1671–3.
[69] Moodley P, Moodley D, Willem SA. Ciprofloxacin resistant Neisseria gonorrhoeae in South Africa. Int J Antimicrob Agents 2004;24(2):192–3.
[70] Heffernan H, Brokenshire M, Woodhouse R, et al. Antimicrobial susceptibility among Neisseria gonorrhoeae in New Zealand in 2002. N Z Med J 2004;117(1191):U817.
[71] Fenton KA, Ison C, Johnson AP, et al. Ciprofloxacin resistance in Neisseria gonorrhoeae in England and Wales in 2002. Lancet 2003;361(9372):1867–9.

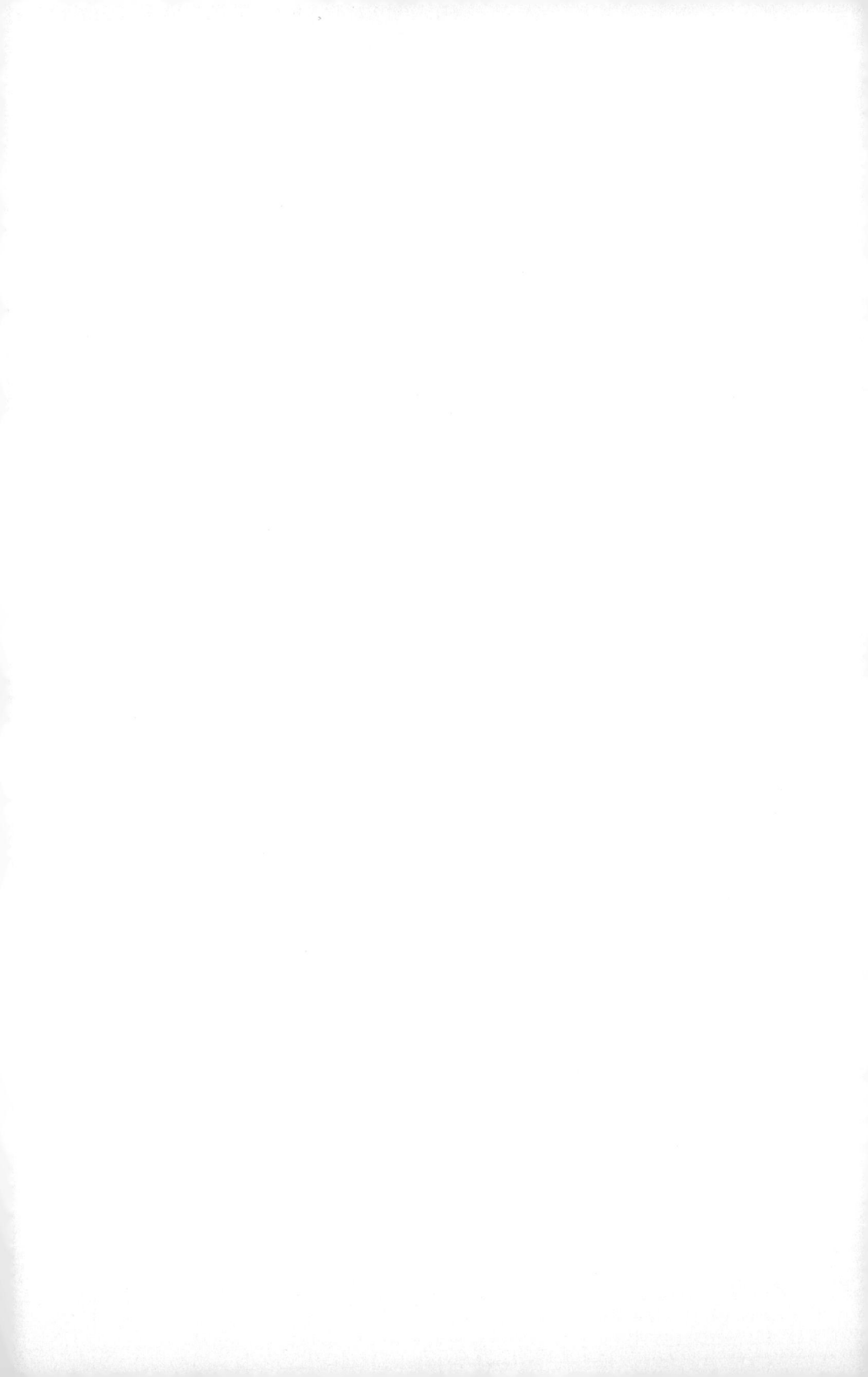

Nucleic Acid Amplification Tests for Gonorrhea and Chlamydia: Practice and Applications

Charlotte A. Gaydos, MS, MPH, DrPH

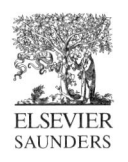

Division of Infectious Diseases, Medicine, Johns Hopkins University School of Medicine, 1159 Ross Research Building, 720 Rutland Avenue, Baltimore, MD 21205, USA

Sexually transmitted infections (STIs) are epidemic among young adults and adolescents, and sequelae among women can include pelvic inflammatory disease, infertility, and cervical cancer [1–6]. Many STIs are asymptomatic and can increase risk for HIV acquisition and transmission [7,8]. Medical costs exceed $5 billion annually [9,10]. Thus, the need to develop acceptable and more easily available techniques for diagnosing STIs in all high-risk populations is significant. Five of the top ten reportable diseases in the United States are sexually transmitted diseases (STDs), with *Chlamydia trachomatis* being the most common (877,478 in 2003) [11]. Infections resulting from *Neisseria gonorrhoeae* are the second most commonly reported notifiable disease in the United States, with 351,104 cases reported in 2003 [11]. This article focuses on these two most common bacterial infections, how the application of nucleic acid molecular amplification tests (NAATs) to the detection of these infections has improved diagnostic capabilities for the clinician and public health practitioner, and the tests' usefulness in reaching individuals at highest risk for having chlamydia and gonorrhea.

The development of NAATs as a diagnostic method has provided new tools that are more sensitive and specific than older traditional culture or nonculture methods for the diagnosis of STIs. These new tests not only improve performance with traditional urogenital specimens but are so sensitive they can use urine and other noninvasive specimens such as vaginal swabs [12–21]. Because physical examinations are not required, use of these specimens has significantly expanded the venues in which individuals can seek screening for STIs. Older approaches to the diagnosis of gonorrhea and chlamydia infections required gynecologic pelvic examinations for women and the use of urethral swabs in men, which are often painful. Previously,

E-mail address: cgaydos@jhmi.edu

symptomatic persons or those in contact with infected patients would be the only persons seeking care for these infections in clinics. Because chlamydia infections are mostly asymptomatic, as are many gonorrhea infections, traditional clinic approaches to diagnoses overlook whole population groups that would not ordinarily be tested. Use of self-obtained specimens, which are tested by the highly sensitive and specific NAATs, has greatly increased the use of nontraditional locations for screening programs because a clinician is not required to obtain the specimens.

Nucleic acid amplification tests for chlamydia

In the early 1990s, the usefulness of polymerase chain reaction (PCR) was recognized for its ability to detect difficult-to-grow pathogens. *C trachomatis* was the first organism for which there was a commercially available PCR assay [22]. Now there are many published studies using several different types of NAATs and new technologies that are commercially available for detecting chlamydia and *N gonorrhoeae* [23–28]. These assays were the first tests able to be used with urine samples because of their greatly expanded sensitivity, and include (1) PCR (Amplicor; Roche Molecular Diagnostics, Indianapolis, Indiana), (2) ligase chain reaction (LCR) (LCX; Abbott Laboratories, Abbott Park, Illinois), (3) transcription mediated amplification (TMA) (Aptima Combo2; GenProbe, San Diego, California), and (4) strand displacement amplification (SDA) (ProbTec; Becton Dickinson, Sparks, Maryland). LCR assays have recently been taken off the market, but many validations and epidemiologic studies have been previously performed [29–32]. These methods offer expanded sensitivities of detection, usually well above 90%, while maintaining high specificity (Fig. 1) [33,34].

Polymerase chain reaction

The PCR test is available as a microwell format, and as an automated method (COBAS [Amplicor, Roche Molecular Diagnostics, Indianapolis, Indiana]). The sensitivity was 89.7% for endocervical samples, 89.2% for female urine specimens, 88.6% for male urethral swabs, and 90.3% for male urines in the clinical trial for chlamydia (Table 1) [25].

Strand displacement amplification

The clinical trial of SDA demonstrated a sensitivity for chlamydia of 92.8% for cervical swabs, 80.5% for female urine, 94.6% for male urethral swabs, and 94.5% for male urine (see Table 1) [27].

Transcription mediated amplification

The originally produced GenProbe Amplified CT assay [35] is no longer produced and has been replaced by the Aptima Combo2 assay, which has

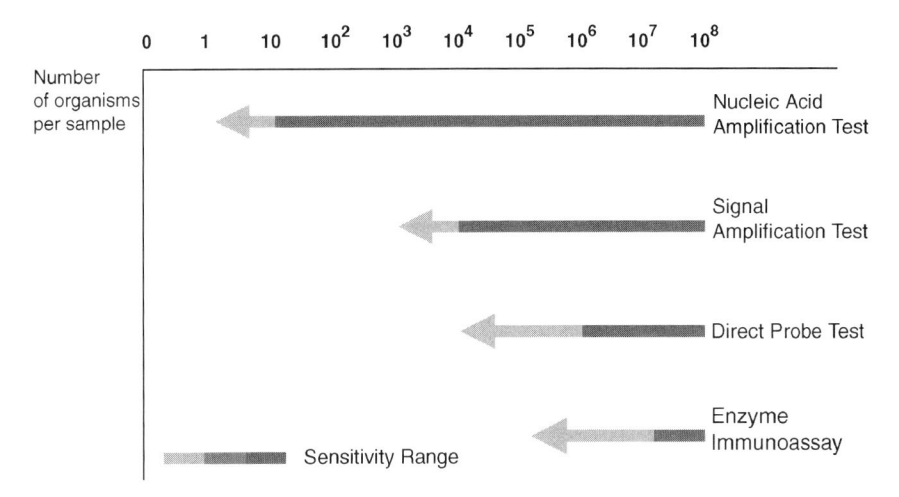

Fig. 1. Relative comparison of sensitivity of various types of tests for detection of chlamydia or gonorrhea.

added hybrid capture technology and simultaneously detects gonorrhea [28]. The sensitivity ranges from 94.2% to 97.0% (see Table 1). The somewhat lower specificities presented in the clinical trial may be artificially low because this assay seems to be slightly more sensitive than other NAATs and confirmation of uniquely positive samples by another NAAT can be problematic. Unique positives can often be confirmed by another primer set using the same assay [28,33,34].

How many comparator tests should be used for measuring the performance of new assays and whether to use the single urogenital site evaluation as opposed to the infected patient as a reference standard are often areas of much discussion in clinical trials [36,37]. NAATs can be used to define the infected patient gold standard (IPGS) to evaluate chlamydia diagnostic tests. It is not clear how many test results run by different NAATs and what combinations of specimens comprise the best IPGS. Martin et al used data from a large multicenter clinical trial [28] for comparing results from three different assays for 1412 women [37]. Using receiver operator-like curves, it was determined that use of any "two-tests-positive-out-of-three" definition resulted in estimates that were as good as or better than using the any "three-of-four-positive" definition or the "at-least-one-specimen-positive-by-each-of-two-comparator-assays" definition, and provided the best combinations of sensitivity and specificity estimates [37].

Inhibitors

Although a high level of sensitivity for detection of chlamydia using NAATs has been achieved, some specimens contain inherent "inhibitors" to

Table 1
Diagnostic tests for the detection of *Chlamydia trachomatis* and *Neisseria gonorrhoeae*

Diagnostic method	*Chlamydia trachomatis* % Sensitivity	*Chlamydia trachomatis* % Specificity	*Neisseria gonorrhoeae* % Sensitivity	*Neisseria gonorrhoeae* % Specificity
Tissue culture	70–85	100	80–95	100
Gram stain				
Males: symptomatic			90–95	95–100
Males: asymptomatic			50–70	95–100
Females			50–70	95–100
Direct fluorescent antibody	80–85	>99	—	—
Enzyme immunoassay	53–76	95	—	—
Hybridization (Pace2)	65–83	99	92.1–96.4	98.8–99.1
Polymerase chain reaction (COBAS)				
Cervical	89.7	99.4	92.4	99.5
Female urine	89.2	99.0	64.8	99.8
Male urine	90.3	98.4	94.1	99.9
Strand displacement amplification				
Cervical	92.8	98.1	96.6	98.9–99.8
Female urine	80.5	98.4	84.9	98.8–99.8
Male urine	94.5	91.4	98.1	96.8–98.7
Male urethral	94.6	94.2	98.1	96.8–98.7
Transcriptional mediated amplification				
Cervical	94.2	97.6	99.2	98.7
Female urine	94.7	98.9	91.3	99.3
Male urine	97.0	99.1	97.1	99.2
Male urethral	95.2	98.2	98.8	98.2

Compared with infected patient status, package inserts, and clinical trials.

amplification, which were first described when chlamydia positive cultures were PCR-negative. Some inhibitors are labile and disappear on retesting or at a 1:10 dilution [38,39]. The prevalence of inhibitors range from 1.8% in female urine and 2.6% in male and female urine samples to 19% for cervical samples in one study [38,39]. In a comparison of agents causing inhibition in PCR, LCR, and TMA, Mahoney et al [40] reported rates of complete inhibition in PCR of 4.9%, in LCR of 2.6%, and in TMA of 7.5%. Agents independently associated with inhibition included beta human choriogonadotropin and crystals for PCR, nitrates for LCR, and hemoglobin, nitrates, and crystals for TMA [40]. The use of amplification controls in commercial NAAT assays can indicate when a specimen contains inhibitors by failure of the nonspecific amplification control to be amplified. When inhibition occurs, steps such as heating or dilution can be performed and the test can then be repeated. The National Chlamydia Laboratory Committee presents a complete discussion of inhibitors on the American Public Health Laboratories (APHL) Web site, www.aphl.org/docs/NCCInhibitorsofAmplification.

New specimen types available for the detection of *Chlamydia trachomatis*

New nucleic acid amplification technology is so powerful that theoretically even one organism can serve as a target for amplification in clinical specimens. Because of this improved sensitivity of detection, alternative urogenital sample types can be used for the detection of chlamydia. First-void or "first-catch" urine from men and women can be used with NAATs with great accuracy. Because urine samples are easily obtained, they offer a great advantage for large public health screening programs where there is no opportunity to obtain a cervical or urethral specimen. Additionally, urine specimens are highly acceptable to individuals who may be asymptomatic and are unwilling to submit to a medical examination. Because a clinician is not required for urine collection, cost savings are also generated when screening large numbers of individuals.

Another type of specimen that has been shown to be sensitive and specific for the detection of chlamydia when amplified tests are used and that has high acceptability is a vaginal or vulvar swab [14,41–43]. Many studies have reported the successful use of vaginal swabs, which can be self-administered or administered by a clinician, but this specimen type is not yet cleared by the US Food and Drug Administration (FDA), except for the Aptima Combo2 assay [14,16,17,44,45].

Although STD and family planning clinics have been the traditional source of specimens for chlamydia screening programs, the usefulness of different specimen types has made alternative venues for screening programs attractive for public health programs. Some of these include schools, prisons, military reception stations, health vans, shopping malls, and even street outreach sites and teen centers [15,46–52].

Culture was originally thought to be the gold standard for the detection of chlamydia in clinical specimens. However, because of the extremely high sensitivity of nucleic acid amplified technology, it is now known that culture may have a sensitivity ranging from only 50% to 85% [53]. Because of its near perfect specificity, however, culture is still recommended for medicolegal cases for detection of chlamydia in investigations of sexual abuse cases [54].

Older methods for the detection of chlamydia include (1) staining of chlamydia inclusion bodies grown in tissue culture cells [55], (2) staining of patient clinical specimens for chlamydia elementary bodies using monoclonal antibodies (direct fluorescent antibody [DFA] staining) [56–58], (3) antigen detection in enzyme immunoassay (EIA) [59–62], or (4) nucleic acid probe hybridization [63–65]. Culture is mostly performed now only by research or state health laboratories, and DFA and EIA can no longer be recommended as accurate enough for the detection of chlamydia in cervical and urethral swabs. None of these methods is sensitive enough to be used for urine or vaginal swabs.

Several rapid point-of-care tests have been marketed. These are designed to be performed while the patient waits for results. The optical immunoassay by Thermo Electron, Boulder, Colorado (previously Biostar) is one example and may be useful when patients are not likely to return for test results [66]. However, these tests have low sensitivities compared with DNA amplification assays (ie, 50%–70%) and cannot be used with noninvasive specimen types. The Digene Hybrid Capture II CT-ID Test (Digene, Silver Spring, Maryland) is another type of hybridization test that does not amplify the nucleic acid, but amplifies the detection signal after hybridization. In one study, this assay performed with a sensitivity of 95.4% and a specificity of 99% with cervical specimens, but it cannot be used with urine samples [67].

Symptomatic patients

When patients are symptomatic and are in contact with a health care provider, they should receive a complete urogenital examination, with samples (cervical swabs for women and either urethral or urine samples for men) taken for diagnostic testing using the most sensitive and specific test available (ie, a NAAT test, recommended by the Centers for Disease Control and Prevention [CDC] as the test of choice) [68].

Asymptomatic patients

When populations of asymptomatic persons are being screened, the use of noninvasive samples such as urine or self-administered vaginal swabs can be recommended. Specimen collection using these methods eliminates the need for a clinician (unless the person is found to be infected) and can be very cost-effective, especially when surveying many people [69–72]. Only a NAAT test can be used with these noninvasive samples to screen asymptomatic persons for chlamydia, as none of the other older tests has the adequate sensitivity.

Necessity for confirmation of positive tests

Because of the potential for false positive tests caused by lower positive predictive values (PPV) of NAATs in low prevalence populations (eg, when the test specificity is less than 100%) [73], the CDC has recommended that a confirmatory test should be done for individuals from populations with a PPV less than 90% who test positive [68]. Approaches that have been suggested, in order of desirability, include (1) testing a second specimen with a different test using a different target; (2) testing the original specimen with a different test that uses a different target or format; (3) repeating the original test on the original specimen with a blocking antibody or competitive probe; or (4) repeating the original test on the original specimen [68]. The necessity of confirmatory testing for NAATs is controversial, and therefore more definitive studies are required before a consensus can be reached by public health officials [34].

Recommendations from professional organizations for chlamydia screening and rescreening

In the United States, the CDC recommends that all sexually active adolescent women should be screened for chlamydia infection at least annually, even if symptoms are not present [74]. Also recommended is annual screening of sexually active women aged 20 to 25 years and older and women with risk factors such as a new sex partner or multiple sex partners [74]. The US Preventive Services Task Force has similar recommendations [75], as do other professional societies and federal agencies [76–78]. St. Lawrence et al [79] reported that despite federal and professional screening recommendations, less than one third of the physicians responding to a national survey routinely screen men or women for STIs. Because the risk for reinfection is high, especially in women [80–82], the CDC recommends that previously infected women constitute a priority for repeat testing and should be rescreened 3 to 4 months after treatment [74]. Even lower genital tract infection with chlamydia has been associated with endometritis and subclinical pelvic inflammatory disease [83,84].

Use of nucleic acid amplification tests and self-administered sampling for chlamydia has influenced the epidemiology of this infection

The dramatic change in diagnostic testing that took place after the introduction of NAATs has resulted in a significant increase in estimates of population prevalence of chlamydia infection [85]. In 2003, 877,478 chlamydia infections from 50 states and the District of Columbia were reported to CDC, increasing from 1987 through 2003 from 78.5 cases per 100,000 population to 304.3 per 100,000 population. [11]. These increases in the national rate may result from increased chlamydia screening programs in general, the increased use of NAATs, and improved reporting, but also may be cause by increasing numbers of new infections [11]. The number of infections detected by NAAT may be up to 80% higher than those found with the use of older tests [53,86]. There has been an increasing prevalence of chlamydia infections in female and male military recruits [19,72,87]. Recent surveys of young adults and adolescents in the Adolescent Health Study in middle and high schools using NAAT technology also indicate substantial prevalence in men and women [71].

In 2003, the chlamydia prevalence in United States family planning clinics where women come to see a clinician was 5.9%, whereas screening of women in nontraditional settings, such as the National Job Training Program, was 9.9% [11].

Data on high reinfection rates in women [80,88,89] and the high prevalence in asymptomatic men in several studies [87,90] indicate that it will be highly improbable to significantly control the chlamydia epidemic without screening men and women in high-risk populations. NAATs have been accurate in screening asymptomatic men, although the burden of bacterial load may be low [71,72,91]. A national household survey sample demonstrated a prevalence of 2.8% [51]; military studies demonstrated a prevalence of 4.7% to 5.3% in male recruits not seeking health care [72,87], and other studies have demonstrated similar prevalence (5.5%) in asymptomatic men attending an STD clinic [90]. Thus, there is increasing public health interest in screening men as a prevention measure to help reduce reservoirs of infection available for transmission to women. One such study in four cities in the United States demonstrated a chlamydia prevalence of 7% in mostly asymptomatic men [92]. Screening and treating infected men could lead to the reduction of chlamydia associated sequelae in women.

A population study of adults aged 18 to 35 years in inner-city homes demonstrated a prevalence of 3% for chlamydia, 5.3% for gonorrhea, and an overall weighted prevalence estimate of 7.9% for either infection, most of which (94.7%) were asymptomatic [93]. Such studies can focus future control efforts toward areas where high burdens of disease exist in asymptomatic and untreated persons not seeking health care.

Other sites where screening has been used for populations who would not ordinarily seek reproductive health care include juvenile correction facilities, where prevalence can reach as high as 28% [85]. Few detention centers routinely screen for chlamydia and gonorrhea. There have been few studies of these STIs in incarcerated women or men in the United States [94–98]. One survey of adolescents reported a prevalence of 28.1% in women and 9.6% in men [97]. Most detention facilities throughout the United States test for genital infections only on the basis of symptoms, but testing of asymptomatic persons is highly desirable as these infections are frequently asymptomatic. The incarcerated population represents a high-risk group for STIs, and should be considered as an important target for public health programs [95,99]. One recent study demonstrated a high prevalence of chlamydia infections (8.0%) in asymptomatic men but a low prevalence for gonorrhea (1.2%) through urine testing with NAATs [100]. A high volunteer rate among the men in detention centers indicated the acceptability and feasibility of a urine-based screening program. Young age (<30 years) and reported condom use with a casual partner were independent predictors of a chlamydia infection in that study [100]. Others have also reported high prevalence for chlamydia in incarcerated men, especially adolescents, but have not separated the prevalence by presence or absence of symptoms [94,95,97]. Because men in detention practice high-risk behaviors that put them at risk for STIs, screening of this population has been recommended as a worthwhile public health intervention of compelling need [96]. Testing men in detention centers who are younger than 30 years may be a useful and easily implemented criterion for the implementation of screening programs. Detention centers provide ideal settings in which to successfully screen and treat men for chlamydia and gonorrhea infections.

Hospital emergency departments have been successful locations for screening programs for young adults who present for reasons other than reproductive health care, and have demonstrated high prevalence of chlamydia using urine screening [101–103]. Thus, widespread screening programs of sexually active individuals using NAATs are justified and supported by recommendations of public health officials [53]. Expanded screening programs to reduce chlamydia prevalence have been effective in areas where the screening programs have been in existence for an extended time [104].

Nucleic acid amplification tests for *Neisseria gonorrhoeae*

Although PCR (Amplicor, Roche Molecular Diagnostics, Branchburg, New Jersey) has been used with sensitivity well above 90% for the detection of gonorrhea in cervical specimens, the clinical trial did not achieve a high enough sensitivity (64.8%) for the detection of gonorrhea in urine samples from women for FDA clearance, although it is highly accurate with male urine (see Table 1) [26]. PCR has accurately detected gonorrhea in the urine of 1291symptomatic men with a sensitivity of 94.1% and a specificity of 99.9%, with a somewhat lower sensitivity (73.1%) in a sample of 721 asymptomatic men [26]. However, PCR has been used successfully with self-administered vaginal swabs from women (see Fig. 1) [44,45].

SDA (ProbeTec, Becton Dickinson, Sparks, Maryland) is approved for detection of gonorrhea in cervical, male urethral, and female and male urine samples and has achieved widespread use in clinical laboratories throughout the United States and Europe (see Fig. 1) [27]. The BD ProbeTec ET system demonstrated a sensitivity of 97.9% for the detection of gonorrhea in male urine from 680 patients [27].

The newest and perhaps most sensitive assay for gonorrhea is the TMA assay (Aptima Combo2, GenProbe, San Diego, California) (see Fig. 1 and Table 1) [28].

Alternative assays for the detection of gonorrhea

Direct smear examination

A direct Gram stain may be performed as soon as the specimen is collected on site, or a smear may be prepared and transported to the laboratory. Urethral smears from men who have symptomatic gonorrhea usually contain intracellular gram-negative diplococci in polymorphonuclear leukocytes. A presumptive diagnosis of gonorrhea requires the presence of intracellular diplococci. The sensitivity of such smears in men is 90% to 95% [105]. However, endocervical smears from women and rectal specimens require careful interpretation because of colonization with other gram-negative coccobacillary organisms. In women, the sensitivity of an endocervical Gram stain is estimated to be 50% to 70% [105].

Culture

The isolation and identification of *N gonorrhoeae* is still the currently accepted gold standard for the diagnosis of gonococcal infections [106]. It is the recommended method for medicolegal investigations of sexual abuse [54]. Specimens should be inoculated onto selective media, such as modified Thayer-Martin, Martin-Lewis, or New York City. The ideal method for transporting organisms for culture is to plate the specimens directly onto the culture medium and immediately incubate the plates in an increased humidity atmosphere of 3% to 5% carbon dioxide at 35°C to 37°C. Confirmatory identification requires that biochemical, fluorescent antibody, chromogenic enzyme substrate, serological, or coagglutination tests be performed to distinguish the isolate from nonpathogenic *Neisseria* spp.

Probe hybridization

The first molecular FDA-approved DNA test for *N gonorrhoeae* was the unamplified probe test (Pace 2, GenProbe, San Diego, California). Sensitivity and specificity are high for the Pace 2 assay. Compared with cultures, sensitivity ranges from 90.8% to 96.3% for women and 99.1% to 99.6% for men [107–111]. Specificity is uniformly high, ranging from 97.5% to 100% for men and women [107–111]. Clinical evaluations of the assay have supported the reported high sensitivity and specificity of the assay [107–111].

Although all of the alternative methods can be used for the detection of gonorrhea and can be used successfully with traditional cervical or urethral swab specimens, none can be used with urine specimens or self-administered vaginal swabs.

One sample: two pathogens and alternative/new testing venues

One of the main advantages of using amplified tests for the detection of STIs is the flexibility of being able to use the same sample type, such as urine or self-administered swabs, for the detection of multiple STIs. Although most outreach screening studies have used NAATs primarily for chlamydia testing, being able to also screen for gonorrhea has distinct advantages, especially in populations and regions that have demonstrated high prevalence for gonorrhea [93,101].

Other diagnostic issues

Because NAATs measure DNA or RNA rather than live organisms, caution should be used in using DNA amplification tests for test-of-cure assays. Residual nucleic acid from cells rendered noninfective by antibiotics may give a positive amplified test for up to 3 weeks after therapy, although the patient may actually be cured of viable organisms [112,113].

Vaginal swabs have performed as well as or better than clinician-obtained endocervical swabs to diagnose either chlamydia or gonococcal infections using DNA amplification assays. There seems to be no difference in detection rates whether the vaginal swab is collected by the patient or the clinician [44]. A vaginal swab that was transported to the laboratory in a "dry" state was demonstrated to be as accurate for the detection of chlamydia and gonorrhea as shipping the swab in the "wet" liquid transport medium recommended by the manufacturer [18]. The ability to transport swabs in a dry state to the laboratory extends the utility of the vaginal swab to be easily mailed in a preaddressed mailing packet from a distant site to a central laboratory for testing.

Requirement for a pelvic examination and cost-effectiveness studies

Although molecular amplification assays are generally more expensive than nonculture tests, cost-effectiveness analyses for women, when done from a societal prospective, have shown NAATs to be more cost-effective in preventing the sequelae associated with chlamydia infections [69,70,114–119]. However, if a female patient has urogenital symptoms or if a pelvic examination is being performed on a patient for reasons other than screening, clinicians should obtain a cervical swab for a NAAT, because cervical swabs have a slightly higher sensitivity than urine specimens. If a woman is not receiving a pelvic examination, such as in a screening program or because a Pap test is not indicated, clinicians should take advantage of the ease of obtaining a urine specimen or even a self-administered vaginal swab for amplification testing. A recent model demonstrated that annual screening for chlamydia in all women aged 15 to 29 years and selective targeting through semiannual screening of those who had a history of infection were cost-effective compared with other well-accepted clinical interventions [120]. Cost-effectiveness studies for screening and treating infected men to prevent chlamydia infections and their sequelae in women are few and have been controversial with some, but not all, showing cost-effectiveness [121,122].

Cost savings by pooling of diagnostic specimens

Using NAATs is often too expensive for many public health programs, although they have been shown to be cost-effective in the prevention of costly sequelae, especially with regard to chlamydia [69,123]. There are methods that have been explored to lower the cost per sample tested, such as pooling the patient samples before testing [124–126]. Pooling techniques are highly sensitive and specific for chlamydia and gonorrhea detection [124–129]. The algorithm that has been developed employs testing four or more samples in one pooled test unit. If the test unit assay is negative, all samples are considered to be negative. Positive pool results lead to retesting all samples in the pool individually to determine which ones are positive. Because most specimens in testing situations are negative, the technique will ultimately save significant costs. Formulas exist to calculate the number of samples to pool to achieve the greatest cost savings for a particular prevalence [125].

Partnering to achieve screening of larger numbers of persons at risk

Increasing awareness of STIs and partnering of outreach public health programs for STIs with programs offered by other large providers of health care, such as managed care organizations and the military, has the potential to provide broader coverage for routine STI screening [50,130–133]. One household cluster survey in low-income women in California demonstrated a prevalence of 3.2% for chlamydia and found that most had received health care within the last year [134]. Approximately 50% of those surveyed were covered by state insurance programs and 62% had received a pelvic examination, yet they had not been screened for chlamydia. The data demonstrated a two- to threefold greater burden of infection than routine surveillance programs indicated.

Summary and the future

Studies have demonstrated that self-collected genital specimens, such as urine or vaginal swabs, can be accurately used to diagnose chlamydia and gonorrhea when they are used with NAATs. Use of these sample collection methods can often reduce or eliminate the need for a clinician and a genital examination, unless an examination is clinically indicated for reasons other than screening. Although there are excellent data for urine and vaginal swabs for chlamydia and gonorrhea, the use of such specimens for the diagnosis of other STIs, such as human papillomavirus, *Trichomonas vaginalis*, and *Mycoplasma genitalium* urogenital infections, needs to be further explored. Further research will be needed and as more commercially available diagnostic kits become available, it will be possible to provide greater diagnostic accuracy to more types of STIs and extend screening programs to reach more individuals at risk.

Self-collected specimens appear to be useful in several clinical and nonclinical situations. They can be obtained when it is desirable to test women or men who are not seeking health care and would not attend a clinic because of the asymptomatic nature of these infections. Adolescents especially are reluctant to seek care for STIs. Among 228 adolescent women enrolled in a self-collection study, nearly 13% of teens who had never previously had a gynecologic examination tested positive for an STI [45]. Among those infected (prevalence of 18% for any STI), 87% did not think they had an STI and half would not have sought STI testing if the study as not offered [45]. These data clearly underscore the necessity to be proactive in screening adolescents for STD.

Urine or the self-collected vaginal swabs should also be useful in screening large numbers of persons for genital tract infections where pelvic examinations and urogenital examinations are impractical or cost-prohibitive, such as with cohorts of college students, job corps applicants, or military recruits. Lastly, for women or men who cannot get an immediate clinic appointment or who are reporting to a clinic for reasons other than a urogenital examination, self-collected swabs or urine may be obtained opportunistically [133]. Self-administered vaginal swabs and the collection of urine appear be acceptable to women and men, as indicated by the high volunteer rate among individuals who were approached for participation in studies [20,21,42,43].

Widespread use of sensitive and specific diagnostic tests for STIs in screening programs for asymptomatic or non–health care-seeking women and men, which are readily available to those at most risk, is an important goal in the strategy for controlling these highly prevalent infections. Future studies are needed to explore acceptability and usefulness of self-collected urine and vaginal swabs and to further define their role in the control of STIs. Continued explorations of ways to reach infected patients easily and diagnose infections inexpensively, and better partner management will help to control the epidemic of STIs in the world. Clinicians and public health officials alike should be encouraged to use amplified tests in their practices and screening programs. Only through increased surveillance, better detection, and treatment of infected patients and their partners can the epidemic of STIs be halted.

References

[1] Hillis SD, Joesoef R, Marchbanks PA, et al. Delayed care of pelvic inflammatory disease as a risk factor for impaired fertility. Am J Obstet Gynecol 1993;168:1503–9.
[2] Westrom LV. Sexually transmitted diseases and infertility. Sex Transm Dis 1994;21(Suppl 2):S32–7.
[3] Westrom L. Effect of pelvic inflammatory disease on fertility. Venereology 1995;8:219–22.
[4] Hillis SD, Wasserheit JN. Screening for chlamydia–a key to the prevention of pelvic inflammatory disease. N Engl J Med 1996;334:1399–401.
[5] Anttila T, Saikku P, Koskela P, et al. Serotypes of Chlamydia trachomatis and risk for development of cervical squamous cell carcinoma. JAMA 2001;285:47–51.
[6] Smith JS, Munoz N, Herrero R, et al. Evidence for Chlamydia trachomatis as a human papillomavirus cofactor in the etiology of invasive cervical cancer in Brazil and the Philippines. J Infect Dis 2002;185:324–31.
[7] Laga M, Manoka A, Kivuvu M, et al. Non-ulcerative sexually transmitted diseases as risk factors for HIV-1 transmission in women: results from a cohort study. AIDS 1993;7:95–102.
[8] Dallabetta G, Neilsen G. Efforts to control sexually transmitted infections as a means to limit HIV transmission: what is the evidence? Curr Infect Dis Rep 2005;7:79–84.

[9] Eng TR, Butler WT. The neglected health and economic impact of STDs. In: Eng TR, Butler WT, editors. The hidden epidemic, confronting sexually transmitted diseases. Washington (DC): National Academy Press; 1997. p. 28–68.
[10] Eng TR. Prevention of sexually transmitted diseases A model for overcoming barriers between managed care and public health. The IOM Workshop on the Role of Health Plans in STD Prevention. Amer J Prev Med 1999;16:60–9.
[11] Centers for Disease Control and Prevention. Sexually transmitted disease surveillance, 2003. Atlanta (GA): US Department of Health and Human Services; 2004.
[12] Gaydos CA, Howell MR, Quinn TC, et al. Use of ligase chain reaction with urine versus cervical culture for detection of Chlamydia trachomatis in an asymptomatic military population of pregnant and nonpregnant females attending Papanicolaou smear clinics. J Clin Microbiol 1998;36:1300–4.
[13] Hook EW III, Ching SF, Stephens J, et al. Diagnosis of Neisseria gonorrhoeae infections in women by using the ligase chain reaction on patient-obtained vaginal swabs. J Clin Microbiol 1997;35(8):2129–32.
[14] Hook EW III, Smith K, Mullen C, et al. Diagnosis of genitourinary Chlamydia trachomatis infections by using the ligase chain reaction on patient-obtained vaginal swabs. J Clin Microbiol 1997;35:2133–5.
[15] Marrazzo JM, White CL, Krekeler B, et al. Community-based urine screening for Chlamydia trachomatis with a ligase chain reaction assay. Ann Intern Med 1997;127:796–803.
[16] Polaneczky M, Quigley C, Pollock L, et al. Use of self-collected vaginal specimens for detection of Chlamydia trachomatis infection. Obstet Gynecol 1998;91:375–8.
[17] Gray RH, Wawer MJ, Girdner J, et al. Use of self-collected vaginal swabs for detection of Chlamydia trachomatis infection. Sex Trans Dis 1998;25:450.
[18] Gaydos CA, Crotchfelt KA, Shah N, et al. Evaluation of dry and wet transported intravaginal swabs in detection of Chlamydia trachomatis and Neisseria gonorrhoeae infections in female soldiers by PCR. J Clin Microbiol 2002;40:758–61.
[19] Gaydos CA, Howell MR, Quinn TC, et al. Sustained high prevalence of Chlamydia trachomatis infections in female army recruits. Sex Transm Dis 2003;30:539–44.
[20] Schachter J, McCormack WM, Chernesky MA, et al. Vaginal swabs are appropriate specimens for diagnosis of genital tract infection with Chlamydia trachomatis. J Clin Microbiol 2003;41:3784–9.
[21] Shafer MA, Moncada J, Boyer CB, et al. Comparing first-void urine specimens, self-collected vaginal swabs, and endocervical specimens to detect Chlamydia trachomatis and Neisseria gonorrhoeae by a nucleic acid amplification test. J Clin Microbiol 2003;41:4395–9.
[22] Jaschek G, Gaydos C, Welsh L, et al. Direct detection of Chlamydia trachomatis in urine specimens from symptomatic and asymptomatic men by using a rapid polymerase chain reaction assay. J Clin Microbiol 1993;31:1209–12.
[23] Bauwens JE, Clark AM, Stamm WE. Diagnosis of Chlamydia trachomatis endocervical infections by a commercial polymerase chain reaction assay. J Clin Microbiol 1993;31:3023–7.
[24] Quinn TC, Welsh L, Lentz A, et al. Diagnosis by AMPLICOR PCR for Chlamydia trachomatis infection in urine samples from women and men attending sexually transmitted disease clinics. J Clin Microbiol 1996;34:1401–6.
[25] Van Der Pol B, Quinn TC, Gaydos CA, et al. Multicenter evaluation of the AMPLICOR and automated COBAS AMPLICOR CT/NG tests for the detection of Chlamydia trachomatis. J Clin Microbiol 2000;38:1105–12.
[26] Martin DH, Cammarata C, Van Der Pol B, et al. Multicenter evaluation of AMPLICOR and automated COBAS AMPLICOR CT/NG tests for Neisseria gonorrhoeae. J Clin Microbiol 2000;38:3544–9.
[27] Van Der Pol B, Ferrero D, Buck-Barrington L, et al. Multicenter evaluation of the BDProbeTec ET System for the detection of Chlamydia trachomatis and Neisseria

gonorrhoeae in urine specimens, female endocervical swabs, and male urethral swabs. J Clin Microbiol 2001;39:1008–16.

[28] Gaydos CA, Quinn TC, Willis D, et al. Performance of the APTIMA Combo 2 assay for detection of Chlamydia trachomatis and Neisseria gonorrhoeae in female urine and endocervical swab specimens. J Clin Microbiol 2003;41:304–9.

[29] Chernesky MA, Jang D, Lee H, et al. Diagnosis of Chlamydia trachomatis infections in men and women by testing first-void urine by ligase chain reaction. J Clin Microbiol 1994; 32:2682–5.

[30] Smith KR, Ching S, Lee H, et al. Evaluation of ligase chain reaction for use with urine for identification of Neisseria gonorrhoeae in females attending a sexually transmitted disease clinic. J Clin Microbiol 1995;33:455–7.

[31] Lee HH, Chernesky MA, Schachter J, et al. Diagnosis of Chlamydia trachomatis genitourinary infection in women by ligase chain reaction assay of urine. Lancet 1995;345: 213–6.

[32] Schachter J, Whidden R, Shaw H, et al. Noninvasive tests for diagnosis of Chlamydia trachomatis infection: application of ligase chain reaction to first-catch urine specimens of women. J Infect Dis 1995;172:1411–4.

[33] Gaydos CA, Theodore M, Dalesio N, et al. Comparison of three nucleic acid amplification tests for detection of Chlamydia trachomatis in urine specimens. J Clin Microbiol 2004;42: 3041–5.

[34] Boyadzhyan B, Yashina T, Yatabe JH, et al. Comparison of the APTIMA CT and GC assays with the ATIMA Combo2 assay, the Abbott LCX assay, and direct florescent-antibody and culture assays for the detection of Chlamydia trachomatis and Neisseria gonorrhoeae. J Clin Microbiol 2004;42:3089–93.

[35] Crotchfelt KA, Pare B, Gaydos C, et al. Detection of Chlamydia trachomatis by the Gen-Probe AMPLIFIED Chlamydia Trachomatis Assay (AMP-CT) in urine specimens from men and women and endocervical specimens from women. J Clin Microbiol 1998;36(2): 391–4.

[36] Moncada J, Schachter J, Hook EW III, et al. The effect of urine testing in evaluations of the sensitivity of the Gen-Probe APTIMA Combo 2 assay on endocervical swabs for Chlamydia trachomatis and Neisseria gonorrhoeae: the infected patient standard reduces sensitivity of single site evaluation. Sex Transm Dis 2003;31:273–7.

[37] Martin DH, Nsuami M, Schachter J, et al. Use of multiple nucleic acid amplification tests to define the infected-patient "gold standard" in clinical trials of new diagnostic tests for Chlamydia trachomatis infections. J Clin Microbiol 2004;42:4749–58.

[38] Bassiri M, Mardh PA, Domeika M. Multiplex AMPLICOR PCR screening for Chlamydia trachomatis and Neisseria gonorrhoeae in women attending non-sexually transmitted disease clinics. The European Chlamydia Group. J Clin Microbiol 1997; 35(10):2556–60.

[39] Verkooyen RP, Luijendijk A, Huisman WM, et al. Detection of PCR inhibitors in cervical specimens by using the AMPLICOR Chlamydia trachomatis assay. J Clin Microbiol 1996; 34(12):3072–4.

[40] Mahony J, Chong S, Jang D, et al. Urine specimens from pregnant and nonpregnant women inhibitory to amplification of Chlamydia trachomatis nucleic acid by PCR, ligase chain reaction, and transcription-mediated amplification: identification of urinary substances associated with inhibition and removal of inhibitory activity. J Clin Microbiol 1998;36:3122–6.

[41] Stary A, Chouieri B, Lee H. Implications of sensitive molecular diagnosis of Chlamydia trachomatis in non-invasive sample types. Presented at the Eleventh Meeting of the International Society for STD Research. New Orleans, LA, August 27–30, 1995.

[42] Newman SB, Nelson MB, Gaydos CA, et al. Female prisoners' preference of collection methods for testing for Chlamydia trachomatis and Neisseria gonorrhoeae infection. Sex Trans Dis 2003;30:306–9.

[43] Hsieh YH, Howell MR, Gaydos JC, et al. Preference among female Army recruits for use of self-administered vaginal swabs or urine to screen for Chlamydia trachomatis genital infections. Sex Transmit Dis 2003;30:769–73.

[44] Rompalo AM, Gaydos CA, Shah N, et al. Evaluation of use of a single intravaginal swab to detect multiple sexually transmitted infections in active-duty military women. Clin Infect Dis 2001;33:1455–61.

[45] Wiesenfeld HC, Lowry DL, Heine RP, et al. Self-collection of vaginal swabs for the detection of Chlamydia, gonorrhea, and trichomonas: opportunity to encourage sexually transmitted disease testing among adolescents. Sex Transm Dis 2001;28:321–5.

[46] Rietmeijer CA, Bull SS, Ortiz CG, et al. Patterns of general health care and STD services use among high-risk youth in Denver participating in community-based urine chlamydia screening. Sex Transm Dis 1998;25:457–63.

[47] Gunn RA, Podschun GD, Fitzgerald S, et al. Screening high-risk adolescent males for Chlamydia trachomatis infection. Obtaining urine specimens in the field. Sex Transm Dis 1998;25:49–52.

[48] Cohen DA, Nsuami M, Etame RB, et al. A school-based Chlamydia control program using DNA amplification technology. Pediatrics 1998;101:E1.

[49] Gaydos CA, Howell MR, Pare B, et al. Chlamydia trachomatis infections in female military recruits. N Engl J Med 1998;339(11):739–44.

[50] Burstein GR, Waterfield G, Joffe A, et al. Screening for gonorrhea and chlamydia by DNA amplification in adolescents attending middle school health centers. Opportunity for early intervention. Sex Transm Dis 1998;25:395–402.

[51] Mertz KJ, McQuillan GM, Levine WC, et al. A pilot study of the prevalence of chlamydial infection in a national household survey. Sex Transm Dis 1998;25:225–8.

[52] Ford CA, Viadro CI, Miller WC. Testing for chlamydial and gonorrheal infections outside of clinical settings: a summary of the literature. Sex Transm Dis 2004;31:38–51.

[53] Schachter J. Chlamydia trachomatis: the more you look, the more you find—how much is there? Sex Transm Dis 1998;25(5):229–31.

[54] Hammerschlag MR. Use of nucleic acid amplification tests in investigating child sexual abuse. Sex Transm Infect 2001;77:153–4.

[55] Centers for Disease Control. Laboratory update: isolation of Chlamydia trachomatis in cell culture. Washington (DC): US Department of Health and Human Services; 1980.

[56] Taylor HR, Agarwala N, Johnson SL. Detection of experimental Chlamydia trachomatis eye infections in conjunctival smears and in tissue cultures by use of fluorescein-conjugated monoclonal antibody. J Clin Microbiol 1984;20:391–5.

[57] Uyeda CT, Welborn P, Ellison-Birang N, et al. Rapid diagnosis of chlamydial infections with MicroTrak direct test. J Clin Microbiol 1984;20:948–50.

[58] Lindner LE, Geerling S, Nettum JA, et al. Identification of chlamydia in cervical smears by immunofluorescence: technique, sensitivity, and specificity. Am J Clin Pathol 1986;85:180–5.

[59] Clark A, Stamm WE, Gaydos C, et al. Multicenter evaluation of the AntigEnz Chlamydia enzyme immunoassay for diagnosis of Chlamydia trachomatis genital infection. J Clin Microbiol 1992;30:2762–4.

[60] Gaydos C, Reichart C, Long J, et al. Evaluation of Syva enzyme immunoassay for detection of Chlamydia trachomatis in genital specimens. J Clin Microbiol 1990;28:1541–4.

[61] Sanders JW, Hook EW, Welsh LE, et al. Evaluation of an enzyme immunoassay for detection of Chlamydia trachomatis in urine of asymptomatic men. J Clin Microbiol 1994;32:24–7.

[62] Chan EL, Brandt K, Horsman GB. A 1-year evaluation of Syva MicroTrak Chlamydia enzyme immunoassay with selective confirmation by direct fluorescent-antibody assay in a high-volume laboratory. J Clin Microbiol 1994;32:2208–11.

[63] Clarke LM, Sierra MF, Daidone BJ, et al. Comparison of the Syva MicroTrak enzyme immunoassay and Gen-Probe PACE 2 with cell culture for diagnosis of cervical Chlamydia

trachomatis infection in a high-prevalence female population. J Clin Microbiol 1993;31: 968–71.
[64] Warren R, Dwyer B, Plackett M, et al. Comparative evaluation of detection assays for Chlamydia trachomatis. J Clin Microbiol 1993;31:1663–6.
[65] Stary A, Teodorowicz L, Horting-Muller I, et al. Evaluation of the Gen-Probe PACE 2 and the Microtrak enzyme immunoassay for diagnosis of Chlamydia trachomatis in urogenital samples. Sex Transm Dis 1994;21:26–30.
[66] Gift TL, Pate MS, Hook EW III, et al. The rapid test paradox: when fewer cases detected lead to more cases treated: a decision analysis of tests for Chlamydia trachomatis. Sex Transm Dis 1999;26:232–40.
[67] Girdner JL, Cullen AP, Salama TG, et al. Evaluation of the Digene Hybrid Capture II CT-ID test for the detection of Chlamydia trachomatis in endocervical specimens. J Clin Microbiol 1999;37:1579–81.
[68] Centers for Disease Control and Prevention. Screening tests to detect Chlamydia trachomatis and Neisseria gonorrhoeae infections–2002. MMWR Recomm Rep 2002; 51(RR-15):1–38.
[69] Howell MR, Quinn TC, Gaydos CA. Screening for Chlamydia trachomatis in asymptomatic women attending family planning clinics. A cost-effectiveness analysis of three strategies. Ann Intern Med 1998;128:277–84.
[70] Howell MR, Quinn TC, Brathwaite W, et al. Screening women for Chlamydia trachomatis in family planning clinics: the cost-effectiveness of DNA amplification assays. Sex Transm Dis 1998;25(2):108–17.
[71] Miller WC, Ford CA, Morris M, et al. Prevalence of chlamydial and gonococcal infections among young adults in the United States. JAMA 2004;291:2229–36.
[72] Arcari CM, Gaydos JC, Howell MR, et al. Feasibility and short-term impact of linked education and urine screening interventions for Chlamydia and gonorrhea in male army recruits. Sex Transm Dis 2004;31:443–7.
[73] Zenilman JM, Miller WC, Gaydos C, et al. LCR testing for gonorrhea and chlamydia in population surveys and other screenings of low prevalence populations: coping with decreased positive predictive value. Sex Transm Infect 2003;79:94–7.
[74] Centers for Disease Control and Prevention. Sexually transmitted diseases treatment guidelines 2002. MMWR Recomm Rep 2002;51(RR-6):1–78.
[75] US Preventive Services Task Force. Screening for chlamydial infection: recommendations and rationale. Am J Prev Med 2001;20(Suppl 3):S90–4.
[76] Crosby RA, DiClemente RJ, Wingood GM, et al. Associations between sexually transmitted disease diagnosis and subsequent sexual risk and sexually transmitted disease incidence among adolescents. Sex Transm Dis 2004;31:205–8.
[77] Workowski KA, Levine WC, Wasserheit JN. US Centers for Disease Control and Prevention guidelines for the treatment of sexually transmitted diseases: an opportunity to unify clinical and public health practice. Ann Intern Med 2002;137:255–62.
[78] Hollblad-Fadiman K, Goldman SM. American College of Preventive Medicine practice policy statement: screening for Chlamydia trachomatis. Am J Prev Med 2003;24:287–92.
[79] St. Lawrence JS, Montano DE, Kasprzyk D, et al. STD screening, testing, case reporting, and clinical and partner notification practices: a national survey of US physicians. Am J Public Health 2002;92:1784–8.
[80] Whittington WL, Kent C, Kissinger P, et al. Determinants of persistent infection and recurrent Chlamydia trachomatis infection in young women: results of a multicenter cohort study. Sex Transm Dis 2001;28:117–23.
[81] Xu F, Schillinger JA, Markowitz LE, et al. Repeat Chlamydia trachomatis infection in women: analysis through a surveillance case registry in Washington State, 1993–1998. Am J Epidemiol 2000;152:1164–70.
[82] Mardh PA, Persson K. Is there a need for rescreening of patients treated for genital chlamydial infections? Int J STD AIDS 2002;13:363–7.

[83] Wiesenfeld HC, Hillier SL, Krohn MA, et al. Lower genital tract infection and endometritis: insight into subclinical pelvic inflammatory disease. Obstet Gynecol 2002; 100:456–63.
[84] Ness RB, Randall H, Richter HE, et al. Condom use and the risk of recurrent pelvic inflammatory disease, chronic pelvic pain, or infertility following an episode of pelvic inflammatory disease. Am J Public Health 2004;94:1327–9.
[85] Centers for Disease Control and Prevention. Sexually Transmitted Disease Surveillance 2000 Supplement, Chlamydia Prevalence Monitoring Project. Atlanta, GA: US Department of Health and Human Services, Centers for Disease Control and Prevention; 2001.
[86] Black CM, Marrazzo JM, Johnson RE, et al. Head-to-head multicenter comparison of DNA probe and nucleic acid amplification tests for Chlamydia trachomatis in women performed with an improved reference standard. J Clin Microbiol 2002;40:3757–63.
[87] Cecil JA, Howell MR, Tawes JJ, et al. Features of Chlamydia trachomatis and Neisseria gonorrhoeae infection in male Army recruits. J Infect Dis 2001;184:1216–9.
[88] Burstein GR, Gaydos CA, Diener-West M, et al. Incident Chlamydia trachomatis infections among inner-city adolescent females. JAMA 1998;280(6):521–6.
[89] Burstein GR, Zenilman JM, Gaydos CA, et al. Predictors of repeat Chlamydia trachomatis infections diagnosed by DNA amplification testing among inner city females. Sex Transm Infect 2001;77:26–32.
[90] Marrazzo JM, Whittington WL, Celum CL, et al. Urine-based screening for Chlamydia trachomatis in men attending sexually transmitted disease clinics. Sex Transm Dis 2001;28: 219–25.
[91] Cheng H, Macaluso M, Vermund SH, et al. Relative accuracy of nucleic acid amplification tests and culture in detecting Chlamydia in asymptomatic men. J Clin Microbiol 2001;39: 3927–37.
[92] Schillinger JA, Dunne EF, Chapin JB, et al. Prevalence of Chlamydia trachomatis infection among men screened in 4 U.S. cities. Sex Transm Dis 2005;32:74–7.
[93] Turner CF, Rogers SM, Miller HG, et al. Untreated gonococcal and chlamydial infection in a probability sample of adults. JAMA 2002;287:726–33.
[94] Oh MK, Smith KR, O'Cain M, et al. Urine-based screening of adolescents in detention to guide treatment for gonococcal and chlamydial infections. Translating research into intervention. Arch Pediatr Adolesc Med 1998;152:52–6.
[95] Centers for Disease Control and Prevention. High prevalence of chlamydial and gonococcal infection in women entering jails and juvenile detention centers—Chicago, Birmingham, and San Francisco, 1998. MMWR Morb Mortal Wkly Rep 1999;48: 793–6.
[96] Glaser JB. Sexually transmitted diseases in the incarcerated. An underexploited public health opportunity. Sex Transm Dis 1998;25:308–9.
[97] Risser JMH, Risser WL, Gefter LR, et al. Implementation of a screening program for chlamydial infection in incarcerated adolescents. Sex Transm Dis 2001;28:43–6.
[98] Mertz KJ, Schwebke JR, Gaydos CA, et al. Screening women in jails for chlamydial and gonococcal infection using urine tests: feasibility, acceptability, prevalence, and treatment rates. Sex Transm Dis 2002;29:271–6.
[99] Skolnick AA. Look behind bars for key to control of STDs. JAMA 1998;279:97–8.
[100] Gaydos CA, Hardick J, Willard N, et al. Screening asymptomatic males for Chlamydia trachomatis and Neisseria gonorrhoeae in a detention center setting. Int J STD AIDS 2001; 12(Suppl 2):83–5.
[101] Mehta SD, Rothman RE, Kelen GD, et al. Unsuspected gonorrhea and chlamydia in patients of an urban adult emergency department: a critical population for STD control intervention. Sex Transm Dis 2001;28:33–9.
[102] Mehta SD, Rothman RE, Kelen GD, et al. Clinical aspects of diagnosis of gonorrhea and Chlamydia infection in an acute care setting. Clin Infect Dis 2001;32:655–9.

[103] Finelli L, Schillinger JA, Wasserheit JN. Are emergency departments the next frontier for sexually transmitted disease screening? Sex Transm Dis 2001;28:40–2.
[104] Mertz KJ, Levine WC, Mosure DJ, et al. Trends in the prevalence of chlamydia infections. The impact of community-wide testing. Sex Transm Dis 1997;24:169–75.
[105] Hook EW III, Handsfield HH. Gonococcal infections in the adult. In: Holmes KK, Mardh P, Sparling PF, et al, editors. Sexually transmitted diseases. New York: McGraw-Hill; 1990. p. 149–65.
[106] Knapp JS, Rice RJ. Neisseria and Branhamella. In: Murray PR, Baron EJ, Pfaller MA, et al, editors. Manual of clinical microbiology. Washington (DC): ASM Press; 1995. p. 324–40.
[107] Iwen PC, Walker RA, Warren KL, et al. Evaluation of nucleic acid-based test (PACE 2C) for simultaneous detection of Chlamydia trachomatis and Neisseria gonorrhoeae in endocervical specimens. J Clin Microbiol 1995;33(10):2587–91.
[108] Stary A, Kopp W, Zahel B, et al. Comparison of DNA-probe test and culture for the detection of Neisseria gonorrhoeae in genital samples. Sex Transm Dis 1993;20(5): 243–7.
[109] Hale YM, Melton ME, Lewis JS, et al. Evaluation of the PACE 2 Neisseria gonorrhoeae assay by three public health laboratories. J Clin Microbiol 1993;31:451–3.
[110] Limberger RJ, Biega R, Evancoe A, et al. Evaluation of culture and the Gen-Probe PACE 2 assay for detection of Neisseria gonorrhoeae and Chlamydia trachomatis in endocervical specimens transported to a state health laboratory. J Clin Microbiol 1992;30: 1162–6.
[111] Vlaspolder F, Mutsaers JA, Blog F, et al. Value of a DNA probe assay (Gen-Probe) compared with that of culture for diagnosis of gonococcal infection. J Clin Mircobiol 1993; 31(1):107–10.
[112] Gaydos CA, Crotchfelt KA, Howell MR, et al. Molecular amplification assays to detect chlamydial infections in urine specimens from high school female students and to monitor the persistence of chlamydial DNA after therapy. J Infect Dis 1998;177:417–24.
[113] Workowski KA, Lampe MF, Wong KG, et al. Long-term eradication of Chlamydia trachomatis genital infection after antimicrobial therapy. Evidence against persistent infection. JAMA 1993;270:2071–5.
[114] Genc M, Mardh A. A cost-effectiveness analysis of screening and treatment for Chlamydia trachomatis infection in asymptomatic women. Ann Intern Med 1996;124:1–15.
[115] Mangione-Smith R, O'Leary J, McGlynn EA. Health and cost-benefits of chlamydia screening in young women. Sex Transm Dis 1999;26:309–16.
[116] Mehta SD, Bishai D, Howell MR, et al. Cost-effectiveness of five strategies for gonorrhea and chlamydia control among female and male emergency department patients. Sex Transm Dis 2002;29:83–91.
[117] Goeree R, Jang D, Blackhouse G, et al. Cost-effectiveness of screening swab or urine specimens for Chlamydia trachomatis from young Canadian women in Ontario. Sex Transm Dis 2001;28:701–9.
[118] Gupta M, Hernon M, Gokhale R, et al. Cost effectiveness analysis of a population based screening programme for asymptomatic Chlamydia trachomatis infection in women. Sex Transm Infect 2002;78:76.
[119] Postma MJ, Welte R, Van den Hoek JA, et al. Comparing cost effectiveness of screening women for Chlamydia trachomatis in systematic and opportunistic approaches. Sex Transm Infect 2002;78:73–4.
[120] Hu D, Hook EW III, Goldie SJ. Screening for Chlamydia trachomatis in women 15 to 29 years of age: a cost-effectiveness analysis. Ann Intern Med 2004;141:501–13.
[121] Blake DR, Gaydos CA, Quinn TC. Cost-effectiveness analysis of screening adolescent males for Chlamydia on admission to detention. Sex Transm Dis 2004;31:85–95.
[122] Ginocchio RH, Veenstra DL, Connell FA, et al. The clinical and economic consequences of screening young men for genital chlamydial infection. Sex Transm Dis 2003;30:99–106.

[123] Howell MR, Gaydos JC, McKee JK Jr, et al. Control of Chlamydia trachomatis in female Army recruits: cost-effective screening and treatment in training cohorts to prevent pelvic inflammatory disease. Sex Transm Dis 1999;26:519–26.

[124] Peeling RW, Toye B, Jessamine P, et al. Pooling of urine specimens for PCR testing: a cost saving strategy for Chlamydia trachomatis control programmes. Sex Transm Infect 1998;74:66–70.

[125] Kacena KA, Quinn SB, Howell MR, et al. Pooling urine samples for ligase chain reaction screening for genital Chlamydia trachomatis infection in asymptomatic women. J Clin Microbiol 1998;36:481–5.

[126] Clark AM, Steece R, Crouse K, et al. Multisite pooling study using ligase chain reaction in screening for genital Chlamydia trachomatis infections. Sex Transm Dis 2001;28:565–8.

[127] Kacena K, Quinn S, Hartman S, et al. Pooling urine samples for the screening of *Neisseria gonorrhoeae* by ligase chain reaction (LCR): accuracy and application. J Clin Microbiol 1998;36:3624–8.

[128] Kapala J, Copes D, Sproston A, et al. Pooling cervical swabs and testing by ligase chain reaction are accurate and cost-saving strategies for diagnosis of Chlamydia trachomatis. J Clin Microbiol 2000;38:2480–3.

[129] Morre SA, Meijer CJ, Munk C, et al. Pooling of urine specimens for detection of asymptomatic Chlamydia trachomatis infections by PCR in a low-prevalence population: cost-saving strategy for epidemiological studies and screening programs. J Clin Microbiol 2000;38:1679–80.

[130] Brodine SK, Shafer MA, Shaffer RA, et al. Asymptomatic sexually transmitted disease prevalence in four military populations: Application of DNA amplification assays for Chlamydia and gonorrhea screening. J Infect Dis 1998;178:1202–4.

[131] Howell MR, McKee KT Jr, Gaydos JC, et al. Point-of-entry screening for C. trachomatis in female army recruits. Who derives the cost savings? Am J Prev Med 2000;19:160–6.

[132] Burstein GR, Snyder MH, Conley D, et al. Adolescent chlamydia testing practices and diagnosed infections in a large managed care organization. Sex Transm Dis 2001;28:477–83.

[133] Ostergaard L, Andersen B, Olesen F, et al. Efficacy of home sampling for screening of Chlamydia trachomatis: randomised study. BMJ 1998;317:26–7.

[134] Klausner JD, McFarland W, Bolan G, et al. Knock-knock: a population-based survey of risk behavior, health care, access, and Chlamydia trachomatis infection among low-income women in the San Francisco Bay area. J Infect Dis 2001;183:1087–92.

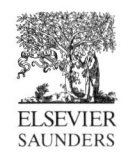

What's New in Bacterial Vaginosis and Trichomoniasis?

Jack D. Sobel, MD

Harper University Hospital, Division of Infectious Diseases, 3990 John R-5 Hudson, Detroit, MI 48201, USA

Trichomoniasis and bacterial vaginosis are often grouped together despite major differences in etiology, pathophysiology, and transmission implications. The reason these two entities are frequently considered together is that they present with elevated vaginal pH, major shifts in vaginal flora, and abnormal vaginal discharge that is characteristically malodorous (Table 1). These conditions share major risk factors, epidemiologic characteristics, and complications, and are treated primarily with the nitroimidazole class of drugs. Perhaps the most poignant reason for considering these conditions together is that they frequently coexist, although few data have been published regarding their concurrence. In one study, *Trichomoniasis vaginalis* was significantly associated with the presence of clue cells on microscopy [1]. Moreover, because there was a greater prevalence of *T vaginalis* in women who had Nugent intermediate Gram stain scores (4–6) and high bacterial vaginosis (BV) scores (7–10), it was suggested that trichomoniasis may predispose to bacterial vaginosis [2]. This article is not intended to be an extensive, inclusive review of either subject, but to emphasize recent advances in epidemiology, diagnosis, and therapy of these two disparate entities.

Trichomoniasis

Epidemiology

Recent data have shown that the annual incidence of trichomoniasis is more than 170 million cases worldwide. In North America, more than 8 million new cases are reported annually with an estimated rate of asymptomatic cases as high as 50% [3–5]. As such, trichomoniasis is the most common sexually transmitted infection in the United States and far

E-mail address: jsobel@med.wayne.edu

Table 1
Characteristics of trichomoniasis and bacterial vaginosis

Characteristic	Trichomoniasis	Bacterial vaginosis
Malodor	Unpleasant	Fishy
Increased pH	+++	+++
Amine test	±	+
Increased PMNs	+++	−
Clue cells	−	++
Abnormal flora	+ to ++	+++
Sexual transmission	+++	± to +
Postmenopausal female	+	Rare
Preterm labor	+	+
PID	+ to ++	+
HIV transmission	+	+
Nitroimidazole therapy	++	++
Clindamycin therapy	−	++
Partner treatment	+++	−
Recurrence	Rare	Common (30%–50%)

Abbreviations: ±, variable/unsure; +, positive; ++, more positive; +++, strongly positive; PID, pelvic inflammatory disease; PMN, polymorphonuclear leukocyte.

exceeds either chlamydia or gonorrhea as a sexually transmitted infection. The prevalence of trichomoniasis in women varies depending on the population studied. Point prevalence studies reveal the following situations: (1) 15% to 54% in sexually transmitted disease (STD) clinics, (2) 10% to 13% in student health clinics, (3) 40% in prenatal clinics, (4) 43% in substance abuse clinics, and (5) 11% to 50% in HIV-infected women [5–7]. Most of these prevalence studies are based on microscopy or culture. The recent availability of polymerase chain reaction (PCR) has made the significant underdiagnosis of trichomoniasis through wet mount and microscopy apparent, leading to many untreated infections. Prevalence rates in men include 10% to 21% in those who have nongonococcal urethritis, 2% to 12% in STD clinic patients, 50% in adolescents at high risk, and 45% in those who have been in contact with infected women [8,9].

Clinical manifestations and complications

Clinical manifestations are shown in Table 2. The complications of trichomoniasis are most evident in nongravid and gravid women. Among pregnant women, at least two studies have shown that trichomoniasis is associated with preterm delivery, premature rupture of membranes, and low birth weight infants [10–12]. There appears to be some controversy as to whether trichomoniasis, either symptomatic or asymptomatic, should be treated during pregnancy in an attempt to reduce the aforementioned adverse outcomes. Remarkably, no published study to date has actually shown that the treatment of trichomoniasis during pregnancy decreases the frequency of adverse outcome in pregnancy. On the contrary, a recent metronidazole treatment trial of asymptomatic trichomoniasis in pregnant

Table 2
Clinical manifestations and sequelae of trichomoniasis

	Women	Men
Asymptomatic	≤50%	>50%
Symptomatic	Vulvovaginal erythema; malodorous, greenish-yellow discharge	Urethritis: urethral irritation (30%–50%) discharge
Complications	Enhanced HIV transmission Increased atypical PID Increased risk of tubal infertility Increased risk of cervical cancer Increased risk of postoperative infection Associated with preterm birth, prematurity	Prostatitis??

Abbreviations: ??, highly controversial; PID, pelvic inflammatory disease.

women not only failed to show that preterm delivery was prevented, but women treated with metronidazole were shown to have a higher rate of preterm delivery than placebo-treated women (19% versus 10.7%) [12]. This study has been heavily criticized because of the definition of asymptomatic trichomoniasis used, delay in therapy, and diagnostic regimen used. Nevertheless, on the basis of this study, the Centers for Disease Control and Prevention (CDC) currently does not recommend routine screening for asymptomatic trichomoniasis during pregnancy or treatment of asymptomatic trichomoniasis during pregnancy. Therefore, it seems practical to treat asymptomatic and symptomatic trichomoniasis before pregnancy.

Several studies have documented evidence that trichomoniasis is associated with enhanced HIV transmission [13–18]. Vaginal trichomoniasis facilitates transmission of HIV infection by increasing susceptibility of an HIV uninfected partner and the infectivity of the infected individual [14]. In case-control and cohort studies, the presence of trichomoniasis was associated with enhanced risk for HIV sera conversion (relative risk 1.9 to 2.26). Of note, Wang et al [13] demonstrated the effects of metronidazole therapy on viral shading in infected patients who had a 4.2-fold reduction in the quantity of free HIV virus in vaginal secretions.

Moodley et al [19] reported a significantly higher rate of pelvic inflammatory disease (PID) among women who have trichomoniasis compared with uninfected women (odds ratio 1.5, $P = .03$). This observation supports other clinical observations of the increased frequency of tubal infertility in women infected with trichomoniasis. Trichomonads may directly access the fallopian tubes or perhaps carry lower genital tract bacterial pathogens to the upper genital tract. Grodstein et al [20] reported that women who had trichomoniasis had a 1.9-fold increased risk of tubal infertility compared with control subjects. Women who had multiple episodes of trichomoniasis had an even higher increased risk (2.5 odds ratio). Similarly, earlier studies by Sherman et al [21] confirmed the association between trichomoniasis and increased risk of tubal infertility. A recent study in Egypt reported a higher rate of culture positive trichomonas infection among a group of 240 infertile women compared with control subjects [22]. Similarly, studies in the United States have found that women colonized with chlamydia were significantly more likely to have symptomatic upper tract disease if they were also colonized with *T vaginalis* [23].

Soper et al [24] reported the association between trichomoniasis and posthysterectomy infection, including cuff cellulitis, cuff abscess, and wound infection. Trichomoniasis may be an additional risk factor for development of cervical neoplasia. A meta-analysis of 22 cohort and two case-control studies found a significant positive association between trichomoniasis and cervical intraepithelial neoplasia (CIN) [26]. Similarly, a Finnish cohort study revealed that infection with *T vaginalis* was associated with a 6.4% risk for developing subsequent CIN [25]. Yap et al [27] recently reported a high prevalence of antibodies to *T vaginalis* in the sera of women who had invasive cervical cancer. This study was supported by a study in Egypt that demonstrated a threefold increase in *T vaginalis* antibodies in Egyptian women who had invasive cervical cancer [28].

Although most men who are infected with *T vaginalis* are entirely asymptomatic, there is growing evidence that this organism acts as a pathogen in the urethra to cause nongonococcal urethritis [29]. Trichomoniasis is also infrequently associated with chronic, nonbacterial prostatitis. The histopathologic techniques reported by Gardner et al [30] demonstrated that *T vaginalis* in the prostate gland was associated with foci of nonspecific acute and chronic inflammation, providing evidence to support the pathogenic nature of trichomoniasis. Skerk et al [31] reported a similar observation in an evaluation of men who had chronic prostatitis. Finally, trichomoniasis may also contribute to male factor infertility by altering sperm motility and viability [32]. A significant improvement in sperm motility, viability, and viscosity was seen after therapy with metronidazole prescribed for 10 days [33].

Diagnosis

Clinical signs and symptoms of trichomoniasis are unreliable and lack sensitivity or specificity in the diagnosis of trichomoniasis [5]. A positive demonstration of the organism is essential for the diagnosis using microscope methodologies. Several new methods are now available that significantly enhance diagnostic capacity (Table 3).

Culture using Diamond's medium, which has been available for several years, is highly effective in identifying *T vaginalis* in up to 95% of infections with high specificity. The disadvantage of the culture method is that it takes several days and is not uniformly available. To enhance availability, a two-chambered plastic bag culture system (InPouch; BioMed Diagnostics, San Jose, California) has been shown to be equivalent to Diamond's medium for

Table 3
Diagnosis of trichomoniasis

	% Sensitivity	% Specificity	Comment
Women			
Wet mount	50–60	>90	Immediate results, insensitive
Culture	85–95	>95	Valuable, not widely available
In-pouch culture	85–95	>95	Useful
Pap smear	50	90	
PCR	>90	>95	
	95	95	Should not be used
Antigen detection (OSOM Trichomonas Rapid Test)	90	>95	High cost, not yet widely available
Affirm VP III			Highly sensitive and specific, expensive
Men			
Wet mount	~30	Low	Rarely useful
Culture: urethral swab	~60	High	Unacceptable sensitivity
Culture: urine sediment	~60	High	Unacceptable
PCR	>90	>90	Expensive, not widely available

Modified from Soper D. Trichomoniasis: under control or undercontrolled? Am J Obstet Gynecol 2004;190:281–90.

the detection of *T vaginalis* [34]. The availability of the recently introduced PCR methodology represents a major advance in diagnosis of symptomatic and asymptomatic trichomoniasis [35]. Recently, Wendel et al [36] compared microscopy, culture, and PCR in evaluating trichomoniasis. Wet mount and culture sensitivities were 52% and 78% respectively, compared with sensitivity of 84% and specificity of 94% for PCR detection of *T vaginalis*. The major advantage of PCR methodology is that it represents an opportunity to eliminate the underdiagnosis of trichomoniasis in practice. Unfortunately, PCR is not yet commercially available but does hold enormous potential, including swabs self-obtained from the introitus.

The Pap smear lacks sensitivity as a diagnostic screening methodology. Moreover, in low-prevalence populations, a report of trichomonads found on Pap cytology frequently represents a false positive result. Therefore, a Pap smear should not be considered a reliable diagnostic method for *T vaginalis* identification. A commercially available DNA probe, which forms part of Affirm VP system (Becton Dickinson, Franklin Lanes, New Jersey), is a highly sensitive and specific method of trichomoniasis diagnosis compared with conventional methodologies. The test, however, does not give an immediate result, requires significant point-of-care expertise, and is best handled by a routine laboratory. OSOM Trichomonas Rapid Test, a new point-of-care antigen-based diagnostic test (Genzyme Diagnostics, Cambridge, Massachusetts), has reported initial high sensitivity and specificity.

Diagnosis of trichomoniasis in men is extremely difficult given the absence of a frequent urethral discharge and difficulties obtaining an adequate urethral specimen [34,37]. Results with traditional microscopy and culture from urethra-obtained specimens have demonstrated low sensitivity. The availability of urine PCR methodologies, however, constitutes a major advance and will be invaluable in clinical research studies.

Treatment

The use of the 5-nitroimidazole class has dominated the effective treatment of trichomoniasis for almost 5 decades. Until recently, metronidazole was the only 5-nitroimidazole available in the United States. The 2002 CDC Sexually Transmitted Disease Treatment Guidelines recommended a single 2-g dose of metronidazole as the drug of choice for trichomoniasis, with an alternative regimen of 500 mg twice a day for 7 days, and treatment of all sexual partners [38]. Metronidazole cure rates are in excess of 90% with the 7-day divided dose or single 2-g dose [39].

Although much has been written about metronidazole resistance in *T vaginalis* isolates, this entity remains extremely uncommon [40]. Low-level resistance is usually defined as an aerobic minimum lethal concentration of 50 to 100 μg/mL [39]. Low-level resistance occurs in 1% to 3% of *T vaginalis* isolates obtained from clinics. These unusual strains are usually recognized by early relapse or failure to respond to single-dose 2-g therapy. Low-level metronidazole resistance can usually be adequately treated by conventional 7-day therapy of 500 mg twice a day [39]. Higher levels of metronidazole resistance, however, will require prolongation of the duration of therapy and an increase in the daily dose [39,40]. The CDC recommends an increase in the daily dose to 2 g/d for 3 to 5 days [38]. Unfortunately, even higher doses of metronidazole will frequently be required. Sobel et al [41] reported a large series of high-level resistance of *T vaginalis* isolates to metronidazole. All patients had failed the regimen recommended by the CDC. A regimen of tinidazole consisting of 2 to 3 g/d by mouth for 14 days was recommended together with an intravaginal tinidazole regimen of 500 mg twice a day. This usually resulted in a total dose of 42 to 56 g of tinidazole prescribed over a 2-week period. Success rate was in excess of 90% for these highly resistant strains. The study, however, failed to determine whether a lower dose of tinidazole would be effective. More recently, Hager and David [42] reported successful therapy in three women who had metronidazole-resistant vaginal trichomoniasis who responded to tinidazole with a total dose of 10 to 15 g only, significantly less than that prescribed by Sobel et al.

Tinidazole, although available worldwide for more than 30 years, has recently been introduced into the United States and is considered a second generation nitroimidazole. Tinidazole demonstrates a minor in vitro advantage over metronidazole against metronidazole-sensitive *T vaginalis*. However, against metronidazole resistant strains of *T vaginalis*, several authors have reported substantially lower minimum inhibitory concentrations for tinidazole compared with metronidazole [43,44]. Several clinical studies support this finding, concluding that the drug of choice for metronidazole-resistant *T vaginalis* is oral tinidazole [41,42]. Although the optimal dosage regime has not yet been determined, it is likely that cure can be obtained by the use of the oral route only. Tinidazole should also be prescribed to the partner of the woman harboring the resistant *T vaginalis*. In addition to the in vitro drug activity, in vivo pharmacokinetics also demonstrate an advantage of tinidazole over metronidazole [41]. A superior safety profile regarding gastrointestinal intolerance and central nervous system complications indicates that tinidazole is better tolerated, particularly when used at higher doses [41].

Bacterial vaginosis

Epidemiology

BV is the most prevalent vaginal disorder in adult women worldwide [45]. It is present in 10% to 20% of white, non-Hispanic women and 30% to 50% of African American women, and it has been found in up to 85% of female sexual workers studied in Africa [45]. Additional epidemiologic studies reveals that the prevalence depends on the subject population. Accordingly, 5% to 26% of pregnant women worldwide [46,47] and 24% to 37% of women attending STD clinics [48,49] have been found to be BV positive. Even higher prevalence rates have been found in lesbian women (24%–51%) [50]. A recent study in young women entering the military in the United States found an overall prevalence of 27% [51]. Most studies in North America have indicated that prevalence is significantly increased in African American women compared with non-Hispanic white women. Even when controlling for variety of behavioral risk factors, race was independently associated with BV, intermediate flora, and a lack of hydrogen peroxide-positive lactobacilli, correlating with the presence of BV-associated anaerobic and facultative aerobic flora [52]. These epidemiologic studies reveal that BV is less likely to occur in women who have used oral contraceptives and condoms consistently. Over the last 2 decades, most epidemiologic studies have been fairly consistent in identifying additional risk-associated factors [45,49,52]. These factors include numbers of sexual partners in the prior 12 months, douching, smoking, and low socioeconomic conditions [52]. Major advances in understanding the pathophysiology of BV are unlikely to occur as a result of annual epidemiologic studies.

Pathophysiology

The pathogenesis of BV remains poorly understood. BV has no single causative agent, although *Gardnerella vaginalis* is present in up to 95% of cases. BV is a complex polymicrobial disorder characterized by decreased lactobacilli and increased colonization by several facultative or strictly anaerobic microorganisms, mainly *G vaginalis*, *Prevotella* spp, *Bacteroides* spp, *Mobiluncus* spp, gram-positive *Coccus* spp, and genital mycoplasmas (eg, *Mycoplasma hominis, Ureaplasma urealyticum*) [45,53].

The microbiologic disruption that forms the foundation of this complex disorder seems indisputable. A critical question relates to the sequence of this disruption. Does loss of protective lactobacilli precede the disturbance of overgrowth of anaerobic vaginal organisms? In this case, a long-term solution to treatment of bacterial vaginosis may relate to restoration of the healthy protective lactobacillus-dominant flora. Alternatively, lactobacillus loss, although protective against other lower genital tract pathogens, may be entirely secondary to the massive disruption in vaginal flora, resulting in incompatible microenvironmental conditions, including an elevated pH, that are nonconducive to lactobacillus persistence. If the latter hypothesis holds, then treatment of the abnormal overgrowth, which is the current management strategy, will continue to be the foundation of future therapy. Little progress has been made in understanding the sequence of pathologic events.

There has also been little progress in further defining and analyzing the vaginal bacterial population overgrowth, which is undoubtedly highly complex. An attempt has now been made to identify unrecognized noncultivatable species. Although several bacteria have been easily grown and implicated in BV, such as *G vaginalis* and *Mobiluncus curtissii*, these species can be found in lower numbers in subjects who do not have bacterial vaginosis, and are therefore not specific markers for disease. Because only a fraction of the bacteria present in the vagina are amenable to propagation in the laboratory, new attempts have been made to study complex microbial bacterial communities without cultivation by the use of molecular methodologies. These methodologies include detection and characterization of ribosomal RNA genes (rDNA), which has the advantage of detecting fastidious or cultivation resistant organisms. In particular, bacterial 16S rRNA genes contain highly conserved regions that can be targeted with PCR primers designed to amplify segments of rDNA from most known bacteria [54]. This methodology might be useful for identifying unrecognized pathogens responsible for the initial disruption. Alternatively, these methods may shed light on new markers for diagnosis and prognosis of bacterial vaginosis [55,56]. Using this new approach, the bacterium *Atopobium vaginae* has recently been recognized in women who have BV. Ferris et al [55] reported that *A vaginae* was present in most (12 out of 22) patients who were BV positive. This bacterium is a strict anaerobe and highly resistant to metronidazole, and perhaps is not the single organism responsible for causing BV, although it may have a role in recurrent or metronidazole-refractory disease [55]. It is likely that these molecular attempts directed at identifying potential new pathogens, particularly when used on a longitudinal basis, may shed additional light on the pathophysiology of this complex syndrome.

In contrast with microbiology, significant progress has been made in understanding the immunologic changes that accompany BV. A growing number of studies have investigated immunoregulatory mechanisms associated with BV in pregnant and nonpregnant women. The systemic immune response is not believed to play a dominant role in the lower genital tract, and studies have focused on local immunoregulatory mechanisms. Traditionally, BV has been so called because of the absence of inflammatory signs traditionally associated with *candida* vaginitis. As such, in the absence of pain, soreness, burning, and dyspareunia, BV has been considered a noninflammatory condition, hence the term *vaginosis* and not *vaginitis*. The lack of major inflammatory signs has correlated with the lack of polymorphonuclear leukocyte (PMN) accumulation in vaginal secretions in BV.

The first report of a vaginal immune response in women who were BV positive was reported in a 1993 study by Cauci et al [57], identifying an IgA response directed at the *G vaginalis* hemolysin (Gvh). Anti-Gvh IgA is considered the only specific vaginal adaptive response characteristic of, but not universally found in, women who have BV. At the same time, Platz-Christensen at al [58] reported high levels of the proinflammatory cytokine IL-1α in vaginal secretions of women who had BV. Several subsequent studies in pregnant and nonpregnant women demonstrated increased levels of IL-1β (approximately 10 to 20 times) in women who were BV positive, implying that the innate immune system is nevertheless responding to abnormal microbial colonization. Similar studies failed to reveal any consistent increase in any other proinflammatory cytokines in women who have BV. Increased IL-1β concentrations in vaginal secretions correlated directly with quantitative cultures of aerobic gram-negative rods and *G vaginalis* found in BV [61]. Remarkably, the cytokine IL-8, a potent chemotactic and PMN activating factor, has generally not been found to be increased in BV and could explain the absence of PMNs in what appears to be an inflammatory environment [59]. Studies by Cauci et al [60] indicated that local factors in BV either inhibit IL-8 elaboration or facilitate IL-8 degradation and thus prevent the mounting of a neutrophil defense in the vagina in women who have BV. These studies defined a small subset of BV-positive women who demonstrated an increase in IL-8–associated accumulation of PMNs. However, an increase in IL-8 is not demonstrated in most women, and accordingly, neutrophils failed to accumulate. (The absence of the IL-8 cytokine response may be the result of degradation of IL-8 as a result of proteases produced by the overgrowth of the anaerobic bacteria [61].)

Despite the anti-Gvh IgA-specific response in some women who have BV, subsets of women who were BV positive have normal or reduced concentrations of IgA. It would appear that premenopausal women who have BV frequently lack detectable levels of anti-Gvh IgA response as a result of extensive degradation of vaginal IgA and IgM, again possibly caused by microbial hydrolytic enzymes (sialidases and prolidases) [62]. Approximately 30% to 40% of women who are BV positive have anti-Gvh IgA in vaginal fluid. Cauci et al [60] reported that levels of anti-Gvh IgA were inversely correlated with sialidase produced mainly by anaerobic rods (*Prevotella* and *Bacteroides* spp) and with high prolidase activity produced predominantly by *G vaginalis* and *Mobiluncus* spp. In another study, Cauci et al [62] emphasized the existence of several patient subgroups of BV. Women who have high levels of anti-Gvh IgA correlate with those who have low concentrations of bacterial hydrolytic enzymes, namely sialidase and prolidase, and represent a less aggressive disturbed environment in the face of an appropriate lower genital tract host response. In contrast, the subgroup of women who have low concentrations or absent anti-Gvh IgA accompanied by high concentrations of sialidase/prolidase represent a more aggressive state with more potential for local and upper genital tract complications. Cauci et al [62] have not detected variations in cytokine or immunoglobulin concentrations based on the anatomic site of sampling. In contrast, Yudin et al [63] reported elevated concentrations of IL-1β, IL-6, and IL-8 obtained from the cervix of women who had BV. The IL-8 concentrations dropped dramatically following successful treatment of BV during pregnancy with oral and intravaginal metronidazole therapy and correlated with establishment of normal vaginal flora [63]. Although Genc et al [64] confirmed the importance of elevated IL-1β concentration in BV, their studies also indicated that a similar effect could be accomplished by diminished concentrations of IL-1β receptor antagonist. Accordingly, any imbalance between pro- and anti-inflammatory cytokines could exist in BV and support the concept of different subgroups of BV at variable risk for developing complications.

Complications of bacterial vaginosis

In pregnant women, BV has been associated with an approximately twofold risk for developing preterm delivery, premature rupture of membranes, and low birth weight [65,66]. A list of obstetric and gynecologic complications of BV is provided in Box 1. BV is associated with chorioamnionitis and there is strong evidence of a causal relationship between ascending intrauterine infection and spontaneous preterm labor and delivery [65–68]. The aforementioned observations were the basis for recommending screening all pregnant women as a strategy to reduce the rate of preterm delivery [69]. However, routine screening is not the present standard of care because of the highly contradictory results of prospective studies of treating pregnant women who have BV. Over the last 10 years, studies have been extremely controversial. Although several studies have shown that antibiotic treatment of BV was associated with reduced preterm delivery, others have failed to do so (Fig. 1) [70–76]. Therefore, screening

Box 1. Complications of bacterial vaginosis

Obstetric
Chorioamnionitis
Premature rupture of membranes
Preterm labor/delivery
Low birth weight
Amniotic fluid infection
Postpartum endometritis

Gynecologic
Tubal infertility
Pelvic inflammatory disease
Postabortal pelvic inflammatory disease
HIV transmission/acquisition/susceptibility
Postsurgical infection
Urinary tract infection
Cervical intraepithelial neoplasia
Mucopurulent endocervicitis
Strong association with STDs (eg, trichomoniasis, gonorrhea, chlamydia, herpes simplex virus, human papillomavirus)

and routine treatment of all gravid women who have BV is currently not recommended but is suggested in high-risk pregnancy where there is a history of previous preterm delivery. Much criticism has been directed against the various study screening methods and the treatment selected,

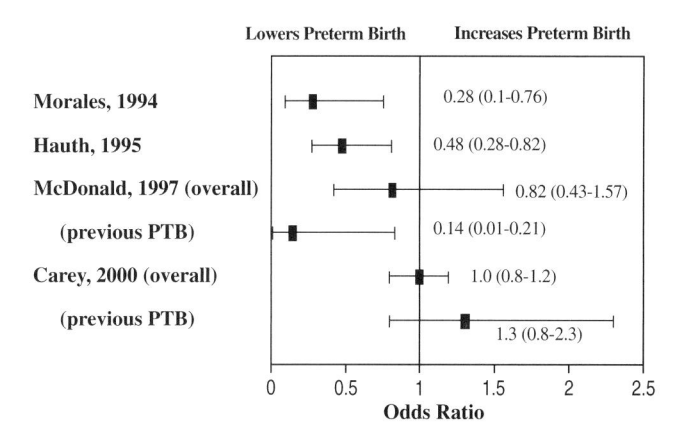

Study	Odds Ratio (95% CI)
Morales, 1994	0.28 (0.1-0.76)
Hauth, 1995	0.48 (0.28-0.82)
McDonald, 1997 (overall)	0.82 (0.43-1.57)
(previous PTB)	0.14 (0.01-0.21)
Carey, 2000 (overall)	1.0 (0.8-1.2)
(previous PTB)	1.3 (0.8-2.3)

Fig. 1. Treatment of bacterial vaginosis to prevent preterm birth. (*Data from* Klein LL, Gibbs RS. Use of microbial cultures and antibiotics in the prevention of infection-associated preterm birth. Am J Obstet Gynecol 2004;190:1493–502.)

including the timing and duration of therapy. Another possibility is that not all women who have BV have the same risk for developing these complications, with only some subgroups at high risk based on a vaginal microenvironmental inflammatory profile. This may explain why some large, interventional cohort studies have failed to show treatment benefit. Only approximately 10% of pregnant women who have BV will experience an adverse pregnancy outcome, and the likelihood of an adverse outcome varies by population studied. In a Danish pregnant women cohort study, Cauci et al [77] demonstrated that vaginal biomarkers, including levels of anti-Gvh IgA and semiquantitative levels of sialidases or prolidases in women who had BV, correlated with increased risk for pregnancy adverse outcome more specifically than diagnosis of BV. In particular, high levels of vaginal anti-Gvh IgA among women who were BV positive were protective for preterm birth and low birth weight. In a recent study, high sialidase activity combined with increased vaginal pH more than five was determined to be a strong risk factor for early preterm birth of less than 32 weeks gestation and very low birth weight (less than 1500 g at birth) [78]. It is also likely that host inflammatory response to the abnormal flora may be profoundly influenced by genetic polymorphism in determining risk within BV subgroups for spontaneous preterm birth [79]. In summary, a more precise definition of the subgroup of women who have BV and are uniquely at risk for preterm delivery will form the basis of future prospective studies to determine optimal antibiotic prevention of this complication.

BV has been strongly associated with PID and histologic endometritis [80–82]. Therefore, women who have BV are more likely to have upper genital tract infection than those who do not. Similarly, women who have PID are more likely to have BV [83]. BV-associated organisms have been isolated from the upper tract of women who have PID and certain organisms, such as anaerobic gram-negative rods, are especially likely to be associated with upper tract infections [84]. Wiesenfeld et al [85] recently reported that subclinical PID is more common in women who have BV, and therefore it is not surprising that women who have tubal infertility are three times more likely to have BV [86].

The cause of mucopurulent cervicitis remains incomplete, with 30% to 50% of patients demonstrating culture negativity for chlamydia, *Neisseria gonorrhoeae*, and herpes simplex. In 1989, Paavonen et al [87] first reported the coexistence of BV and mucopurulent cervicitis. In 1995, Schwebke et al [88] further increased the suspicion of BV contributing to cervicitis in a treatment trial in which doxycycline and metronidazole gel was found to be superior to doxycycline alone in eradicating cervicitis in the presence of concurrent BV. In a further study reported in 2002, Schwebke and Weiss [89] compared doxycycline-ofloxacin with doxycycline-ofloxacin plus metronidazole gel in women who had concurrent cervicitis and BV. The investigators concluded that BV was associated with cervical inflammation and that resolution of cervicitis occurred significantly more often among women who had BV and cervicitis who received the metronidazole-containing regimen, and that they also experienced resolution of BV.

Multiple epidemiologic studies in the United States, Asia, and Africa indicate a firm association between BV, a lactobacillus depleted flora, and HIV infection [90–93]. The seroprevalence of HIV is increased in women who have BV, and the prevalence of BV is similarly increased in women who are seropositive for HIV. BV is thought to facilitate HIV transmission to male sexual partners, with BV also increasing a woman's susceptibility to HIV acquisition. It is thought that BV significantly increases the vaginal HIV RNA load as a consequence of the high levels of TNF-α and IL-1β, hence facilitating transmission [92]. Similarly, in vitro tissue cultures have shown vaginal anaerobes and *G vaginalis* in HIV expression in epithelial and monocytoid cells [94]. Longitudinal studies indicate that BV is not only more common in women who are infected with HIV but is also more likely to persist. Although response rates to appropriate therapy appear to be unaltered, there have been no definitive studies showing that treatment and eradication of BV with appropriate systemic or topical therapy diminishes the risk of HIV transmission or HIV acquisition. Nevertheless, given the prevalence of BV in countries where heterosexual transmission is the dominant method of HIV spread, eradication of symptomatic and asymptomatic BV offers a unique opportunity to decrease HIV transmission.

Diagnosis

In clinical practice, the most widely used method for rapid diagnosis of BV is the use of Amsel criteria, which entail pH measurement, performance of an amine test, and a wet mount microscopy [83]. Unfortunately, although these criteria are extremely useful in diagnosing symptomatic and asymptomatic BV, this method is unreliable because of the lack of microscopy-related skills and availability of pH paper in most doctors' offices. Unfortunately, thousands of women who complain daily of a malodorous discharge are invariably empirically diagnosed with BV without confirmation. A rapid, inexpensive point-of-care diagnostic test is, therefore, urgently required. Although the Gram stain offers high sensitivity and specificity, it is not immediately available and remains largely a research and confirmatory tool. Nevertheless, various commercial laboratory tests are now available and are demonstrated in Box 2. Unfortunately, not all listed tests are available in North America, such as the vaginal acetic acid test [95]. Of greatest value is pH measurement by any method together with a sialidase test [96]. A simple, inexpensive test that could be performed by a symptomatic patient on a self-obtained swab, be processed at home, and provide an immediate response is urgently needed.

> **Box 2. Diagnosis of bacterial vaginosis**
>
> Amsel criteria: depends on practitioner's microscopy skills
> Gram stain: highly reliable, inexpensive, not practical for immediate results
> Affirm VP III DNA probe (Becton Dickinson Co, Franklin Lakes, New Jersey): highly sensitive and specific; expensive, moderate delay for results
> Quickvue Advance pH and Amines test (Quidel Corp, San Diego, California): rapid, reasonably sensitive and specific, inexpensive
> Quickvue Advance G. vaginalis test (Quidel Corp): rapid, highly sensitive and specific
> OSOM BV_{BLUE} (sialidase; Genzyme Diagnostics, Cambridge, Massachusetts): rapid, highly sensitive and specific
> Vaginal acetic acid (Osmetech UK): not available
> pH Screening:
> - Swab/nitrazine paper: lacks specificity
> - Glove paper: not available in United States
> - pHEM-ALERT (Gynex Corp, Redmond, Washington): designed for over-the-counter use
> - VI-SENSE (Common Sense, Cesaria, Israel): panty liner with pH indicator strip; available in Europe only

Treatment

The 2002 CDC recommendations for BV include metronidazole, 500 mg orally twice a day for 7 days; metronidazole gel, 0.75% intravaginally daily for 5 days; or clindamycin cream, 2% intravaginally for 7 days [38]. Alternative therapy includes metronidazole, 2 g single dose orally, or clindamycin, 300 mg orally twice a day for 7 days. Depending on the definition of cure, clinical cure rates vary from 70% to 90% as defined at 21 to 28 days after therapy [97,98]. There seems to be equal effectiveness of the oral and topical routes of therapy, and nitroimidazole and clindamycin regimens appear to be equally efficacious. The main advantage of the topical regimen is reduced gastrointestinal symptomatology. Vaginal therapy is more inconvenient and is associated with a high risk for vaginal candidiasis (10%–30%), even though 3-day suppositories of clindamycin are now available. A topical single-dose adhesive clindamycin preparation has recently been introduced. Tinidazole, recently approved for use in trichomoniasis, can be used for BV but is not yet approved for this indication. Several studies have indicated at least equivalent therapeutic efficacy compared with metronidazole, with some evidence of possible superior activity. However, additional studies will be required to support this claim.

The most important complication of BV in nongravid women is undoubtedly recurrence of the clinical syndrome. Frequency of recurrence varies from 30% within 30 days to approximately 30% within 3 months [97]. All the aforementioned regimens are associated with a high recurrence rate. The cause of recurrent BV is largely unknown. Theories include failure of vaginal acidification, failure to reduce numbers of *G vaginalis* and anaerobic flora, failure to recolonize the vagina with protective *lactobacillus* spp, antimicrobial resistance of overgrowing microorganisms, or persistence of the initial unrecognized precipitating or trigger pathogen. Finally, reinfection or recolonization with the triggering pathogen or agent may be responsible. Studies aimed at vaginal acidification have not reduced the recurrence rate. Similarly, although clindamycin resistance has been seen in vaginal anaerobic flora, metronidazole resistance has not yet been reported [99]. With regard to reinfection, most studies have failed to show any benefit in the treatment of male partners of women who have recurrent BV.

Management of recurrent BV is controversial and largely unexplored. Most practitioners repeat therapy, avoiding short-course regimen and possibly switching from one class of antimicrobials to another and including a trial of tinidazole therapy [100]. There is no evidence that combination therapies benefit. Vaginal lactobacillus replacement is an attractive solution but remains a clinical research endeavor. The use of commercially obtainable unstandardized lactobacillus preparations is not recommended. Therefore, in the absence of any available effective therapy for recurrent disease, clinicians rely mainly on the use of maintenance antimicrobial suppressive therapy. After an initial pilot study showing reasonable efficacy of maintenance metronidazole vaginal gels, 0.75%, a large multicenter study was recently completed that showed considerable efficacy achieving in excess of 70% protective efficacy on a twice-weekly regimen of metronidazole vaginal gel [101]. Nevertheless, a considerable number of women relapsed on cessation of the suppressive therapy.

Summary

The use of biochemical profiles and new molecular microbiologic methodologies is transforming our understanding of BV. Most important is the recognition of different subgroups of women who have BV who are at variable risk of certain obstetric and gynecologic complications. New diagnostic tests may soon be available that will allow women to test self-obtained specimens. Treatment of BV has lagged, although innovative methods appear to be helpful in managing recurrent diseases.

References

[1] Schneider H, Coetzee DJ, Fehler HG, et al. Screening for sexually transmitted diseases in rural South African women. Sex Transm Infect 1998;74(Suppl 1):S147–52.

[2] Moodley P, Connolly C, Sturm AW. Interrelationships among human immunodeficiency virus type 1 infection, bacterial vaginosis, trichomoniasis, and the presence of yeasts. J Infect Dis 2002;185:69–73.
[3] World Health Organization. An overview of selected curable sexually transmitted diseases. Geneva (Switzerland): WHO Global program on AIDS; 1995. p. 2–27.
[4] Fouts AC, Kraus SJ. Trichomonas vaginalis: reevaluation of its clinical presentation and laboratory diagnosis. J Infect Dis 1980;141:137–43.
[5] Soper D. Trichomoniasis: under control or undercontrolled? Am J Obstet Gynecol 2004;190:281–90.
[6] Bowden FJ, Garnett GP. Trichomonas vaginalis epidemiology: parameterising and analysing a model of treatment interventions. Sex Transm Infect 2000;76:248–56.
[7] Sorvillo F, Smith L, Kerndt P, et al. Trichomonas vaginalis, HIV, and African-Americans. Emerg Infect Dis 2001;7:927–32.
[8] Saxena SB, Jenkins RR. Prevalence of Trichomonas vaginalis in men at high risk for sexually transmitted diseases. Sex Transm Dis 1991;18:138–42.
[9] Weston TE, Nicol CS. Natural history of trichomonal infection in males. Br J Vener Dis 1963;39:251–7.
[10] Cotch MF, Pastorek JG II, Nugent RP, et al. Trichomonas vaginalis associated with low birth weight and preterm delivery. The Vaginal Infections and Prematurity Study Group. Sex Transm Dis 1997;24:353–60.
[11] Minkoff H, Grunebaum AN, Schwarz RH, et al. Risk factors for prematurity and premature rupture of membranes: a prospective study of the vaginal flora in pregnancy. Am J Obstet Gynecol 1984;150:965–72.
[12] Klebanoff MA, Carey JC, Hauth JC, et al. National Institute of Child Health and Human Development Network of Maternal-Fetal Medicine Units. Failure of metronidazole to prevent preterm delivery among pregnant women with asymptomatic Trichomonas vaginalis infection. N Engl J Med 2001;345:487–93.
[13] Wang CC, McClelland RS, Reilly M, et al. The effect of treatment of vaginal infections on shedding of human immunodeficiency virus type 1. J Infect Dis 2001;183:1017–22.
[14] Sorvillo F, Kerndt P. Trichomonas vaginalis and amplification of HIV-1 transmission. Lancet 1998;351:213–4.
[15] Dallabetta GA, Miotti PG, Chiphangwi JD, et al. High socioeconomic status is a risk factor for human immunodeficiency virus type 1 (HIV-1) infection but not for sexually transmitted diseases in women in Malawi: implications for HIV-1 control. J Infect Dis 1993;167:36–42.
[16] Laga M, Alary M, Nzila N, et al. Condom promotion, sexually transmitted diseases treatment, and declining incidence of HIV-1 infection in female Zairian sex workers. Lancet 1994;344:246–8.
[17] Cameron DW, Padian NS. Sexual transmission of HIV and the epidemiology of other sexually transmitted diseases. AIDS 1990;4(Suppl 1):S99–103.
[18] Cu-Uvin S, Hogan JW, Warren D, et al. Prevalence of lower genital tract infections among human immunodeficiency virus (HIV)-seropositive and high-risk HIV-seronegative women. HIV Epidemiology Research Study Group. Clin Infect Dis 1999;29:1145–50.
[19] Moodley P, Wilkinson D, Connolly C, et al. Trichomonas vaginalis is associated with pelvic inflammatory disease in women infected with human immunodeficiency virus. Clin Infect Dis 2002;34:519–22.
[20] Grodstein F, Goldman MB, Ryan L, et al. Relation of female infertility to consumption of caffeinated beverages. Am J Epidemiol 1993;137:1353–60.
[21] Sherman KJ, Daling JR, Weiss NS. Sexually transmitted diseases and tubal infertility. Sex Transm Dis 1987;14:12–6.
[22] El-Shazly AM, El-Naggar HM, Soliman M, et al. A study on Trichomoniasis vaginalis and female infertility. J Egypt Soc Parasitol 2001;31(2):545–53.

[23] Paisarntantiwong R, Brockmann S, Clarke L, et al. The relationship of vaginal trichomoniasis and pelvic inflammatory disease among women colonized with Chlamydia trachomatis. Sex Transm Dis 1995;22:344–7.

[24] Soper DE, Bump RC, Hurt WG. Bacterial vaginosis and trichomoniasis vaginitis are risk factors for cuff cellulitis after abdominal hysterectomy. Am J Obstet Gynecol 1990;63:1016–21.

[25] Zhang ZF, Begg CB. Is Trichomonas vaginalis a cause of cervical neoplasia? Results from a combined analysis of 24 studies. Int J Epidemiol 1994;23:682–90.

[26] Viikki M, Pukkala E, Nieminen P, et al. Gynaecological infections as risk determinants of subsequent cervical neoplasia. Acta Oncol 2000;39:71–5.

[27] Yap EH, Ho TH, Chan YC, et al. Serum antibodies to Trichomonas vaginalis in invasive cervical cancer patients. Genitourin Med 1995;71:402–4.

[28] Sayed el-Ahl SA, el-Wakil HS, Kamel NM, et al. A preliminary study on the relationship between Trichomonas vaginalis and cervical cancer in Egyptian women. J Egypt Soc Parasitol 2002;32:167–78.

[29] Krieger JN, Alderete JD. Trichomoniasis vaginalis and trichomoniasis. In: Holmes KK, Sparling PF, Mardh P, et al, editors. Sexually transmitted diseases. 3rd edition. New York: McGraw-Hill; 1999. p. 587–604.

[30] Gardner WA Jr, Culberson DE, Bennett BD. Trichomonas vaginalis in the prostate gland. Arch Pathol Lab Med 1986;110:430–2.

[31] Skerk V, Schonwald S, Krhen I, et al. Aetiology of chronic prostatitis. Int J Antimicrob Agents 2002;19:471–4.

[32] Martinez-Garcia F, Regadera J, Mayer R, et al. Protozoan infections in the male genital tract. J Urol 1996;156:340–9.

[33] Jarecki-Black JC, Lushbaugh WB, Golosov L, et al. Trichomonas vaginalis: preliminary characterization of a sperm motility inhibiting factor. Ann Clin Lab Sci 1988;18:484–9.

[34] Borchardt KA, al-Haraci S, Maida N. Prevalence of Trichomonas vaginalis in a male sexually transmitted disease clinic population by interview, wet mount microscopy, and the InPouch TV test. Genitourin Med 1995;71:405–6.

[35] Schwebke JR, Lawing LF. Improved detection by DNA amplification of Trichomonas vaginalis in males. J Clin Microbiol 2002;40:3681–3.

[36] Wendel KA, Erbelding EJ, Gaydos CA, et al. Trichomonas vaginalis polymerase chain reaction compared with standard diagnostic and therapeutic protocols for detection and treatment of vaginal trichomoniasis. Clin Infect Dis 2002;35:576–80.

[37] Joyner JL, Douglas JM Jr, Ragsdale S, et al. Comparative prevalence of infection with Trichomonas vaginalis among men attending a sexually transmitted diseases clinic. Sex Transm Dis 2000;27:236–40.

[38] Sexually transmitted diseases treatment guidelines 2002. Centers for Disease Control and Prevention. MMWR Recomm Rep 2002;51:44–5.

[39] Lossick JG, Kent HL. Trichomoniasis: trends in diagnosis and management. Am J Obstet Gynecol 1991;165:1217–22.

[40] Ahmed-Jushuf IH, Murray AE, McKeown J. Managing trichomonal vaginitis refractory to conventional treatment with metronidazole. Genitourin Med 1988;64:25–9.

[41] Sobel JD, Nyirjesy P, Brown W. Tinidazole therapy for metronidazole-resistant vaginal trichomoniasis. Clin Infect Dis 2001;33:1341–6.

[42] Hager WD. Treatment of metronidazole-resistant Trichomonas vaginalis with tinidazole: case reports of three patients. Sex Transm Dis 2004;31:343–5.

[43] Crowell AL, Sanders-Lewis KA, Secor WE. In vitro metronidazole and tinidazole activities against metronidazole-resistant strains of Trichomonas vaginalis. Antimicrob Agents Chemother 2003;47:1407–9.

[44] Narcisi EM, Secor WE. In vitro effect of tinidazole and furazolidone on metronidazole-resistant Trichomonas vaginalis. Antimicrob Agents Chemother 1996;40:1121–5.

[45] Eschenbach DA. History and review of bacterial vaginosis. Am J Obstet Gynecol 1993;169: 441–5.
[46] Goldenberg RL, Klebanoff MA, Nugent R, et al. Bacterial colonization of the vagina during pregnancy in four ethnic groups. Vaginal Infections and Prematurity Study Group. Am J Obstet Gynecol 1996;174:1618–21.
[47] Riduan JM, Hillier SL, Utomo B, et al. Bacterial vaginosis and prematurity in Indonesia: association in early and late pregnancy. Am J Obstet Gynecol 1993;169:175–8.
[48] Hallen A, Pahlson C, Forsum U. Bacterial vaginosis in women attending STD clinic: diagnostic criteria and prevalence of Mobiluncus spp. Genitourin Med 1987; 63:386–9.
[49] Smart S, Singal A, Mindel A. Social and sexual risk factors for bacterial vaginosis. Sex Transm Infect 2004;80:58–62.
[50] Marrazzo JM, Koutsky LA, Eschenbach DA, et al. Characterization of vaginal flora and bacterial vaginosis in women who have sex with women. J Infect Dis 2002;185:1307–13.
[51] Yen S, Shafer MA, Moncada J, et al. Bacterial vaginosis in sexually experienced and non-sexually experienced young women entering the military. Obstet Gynecol 2003;102:927–33.
[52] Ness RB, Hillier S, Richter HE, et al. Can known risk factors explain racial differences in the occurrence of bacterial vaginosis? J Natl Med Assoc 2003;95:201–12.
[53] Thorsen P, Jensen IP, Jeune B, et al. Few microorganisms associated with bacterial vaginosis may constitute the pathologic core: a population-based microbiologic study among 3596 pregnant women. Am J Obstet Gynecol 1998;178:580–7.
[54] Ward DM, Bateson MM, Weller R, et al. Ribosomal RNA analysis of microorganisms as they occur in nature. In: Marshall KC, editor. Advances in microbial ecology, vol. 12. New York: Plenum Press; 1992. p. 219–86.
[55] Ferris MJ, Masztal A, Aldridge KE, et al. Association of Atopobium vaginae, a recently described metronidazole resistant anaerobe, with bacterial vaginosis. BMC Infect Dis 2004; 4:5.
[56] Verstraelen H, Verhelst R, Claeys G, et al. Culture-independent analysis of vaginal microflora: the unrecognized association of Atopobium vaginae with bacterial vaginosis. Am J Obstet Gynecol 2004;191:1130–2.
[57] Cauci S, Monte R, Ropele M, et al. Pore-forming and haemolytic properties of the Gardnerella vaginalis cytolysin. Mol Microbiol 1993;9:1143–55.
[58] Platz-Christensen JJ, Mattsby-Baltzer I, Thomsen P, et al. Endotoxin and interleukin-1 alpha in the cervical mucus and vaginal fluid of pregnant women with bacterial vaginosis. Am J Obstet Gynecol 1993;169:1161–6.
[59] Cauci S, Guaschino S, De Aloysio D, et al. Interrelationships of interleukin-8 with interleukin-1beta and neutrophils in vaginal fluid of healthy and bacterial vaginosis positive women. Mol Hum Reprod 2003;9:53–8.
[60] Cauci S, Driussi S, De Santo D, et al. Prevalence of bacterial vaginosis and vaginal flora changes in peri- and postmenopausal women. J Clin Microbiol 2002;40:2147–52.
[61] Cauci S. Vaginal immunity in bacterial vaginosis. Curr Infect Dis Rep 2004;6:450–6.
[62] Cauci S, Driussi S, Guaschino S, et al. Correlation of local interleukin-1beta levels with specific IgA response against Gardnerella vaginalis cytolysin in women with bacterial vaginosis. Am J Reprod Immunol 2002;47:257–64.
[63] Yudin MH, Landers DV, Meyn L, et al. Clinical and cervical cytokine response to treatment with oral or vaginal metronidazole for bacterial vaginosis during pregnancy: a randomized trial. Obstet Gynecol 2003;102:527–34.
[64] Genc MR, Witkin SS, Delaney ML, et al. A disproportionate increase in IL-1beta over IL-1ra in the cervicovaginal secretions of pregnant women with altered vaginal microflora correlates with preterm birth. Am J Obstet Gynecol 2004;190:1191–7.
[65] Hillier SL, Krohn MA, Cassen E, et al. The role of bacterial vaginosis and vaginal bacteria in amniotic fluid infection in women in preterm labor with intact fetal membranes. Clin Infect Dis 1995;20(Suppl 2):S276–8.

[66] Goldenberg RL, Culhane JF. Infection as a cause of preterm birth. Clin Perinatol 2003;30: 677–700.
[67] McGregor JA, French JI. Bacterial vaginosis in pregnancy. Obstet Gynecol Surv 2000;55(5 Suppl 1):S1–19.
[68] Hillier SL, Martius J, Krohn M, et al. A case-control study of chorioamnionic infection and histologic chorioamnionitis in prematurity. N Engl J Med 1988;319:972–8.
[69] Koumans EH, Markowitz LE, Hogan V; CDC BV Working Group. Indications for therapy and treatment recommendations for bacterial vaginosis in nonpregnant and pregnant women: a synthesis of data. Clin Infect Dis 2002;35(Suppl 2):S152–72.
[70] Klein LL, Gibbs RS. Use of microbial cultures and antibiotics in the prevention of infection-associated preterm birth. Am J Obstet Gynecol 2004;190:1493–502.
[71] Leitich H, Brunbauer M, Bodner-Adler B, et al. Antibiotic treatment of bacterial vaginosis in pregnancy: a meta-analysis. Am J Obstet Gynecol 2003;188:752–8.
[72] Hauth JC, Goldenberg RL, Andrews WW, et al. Reduced incidence of preterm delivery with metronidazole and erythromycin in women with bacterial vaginosis. N Engl J Med 1995;333:1732–6.
[73] McDonald HM, O'Loughlin JA, Vigneswaran R, et al. Impact of metronidazole therapy on preterm birth in women with bacterial vaginosis flora (Gardnerella vaginalis): a randomised, placebo controlled trial. Br J Obstet Gynaecol 1997;104:1391–7.
[74] Morales WJ, Schorr S, Albritton J. Effect of metronidazole in patients with preterm birth in preceding pregnancy and bacterial vaginosis: a placebo-controlled, double-blind study. Am J Obstet Gynecol 1994;171:345–7.
[75] Brocklehurst P, Hannah M, McDonald H. Interventions for treating bacterial vaginosis in pregnancy. Cochrane Database Syst Rev 2000;(2):CD000262.
[76] Carey JC, Klebanoff MA, Hauth JC, et al. Metronidazole to prevent preterm delivery in pregnant women with asymptomatic bacterial vaginosis. National Institute of Child Health and Human Development Network of Maternal-Fetal Medicine Units. N Engl J Med 2000; 342:534–40.
[77] Cauci S, Thorsen P, Schendel DE, et al. Determination of immunoglobulin A against Gardnerella vaginalis hemolysin, sialidase, and prolidase activities in vaginal fluid: implications for adverse pregnancy outcomes. J Clin Microbiol 2003;41:435–8.
[78] Cauci S, McGregor J, Thorsen P, et al. Combination of vaginal pH with vaginal sialidase and prolidase activities for prediction of low birth weight and preterm birth. Am J Obstet Gynecol 2005;192:489–96.
[79] Macones GA, Parry S, Elkousy M, et al. A polymorphism in the promoter region of TNF and bacterial vaginosis: preliminary evidence of gene-environment interaction in the etiology of spontaneous preterm birth. Am J Obstet Gynecol 2004;190:1504–8.
[80] Korn AP, Bolan G, Padian N, et al. Plasma cell endometritis in women with symptomatic bacterial vaginosis. Obstet Gynecol 1995;85:387–90.
[81] Paavonen J, Teisala K, Heinonen PK, et al. Microbiological and histopathological findings in acute pelvic inflammatory disease. Br J Obstet Gynaecol 1987;94:454–60.
[82] Peipert JF, Ness RB, Blume J, et al. Pelvic Inflammatory Disease Evaluation and Clinical Health Study Investigators. Clinical predictors of endometritis in women with symptoms and signs of pelvic inflammatory disease. Am J Obstet Gynecol 2001;184:856–63.
[83] Eschenbach DA, Hillier S, Critchlow C, et al. Diagnosis and clinical manifestations of bacterial vaginosis. Am J Obstet Gynecol 1988;158:819–28.
[84] Hillier SL, Kiviat NB, Hawes SE, et al. Role of bacterial vaginosis-associated microorganisms in endometritis. Am J Obstet Gynecol 1996;175:435–41.
[85] Wiesenfeld HC, Hillier SL, Krohn MA, et al. Lower genital tract infection and endometritis: insight into subclinical pelvic inflammatory disease. Obstet Gynecol 2002; 100:456–63.
[86] Wilson JD, Ralph SG, Rutherford AJ. Rates of bacterial vaginosis in women undergoing in vitro fertilisation for different types of infertility. BJOG 2002;109:714–7.

[87] Paavonen J, Roberts PL, Stevens CE, et al. Randomized treatment of mucopurulent cervicitis with doxycycline or amoxicillin. Am J Obstet Gynecol 1989;161:128–35.
[88] Schwebke JR, Schulien MB, Zajackowski M. Pilot study to evaluate the appropriate management of patients with coexistent bacterial vaginosis and cervicitis. Infect Dis Obstet Gynecol 1995;3:119–22.
[89] Schwebke JR, Weiss HL. Interrelationships of bacterial vaginosis and cervical inflammation. Sex Transm Dis 2002;29:59–64.
[90] Martin HL, Richardson BA, Nyange PM, et al. Vaginal lactobacilli, microbial flora, and risk of human immunodeficiency virus type 1 and sexually transmitted disease acquisition J Infect Dis 1999;180:1863–8.
[91] Alvarez-Olmos MI, Barousse MM, Rajan L, et al. Vaginal lactobacilli in adolescents: presence and relationship to local and systemic immunity, and to bacterial vaginosis. Sex Transm Dis 2004;31:393–400.
[92] Cohen CR, Duerr A, Pruithithada N, et al. Bacterial vaginosis and HIV seroprevalence among female commercial sex workers in Chiang Mai, Thailand. AIDS 1995;9:1093–7.
[93] Sewankambo N, Gray RH, Wawer MJ, et al. HIV-1 infection associated with abnormal vaginal flora morphology and bacterial vaginosis. Lancet 1997;350:546–50.
[94] Hashemi FB, Ghassemi M, Faro S, et al. Induction of human immunodeficiency virus type 1 expression by anaerobes associated with bacterial vaginosis. J Infect Dis 2000;181: 1574–80.
[95] Chaudry AN, Travers PJ, Yuenger J, et al. Analysis of vaginal acetic acid in patients undergoing treatment for bacterial vaginosis. J Clin Microbiol 2004;42:5170–5.
[96] Myziuk L, Romanowski B, Johnson SC. BVBlue test for diagnosis of bacterial vaginosis J Clin Microbiol 2003;41:1925–8.
[97] Hay PE. Therapy of bacterial vaginosis. J Antimicrob Chemother 1998;41:6–9.
[98] Kane KY, Pierce R. Clinical inquiries. What are the most effective treatments for bacterial vaginosis in nonpregnant women? J Fam Pract 2001;50:399–400.
[99] Beigi RH, Austin MN, Meyn LA, et al. Antimicrobial resistance associated with the treatment of bacterial vaginosis. Am J Obstet Gynecol 2004;191:1124–9.
[100] Baylson FA, Nyirjesy P, Weitz MV. Treatment of recurrent bacterial vaginosis with tinidazole. Obstet Gynecol 2004;104:931–2.
[101] Sobel JD, Schwebke J, Ferris D, et al. A clinical trial to evaluate efficacy of maintenance therapy with 0.75% metronidazole gel (MVG) to prevent recurrent bacterial vaginosis (BV). Presented at the World Vaginitis Conference. Costa Rica, January 10–13, 2004.

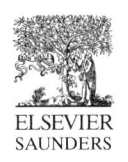

Is *Mycoplasma genitalium* a Cause of Pelvic Inflammatory Disease?

Jonathan D.C. Ross, MB, ChB, MD, FRCP

Whittall Street Clinic, Whittall Street, Birmingham B4 6DH, UK

In most cases of PID, a lower genital tract gonococcal or chlamydial infection cannot be found. This lack of detection is in part caused by prior antibiotic therapy or delay in diagnosis of PID, which may contribute to decreased ascertainment. However, this is believed to only represent a few cases where no lower tract pathogen is found, and has stimulated investigation into other potential organisms or cofactors. Can *Mycoplasma genitalium* fill this gap, and what are the implications for management if it does?

M genitalium is a small bacterium comprising only 580 kilobases. This restricted amount of genetic material limits the number of metabolic processes that the organism can sustain. Therefore, it has fastidious growth requirements, and culture of *M genitalium* has proven difficult to initiate and sustain. Developments in molecular approaches to diagnosis have allowed investigators to learn more about the importance of the organism. On electron microscopy, *M genitalium* is revealed to be a flask-shaped organism with a narrow terminal end containing the adhesin protein that is responsible for cell attachment, and which also functions as a target for polymerase chain reaction (PCR) primers.

To establish whether there is a link between *M genitalium* and PID, it must first be determined whether *M genitalium* is a sexually acquired infection in women.

Mycoplasma genitalium as a sexually acquired infection in women

Most of the evidence linking *M genitalium* to disease comes from men who have urethritis, where descriptive and case-control studies have clearly shown that *M genitalium* is more likely in men who have urethritis

---

The author has received payment from Bayer as a consultant.
E-mail address: jonathan.ross@hobtpct.nhs.uk

compared with asymptomatic controls, and that treatment leading to eradication of mycoplasma is associated with clinical cure. Overall, *M genitalium* can be detected in 20% of men who have urethritis compared with 8% of those who do not [1]. *M genitalium* has also been associated with the development of an antibody response following acute urethritis [2].

Animal inoculation studies have also demonstrated that *M genitalium* can cause urethritis in nonhuman primates [1]. *M genitalium* can be detected in the genital tract of between 2% and 38% of women screened, with the higher rates being reported from those who have genital symptoms, have attended an STD clinic, or are contacts of men who have urethritis. One partner study found *M genitalium* in a third of the female partners of infected men, compared with none of those who had uninfected male partners [3]. Lower rates occur in asymptomatic women, supporting the concept that *M genitalium* is sexually transmitted [4–10]. *M genitalium* has been associated with cervicitis in between 8% and 50% of infected women [6,9,11,12], and only one study by Casin et al [13] revealed no significant association (Table 1). In this study, Casin et al used a control group comprised symptomatic women who had vaginal discharge, whereas the other studies used controls who were asymptomatic, and this fact may have reduced the power of this one study to detect a difference. The largest of these studies suggested that *M genitalium* is associated with a threefold increased risk of cervicitis, which was in the same order of magnitude as *N gonorrhoeae* and *C trachomatis* [11]. It is not just the presence of *M genitalium* that may be important but also the quantity. Men who have urethritis have much higher concentrations of *M genitalium* in the urethra compared with those who have asymptomatic infection [14]. The relevance of this in women requires further study.

Mycoplasma genitalium and pelvic inflammatory disease

The increasing evidence that *M genitalium* is a sexually transmitted cause of urethritis in men and that it has been associated with cervicitis prompts its

Table 1
Studies analyzing the association between *Mycoplasma genitalium* and cervicitis in infected women

Studies	*M genitalium* infection with cervicitis	*M genitalium* infection without cervicitis
Significant association		
Falk et al [9] (N = 22)	50%	24%
Anagrius and Lore [12] (N = 257)	13%	3%
Uno et al [6] (N = 144)	8%	0%
Manhart et al [11] (N = 719)	48%	29%
Nonsignificant association		
Casin et al [13] (N = 170)	42%	32%

nomination as a potential factor in the development of PID. The microbiologic characteristics of the organism are also supportive. In vitro, it is clear that *M genitalium* can adhere to fallopian tube epithelial cells in cell culture and that invasion of epithelial cells may occur, leading to up-regulation of cytokine expression that is associated with an inflammatory response [15]. Infection of cell lines with other mycoplasmas is often indolent and chronic, with infection persisting for several months, suggesting that mycoplasma may cause a low-grade, subclinical infection. There is also laboratory evidence that mycoplasma can adhere to sperm, which may then transport infection to the upper genital tract [16].

Unlike gonorrhoea or chlamydia, good animal models are available for *M genitalium* and show that inoculation of the vagina in chimpanzees leads to a prolonged infection over several months, associated with an inflammatory discharge and systemic antibody response [17]. The spread from the lower to the upper genital tract has been demonstrated in baboons where inoculation of the cervix led to endometritis and salpingitis [18]. The potential for upper genital tract infection is also supported by the development of adnexitis and a systemic antibody response following direct inoculation of the oviduct in grivet monkeys and marmosets [18,19].

The animal data are intriguing, but inoculation studies of this sort would obviously be unethical in humans. Therefore, more indirect evidence to link *M* genitalium to PID must be sought, such as the antibody response to infection. Unfortunately such evidence is somewhat conflicting. One study of 31 women suggests that over a third of women who have PID will develop serologic evidence of mycoplasma infection following acute pelvic infection [20]. A second study, reported a few years later but from a similar geographic area and using a similar serologic assay, found that only one out of 46 women who had acute salpingitis on laparoscopy had an antibody response to *M genitalium* [21]. Serologic data are also available for women under investigation for infertility that link *M genitalium* to tubal damage. Over 20% of those who had tubal infertility had evidence of prior *M genitalium* infection, compared with only 6% of those who had other causes of infertility [22]. The potential exists for cross-reaction between serologic assays for *M genitalium* and *Mycoplasma pneumonia*, but later studies, including those assessing the link with tubal infertility, effectively excluded this possibility by confirming positive results by immunoblotting using a cloned fragment of the *M genitalium*-specific adhesin protein.

More direct evidence of the involvement of *M genitalium* in PID can be obtained by looking for the organism in the genital tract of women who have acute infection. *M genitalium* has been detected in the endometrium of women in two studies. The first study found *M genitalium* in seven out of 58 (12%) Kenyan women who had a history of pelvic pain and evidence of histologic endometritis [23]. Of possible importance is that a third of these women were also HIV positive. Secondly, data are available from a large American treatment trial of women who had mild to moderate PID, in whom a subset of women were tested for *M genitalium* using an endometrial sample. An initial report shows infection in four out of 50 (8%) of these women [24]. There is also a single case of successful detection in the fallopian tube, representing 1% of those studied in an African cohort [25]. In this study, the women had clinically severe PID requiring hospitalization.

Implications for management of pelvic inflammatory disease

The routine detection of the organism is limited by the lack of a commercial test kit. Existing "in-house" or "home-brew" PCRs may vary in their sensitivity and specificity and, compared with culture, some only detect around half of infections [26]. The target sequences vary between different assays, making cross-study comparisons difficult. It is also not clear what the optimal specimen is for detection of the organism. In some studies, a urethral swab has the highest isolation rate, whereas in others a vaginal swab is better (Fig. 1) [13,27]. A combination of specimens may be required (eg, cervical swab plus first-pass urine).

Therapy

If *M genitalium* is detected or strongly suspected, then the question becomes what therapy will be most effective. The organism lacks a cell wall, and therefore penicillins or cephalosporins are unlikely to be useful. Culture of the organism takes several weeks or months and this slow growth rate may require a prolonged course of therapy to ensure eradication. In addition, the intracellular nature of infection indicates a need to maintain drug levels within the cytoplasm, and plasma levels of antibiotic may be less important.

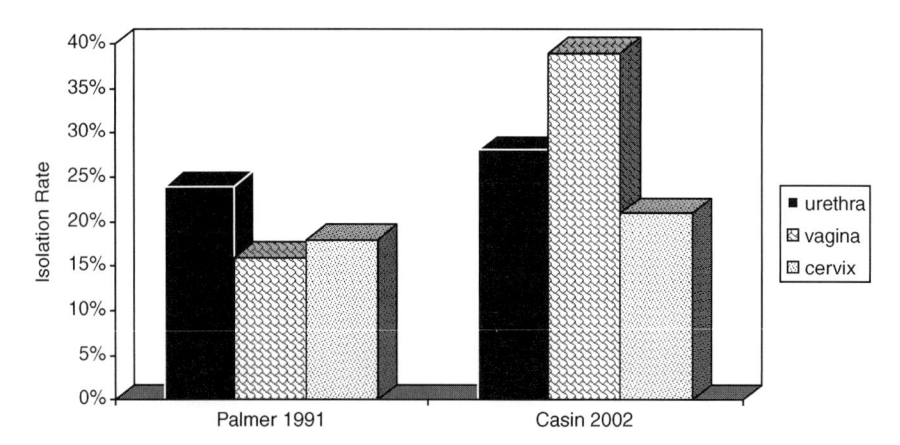

Fig. 1. *Mycoplasma genitalium* isolation rates for different specimens.

In vitro sensitivity testing is restricted by the limited number of culture lines available for testing. Genotyping suggests that there are several different subtypes of *M genitalium*, and a leap of faith is required to assume that all of these different strains will have the same sensitivity pattern as the small number of cultured isolates. With these limitations in mind, in vitro sensitivity testing suggests that macrolides and tetracyclines may be effective, with a more variable response for quinolones [28]. In theory, quinolones should be the drugs of choice because they are bacteriocidal rather than bacteriostatic, but the use of levofloxin has been associated with only a transient reduction in the concentration of *M genitalium*, followed by a recurrence of symptoms over the subsequent few weeks in men presenting initially with urethritis [29]. Some of the newer quinolones, such as sparfloxacin and moxifloxacin, have lower minimum inhibitory concentrations against *M genitalium*, but have yet to be assessed in clinical trials [30].

Most clinical trial evidence for the treatment of *M genitalium* comes from men who have urethritis. The response to tetracyclines has been somewhat variable, and more recent studies in particular suggest microbiologic clearance only occurs in between 30% and 40% of patients [31,32]. The macrolides show the most promising results, particularly using azithromycin either as a stat dose or over 5 days (Fig. 2) [33]. In one of the few studies in women, azithromycin has also been highly effective in eradicating *M genitalium*, whereas the use of doxycycline or lymecycline has been associated with a 50% failure rate as assessed by persistent or recurrent detection of the organism [32].

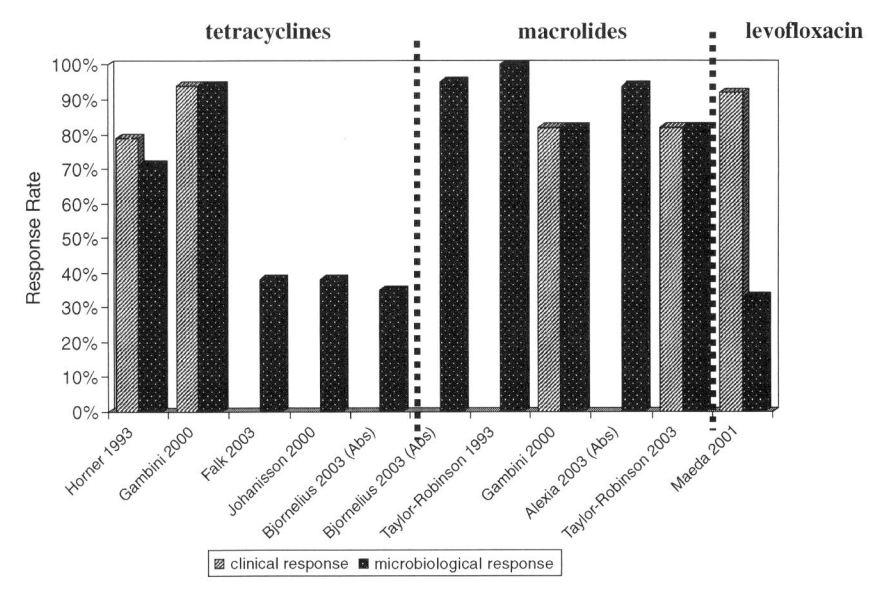

Fig. 2. Clinical and microbiological effectiveness of antibiotics against mycoplasma.

Summary

The evidence for *M genitalium* as a sexually acquired infection in women is strong, and the organism has been associated with cervicitis and urethritis. In vitro evidence supports the concept that *M genitalium* causes inflammation in the fallopian tube epithelium, and animal studies have demonstrated the potential for infection to spread from the lower to the upper genital tract. Serologic data in humans who have PID are somewhat conflicting, but studies in infertile women suggest a link between *M genitalium* and tubal damage. The organism has also been isolated in the endometrium and fallopian tubes of women who have PID.

The evidence is therefore accumulating that *M genitalium* is a cause of PID, and the assessment of reliable tests to further investigate the importance of this organism and its relevance in designing future treatment strategies is urgently needed.

References

[1] Taylor-Robinson D. Mycoplasma genitalium—an up-date. Int J STD AIDS 2002;13:145–51.
[2] Taylor-Robinson D, Furr PM, Hanna NF. Microbiological and serological study of non-gonococcal urethritis with special reference to Mycoplasma genitalium. Genitourin Med 1985;61:319–24.
[3] Keane FE, Thomas BJ, Gilroy CB, et al. The association of Chlamydia trachomatis and Mycoplasma genitalium with non-gonococcal urethritis: observations on heterosexual men and their female partners. Int J STD AIDS 2000;11:435–9.
[4] Samra Z, Soffer Y, Pansky M. Prevalence of genital chlamydia and mycoplasma infection in couples attending a male infertility clinic. Eur J Epidemiol 1994;10:69–73.
[5] Savio ML, Caruso A, Allegri R, et al. Detection of Mycoplasma genitalium from urethral swabs of human immunodeficiency virus-infected patients. New Microbiol 1996;19:203–9.
[6] Uno M, Deguchi T, Komeda H, et al. Mycoplasma genitalium in the cervices of Japanese women. Sex Transm Dis 1997;24:284–6.
[7] Maeda SI, Tamaki M, Nakano M, et al. Detection of Mycoplasma genitalium in patients with urethritis. J Urol 1998;159:405–7.
[8] Tsunoe H, Tanaka M, Nakayama H, et al. High prevalence of Chlamydia trachomatis, Neisseria gonorrhoeae and Mycoplasma genitalium in female commercial sex workers in Japan. Int J STD AIDS 2000;11:790–4.
[9] Falk L, Skov Jensen J. Mycoplasma genitalium prevalence, symptoms, signs and treatment efficacy among attendees at a Swedish STD outpatient clinic. Int J STD AIDS 2001;12:107.
[10] Labbe AC, Frost E, Deslandes S, et al. Mycoplasma genitalium is not associated with adverse outcomes of pregnancy in Guinea-Bissau. Sex Transm Infect 2002;78:289–91.
[11] Manhart LE, Critchlow CW, Holmes KK, et al. Mucopurulent cervicitis and Mycoplasma genitalium. J Infect Dis 2003;187:650–7.
[12] Anagrius C, Lore B. [Chlamydia-like symptoms can have another etiology. Mycoplasma genitalium—an important and common sexually transmitted disease]. Lakartidningen 2002;99:4854–5 [in Swedish].
[13] Casin I, Vexiau-Robert D, De La Salmoniere P, et al. High prevalence of Mycoplasma genitalium in the lower genitourinary tract of women attending a sexually transmitted disease clinic in Paris, France. Sex Transm Dis 2002;29:353–9.

[14] Yoshida T, Deguchi T, Ito M, et al. Quantitative detection of Mycoplasma genitalium from first-pass urine of men with urethritis and asymptomatic men by real-time PCR. J Clin Microbiol 2002;40:1451–5.
[15] Zhang S, Wear DJ, Lo SC. Mycoplasmal infections alter gene expression in cultured human prostatic and cervical epithelial cells. FEMS Immunol Med Microbiol 2000;27:43–50.
[16] Svenstrup HF, Fedder J, Abraham-Peskir J, et al. Mycoplasma genitalium attaches to human spermatozoa. Hum Reprod 2003;18(10):2103–9.
[17] Tully JG, Taylor-Robinson D, Rose DL. Urogenital challenge of primate species with Mycoplasma genitalium and characteristics of infection induced in chimpanzees. J Infect Dis 1986;153:1046–54.
[18] Taylor-Robinson D, Furr PM, Tully JG, et al. Animal models of Mycoplasma genitalium urogenital infection. Isr J Med Sci 1987;23:561–4.
[19] Moller BR, Taylor-Robinson D, Furr PM, et al. Acute upper genital-tract disease in female monkeys provoked experimentally by Mycoplasma genitalium. Br J Exp Pathol 1985;66: 417–26.
[20] Moller BR, Taylor-Robinson D, Furr PM. Serological evidence implicating Mycoplasma genitalium in pelvic inflammatory disease. Lancet 1984;1:1102–3.
[21] Lind K, Kristensen GB. Significance of antibodies to Mycoplasma genitalium in salpingitis. Eur J Clin Microbiol 1987;6:205–7.
[22] Clausen HF, Fedder J, Drasbek M, et al. Serological investigation of Mycoplasma genitalium in infertile women. Hum Reprod 2001;16:1866–74.
[23] Cohen CR, Manhart LE, Bukusi EA, et al. Association between Mycoplasma genitalium and acute endometritis. Lancet 2002;359:765–6.
[24] Haggerty CL, Ness RB. M. genitalium in the endometrium of women with pelvic inflammatory disease. Proceedings of the 2003 ISSTDR Conference. Ottawa, July 28–31, 2003. Poster 0086.
[25] Cohen CR, Mugo NR, Astete S, et al. Detection of Mycoplasma genitalium in laparoscopically diagnosed acute salpingitis in Nairobi, Kenya. 2003 ISSTDR Conference. Ottawa, July 28–31, 2003. Abstract 0420.
[26] Baseman JB, Cagle M, Korte JE, et al. Diagnostic assessment of Mycoplasma genitalium in culture-positive women. J Clin Microbiol 2004;42(1):203–11.
[27] Palmer HM, Gilroy CB, Claydon EJ, et al. Detection of Mycoplasma genitalium in the genitourinary tract of women by the polymerase chain reaction. Int J STD AIDS 1991;2: 261–3.
[28] Renaudin H, Tully JG, Bebear C. In vitro susceptibilities of Mycoplasma genitalium to antibiotics. Antimicrob Agents Chemother 1992;36:870–2.
[29] Deguchi T, Yoshida T, Yokoi S, et al. Longitudinal quantitative detection by real-time PCR of Mycoplasma genitalium in first-pass urine of men with recurrent nongonococcal urethritis. J Clin Microbiol 2002;40:3854–6.
[30] Bebear CM, Renaudin H, Boudjadja A, et al. In vitro activity of BAY 12–8039, a new fluoroquinolone against mycoplasmas. Antimicrob Agents Chemother 1998;42:703–4.
[31] Johannisson G, Enstrom Y, Lowhagen GB, et al. Occurrence and treatment of Mycoplasma genitalium in patients visiting STD clinics in Sweden. Int J STD AIDS 2000;11:324–6.
[32] Falk L, Fredlund H, Jensen JS. Tetracycline treatment does not eradicate Mycoplasma genitalium. Sex Transm Infect 2003;79:318–9.
[33] Gambini D, Decleva I, Lupica L, et al. Mycoplasma genitalium in males with nongonococcal urethritis: prevalence and clinical efficacy of eradication. Sex Transm Dis 2000;27:226–9.

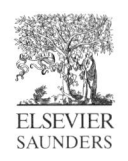

Developments in STD/HIV Interactions: The Intertwining Epidemics of HIV and HSV-2

Steven J. Reynolds, MD, MPH, FRCP(C)[a,b,*], Thomas C. Quinn, MD, MSc[a,b]

[a]Division of Infectious Diseases, Johns Hopkins University School of Medicine, Ross 1159, 720 Rutland Avenue, Baltimore, MD 21205, USA
[b]Laboratory of Immunoregulation, National Institute of Allergy and Infectious Diseases, National Institutes of Health, Bethesda, MD 20892, USA

More than 75 million people worldwide have been infected with HIV over the past 2 decades despite ambitious global prevention programs. Currently 40 million people are living with HIV and over 35 million have died from AIDS. The spread of HIV has been primarily through sexual intercourse with a lesser proportion of cases attributable to intravenous drug use and contaminated blood transfusions. The alarming numbers camouflage the fact that the HIV virus is spread inefficiently through sexual intercourse, perhaps as infrequently as 1 out of 1000 sexual exposures [1]. Sexually transmitted diseases (STDs), particularly ulcerative genital diseases, increase infectiousness and susceptibility to HIV infections. Data from international and domestic studies point increasingly to the role of herpes simplex virus type 2 (HSV-2) as a primary cofactor in facilitating the spread of HIV infection. This article reviews the recent developments in this important interaction and the potential impact of different intervention strategies targeting HSV-2.

Effective control of the current HIV pandemic will only be achievable through a complete understanding of the biologic determinants of HIV transmission. Strong evidence supports the hypothesis that ulcerative and nonulcerative STDs promote HIV transmission by increasing susceptibility and infectiousness. HIV has been detected frequently in genital ulcer exudates [2,3], potentially contributing to the increased infectiousness

* Corresponding author.
E-mail address: sreynol6@jhmi.edu (S.J. Reynolds).

among individuals who have ulcers. In a recent meta-analysis, the presence of HSV-2 antibodies conferred a 2.1-fold increased risk for HIV acquisition among individuals analyzed in nine cohort and nested case-control studies (Fig. 1) [4]. Recent evidence has also highlighted the closely overlapping epidemics of HIV and HSV-2 in Africa, Asia, and the Americas. Of all the

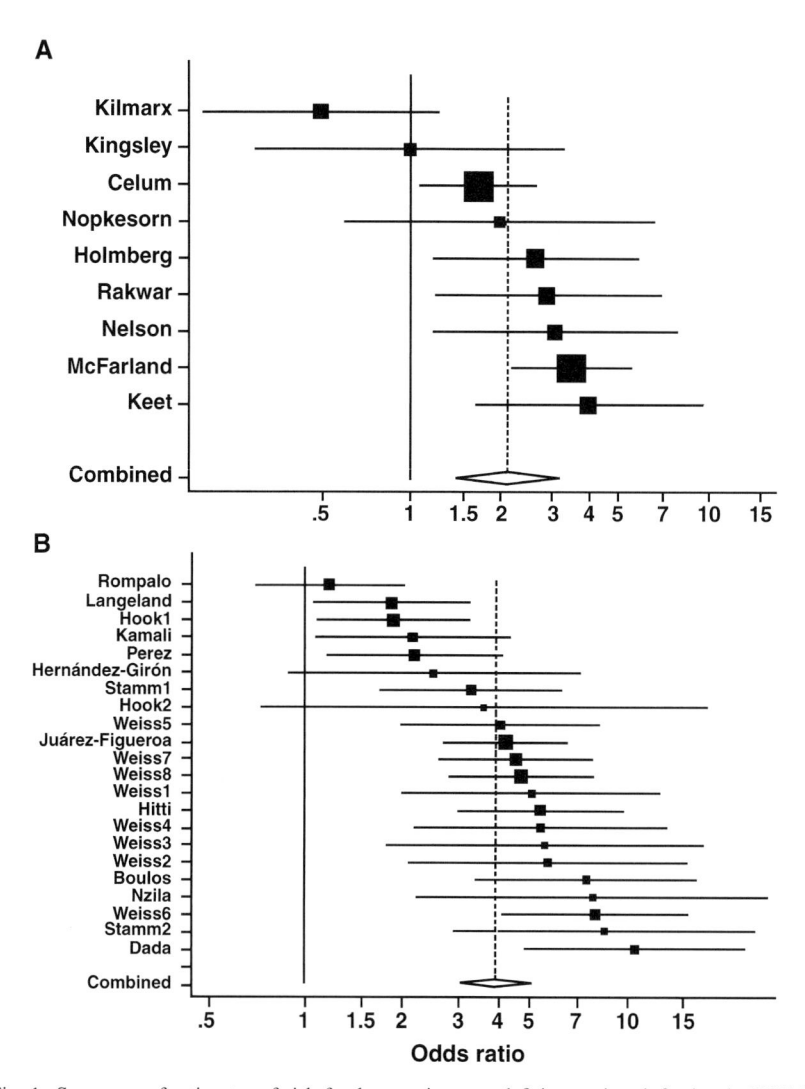

Fig. 1. Summary of estimates of risk for human immunodeficiency virus infection in HSV-2–infected persons, by study design. (*A*) Longitudinal and nested case-control studies. (*B*) Case-control and cross-sectional studies. Studies are identified by first author. Arabic numeral after first author's name indicates that there is more than one study in that particular report. (*From* Wald A, Link K. Risk of human immunodeficiency virus infection in herpes simplex virus type2-seropositive persons: a meta-analysis. J Infect Dis 2002;185(1):45–52; with permission.)

STDs implicated in the spread of HIV, there appears to be a true epidemiologic synergy between HIV and HSV-2 [5].

The emerging role of herpes simplex virus type 2 in the spread of HIV

Because of the silent epidemic of HSV-2 that has been spreading throughout North America, Europe, and most parts of the developing world, the interaction between HIV and HSV-2 is of alarming concern. The latest figures from the United States show that one in four sexually active adults has been infected with HSV-2, and the prevalence of this infection rose by 31% between 1978 and 1990 [6]. Prevalence figures from South America have revealed even higher rates of HSV-2 particularly among the homosexual population where HIV is also a major problem [7]. Alarmingly high rates of HSV-2 have been measured in various settings in sub-Saharan Africa, with rates ranging from >40% among antenatal attendees to 60% to 90% among female sex workers [8,9].

Herpes simplex virus type 2 increases the risk for HIV acquisition

In the recent meta-analysis by Wald and Link [4] of 31 studies examining the association between HSV-2 infection and the risk for HIV acquisition, the risk for HIV infection was elevated in all subgroups examined, including women (odds ratio [OR] = 4.5, 95% CI, 3.8–7.4); men who have sex with men (OR = 4.3, 95% CI, 2.4–7.6); heterosexual men (OR = 5.1, 95% CI, 3.2–8.4); and across different geographic regions, including developing countries (OR = 5.3, 95% CI, 3.8–7.4) and developed countries (OR = 2.9, 95% CI, 1.7–4.7). The consistency of this association across risk groups and geographic areas suggests it is unlikely that the association is solely because of unmeasured confounding by risk behavior. Recent studies suggest that incident HSV-2 infection raises the risk for HIV acquisition even more than prevalent HSV-2. A study from rural Tanzania revealed that among adults who seroconverted for HSV-2 within the prior 2 years, the odds ratio of HIV acquisition was 13.2 (95% CI, 5.0–34.9) among men and 2.4 (95% CI, 0.8–6.9) among women [10]. In a prospective study of 2732 patients attending sexually transmitted and reproductive tract infection clinics in Pune, India, the hazard ratio of HIV infection among participants who acquired HSV-2 within the prior 6 months was 3.81 (95% CI, 1.81–8.03) compared with those who were HSV-2 seropositive at the beginning of the study and had a hazard ratio of 1.67 (95% CI, 1.22–2.30) (Fig. 2) [11]. Clinical and subclinical reactivation of HSV is more frequent in the first year following acquisition, which may offer a biologic explanation for these findings [12,13].

Results from the Rakai Health Sciences Program STD intervention trial has provided additional compelling evidence supporting the critical role that HSV-2 plays in HIV acquisition. In a subanalysis of monogamous

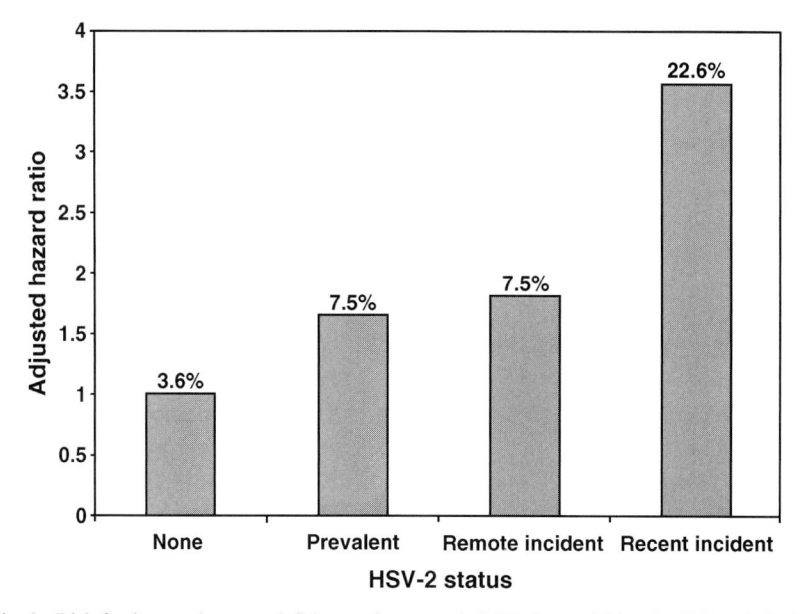

Fig. 2. Risk for human immunodeficiency virus type 1 (HIV-1) acquisition by HSV-2 infection status in a cohort of patients at three sexually transmitted infection clinics and one reproductive tract infection clinic in Pune, India, May 1993 through April 2000. HIV-1 incidence per 100 person-years is given above each column. (*From* Reynolds SJ, Risbud AR, Shepherd ME, et al. Recent herpes simplex virus type 2 infection and the risk of human immunodeficiency virus type 1 acquisition in India. J Infect Dis 2003;187(10):1513–21; with permission.)

HIV-discordant couples, the per-contact probability of HIV acquisition was five times greater if the susceptible partner was HSV-2 seropositive compared with partners who were HSV-2 seronegative (0.002 versus 0.0004, $P = .01$). The risk for HIV acquisition was found to be increased in symptomatic and asymptomatic HSV-2 seropositive susceptible partners, suggesting that subclinical HSV-2 infection may also be an important factor in the increased susceptibility to HIV (Table 1) [1].

Table 1
Per-contact probability of HIV-1 acquisition in HIV-1–discordant couples by HSV-2 serology

Couple status	Per-contact probability
Overall	0.0011
Susceptible HIV-1 partner HSV-2 seropositive	0.002
Susceptible HIV-1 partner HSV-2 seronegative	0.004 ($P = 01$)
Susceptible HIV-1 partner HSV-2 seropositive with symptomatic GUD	0.0031
Susceptible HIV-1 partner HSV-2 seropositive without GUD	0.0019
Susceptible HIV-1 partner HSV-2 seronegative without GUD	0.0004 ($P = 0.01$)

Data from Corey L, Wald A, Celum CL, et al. The Effects of herpes simplex virus-2 on HIV-1 acquisition and transmission: a review of two overlapping epidemics. J Acquir Immune Defic Syndr 2004;35(5):435–45.

Several biologic observations support the epidemiologic observations regarding an association between these two viruses. HSV-2 infection may increase the risk for HIV acquisition at the cellular level through an influx of CD4+ lymphocytes that has been observed in the context of recurrent HSV-2 infection [14,15]. HSV-2 may also increase susceptibility to HIV through the ability of HSV-2 to up-regulate HIV replication [16]. These findings coupled with the portal of entry offered by mucosal disruption during clinically apparent genital HSV-2 episodes may increase the likelihood of HIV acquisition in an exposed individual.

Herpes simplex virus type 2 and the risk for HIV transmission

In addition to an effect on acquisition, HSV-2 may also facilitate HIV transmission from a dually infected individual to an exposed seronegative partner. Several studies have shown that HSV reactivation is associated with an increased replication of HIV on mucosal surfaces [17–19]. A recent study from Rakai Health Sciences Program in Uganda also revealed that HIV/HSV-2 seropositive individuals have higher viral loads than HSV-2 seronegative individuals, which could indirectly have an effect on HIV transmission [20]. Data from the Rakai study found that the probability of HIV transmission did not differ significantly between HSV-2 seropositive and seronegative index cases but this study was limited in statistical power because of the high prevalence of HSV-2 antibodies in the HIV-positive index partner [1]. Future intervention studies of HSV-2 suppression to prevent HIV transmission will hopefully answer this important public health question.

The role of herpes simplex virus type 2 in explaining the current outcomes of sexually transmitted disease intervention trials

Three major community intervention trials have been conducted in Uganda and Tanzania to evaluate the effect of STD treatment for the prevention of HIV infection. The results of these studies have been debated extensively in the literature because of their discrepant findings on HIV incidence [21,22]. Although the Mwanza trial of STD syndromic treatment found a 38% reduction in HIV incidence in the treatment arm receiving enhanced syndromic management, the Rakai study of STD mass treatment and the Masaka study of information, education, and communication with and without syndromic treatment failed to reveal a significant reduction in HIV incidence in their respective treatment arms [23–25]. A subsequent study was performed in Kenya among sex workers who were randomized to receive monthly antibiotic chemoprophylaxis with Azithromycin or placebo. The study arm had a substantially reduced incidence of STDs but no reduction in HIV incidence [26].

Many hypotheses have been proposed to explain the lack of effect on HIV incidence observed in most of these studies. In their review of the discrepant results of the Mwanza and Rakai studies, the investigators propose that several factors unrelated to the differences in study designs could potentially explain the observed differences in outcomes. The Mwanza epidemic was in its earlier stages at the time of the intervention study, with low incidence (<1 per 100 person-years) and low but rising prevalence (4%). By contrast, the Rakai district had reached a mature generalized stage with high incidence (1.5–2.0 per 100 person-years) and stable high prevalence (16%). The investigators argue that in mature epidemics where HIV is prevalent relative to other STDs, the importance of other STDs as factors influencing HIV transmission may be limited [21]. The investigators also hypothesize that the Mwanza study design was more suited to treating symptomatic STDs compared with asymptomatic STDs and that symptomatic STDs may play a greater role in HIV transmission because of increased inflammation. The Rakai study design involving episodic mass treatment also opened up the possibility of reintroduction of new STDs during the intermittent period, which could contribute to HIV incidence in the treatment arm. The study found substantial STD prevalence at the end of each 10-month follow-up period that may have been caused by high rates of reintroduction of STDs. Other opinions regarding the results of these trials have been debated extensively, including the view that differences in sexual behavior may account for the reduction in HIV incidence observed in the Mwanza study [22]. A recent modeling study performed by the investigators of the Mwanza, Rakai, and Masaka trials concluded that population differences in sexual behavior, curable STD rates, and epidemic stages could explain the differences observed between these intervention trials. This conclusion supports the view that STD management remains a key HIV prevention strategy among populations that have high rates of curable STDs and possibly among those early in the stages of the HIV epidemic [27]. A follow-up analysis of the Rakai, Masaka, and Mwanza trials using a simulation model to assess the various hypotheses to explain the different outcomes of these trials concluded that the differences could be explained by low rates of curable cofactor STDs, which were caused, in turn, by reduction in risk behaviors before the trails and also partially explained by the advanced stage of the HIV epidemic in Uganda [28]. Other hypotheses, such as differences in study design and differences between interventions and population mobility, did not result in the observed differences when factored into their simulation model. What is clear from the debate is that STD treatment for HIV prevention is extremely complex in the mode of delivery and pathogens covered and requires different approaches in different populations.

The emergence of HSV-2 as a key factor in the spread of HIV has also entered into the debate over the negative results seen in the Rakai STD intervention trial. HSV-2 was detected by polymerase chain reaction in 45% of genital ulcers found in the Rakai trial. The Mwanza study did not have comparable data, but some data from the Mwanza STD clinic suggests that rates of HSV-associated genital ulcers were lower (<10%) in Mwanza [21].

Rates of HSV-2 reactivation are greater with advanced immunosuppression, and therefore one might expect higher rates of HSV-2–associated genital ulcer disease in mature epidemics, which could potentially play a major role in HIV transmission [29]. Untreated HSV-2 could theoretically explain in part the lack of impact of STD control on HIV incidence observed in Rakai. When factored into the simulation model discussed earlier, the effect of HIV infection on herpes did not considerably increase HSV-2 seroprevalence in Uganda consistent with the clinical trial data [28,30].

To add to the current debate, a recent study from Kenya, which provided monthly antibiotic chemoprophylaxis for bacterial STDs to Kenyan sex workers, demonstrated an incidence reduction of STDs but not of HIV [26]. Although analysis of HSV-2 and its interactions with HIV was not a predefined study endpoint, the investigators did observe a high baseline prevalence of HSV-2 infection (72.7%) that did not differ across treatment or placebo groups. In a multivariate analysis using Cox regression, the relative risk for HIV acquisition associated with prevalent HSV-2 infection was 6.3 (95% CI, 1.5–27.1). Although not designed to study this association, untreated HSV-2 infections in this study could partially explain the lack of effect of monthly antibiotic chemoprophylaxis on the study endpoint (HIV infection).

The next step: the potential role of herpes simplex virus type 2 in HIV prevention

The emerging role of HSV-2 in the current HIV pandemic has led to the possibility of using HSV-2 treatment strategies in the prevention of HIV transmission and acquisition. Antiviral medication can suppress the symptomatic and asymptomatic reactivation of HSV-2 in immunocompetent and immunocompromised individuals. Daily acyclovir therapy has been shown to reduce viral shedding from 9.9% of days to 0.5% of days in immunocompetent women [31]. Acyclovir has also been shown to prevent clinical recurrences of HSV in immunocompromised patients, and additional studies with famciclovir have shown dramatic decreases (from 11% to 1%) in viral shedding in immunocompromised individuals [32–34]. If genital herpes is a key risk factor for HIV acquisition, as supported by the wealth of epidemiologic studies, an important question is whether suppression of HSV-2 in sexually active, HIV-negative individuals reduces the risk for HIV acquisition. During subclinical and clinically apparent episodes of HSV-2 infection, the per-contact–enhancing effects on the risk for HIV acquisition may be considerable. The proportion of incident HIV-1 cases attributable to HSV-2 would be dependent on the prevalence of HSV-2 in the population. Given the high prevalence of HSV-2 in areas hardest hit by the HIV pandemic, HSV-2 may be a key factor in the dynamics of HIV acquisition.

An additional benefit to an intervention aimed at suppressing HSV-2 reactivation among those who have prevalent infection would be the potential decrease in incidence of new HSV-2 infections, as supported by recent studies looking at the role of HSV-2 suppression to prevent the transmission of HSV-2 [35]. The question of whether suppression of chronic HSV-2 among seropositive individuals will reduce the risk for HIV-1 acquisition is currently being addressed in a multicenter clinical trial of high-risk HIV-negative individuals who have HSV-2 infection under the HIV Prevention Trials Network Study 039 [36].

A second potential prevention strategy is supported by the knowledge that HIV/HSV-2–coinfected individuals experience HSV-2 reactivation more frequently than HIV-negative individuals (46% versus 31%) [37]. HIV-infected individuals who have herpetic ulcers have also been found to have high HIV RNA viral copy numbers from ulcer exudates [17,38]. Reduced lesional HIV-1 viral RNA was found in studies where episodic treatment for HSV-2 recurrences was provided [33]. Rates of reactivation of HSV-2 have been found at all levels of CD4 cell counts among HIV-infected individuals [37]. It is clear from this evidence that HIV-1 alters the natural history of HSV-2 infection, resulting in more frequent reactivation and shedding of HSV-2, leading to the potential for increased transmission of HSV-2 and possibly HIV-1. Interventions aimed at suppressive treatment of HIV/HSV-2–coinfected individuals with antiviral agents to suppress HSV-2 could represent a potential additional HIV prevention strategy. This question is also being addressed in a Gates-funded study of HSV-2/HIV discordant couples [36].

The potential impact of herpes simplex virus type 2 treatment on HIV disease progression and outcomes

HSV-2 has been shown to up-regulate HIV-1 replication at the cellular level [16]. Management of HSV-2 is particularly important in HIV-positive individuals who may experience severe, frequent, prolonged outbreaks as their level of immunosuppression advances. Episodic or chronic suppressive therapy has been shown to be effective in controlling HSV disease in HIV-infected individuals [33,39,40]. Beyond symptomatic improvement, treating HSV-2/HIV seropositive individuals may also affect HIV disease progression because of the indirect effect of HSV-2 recurrences on HIV viral load. HIV-infected individuals who have HSV-2 recurrences have been shown to have a median increase in HIV-1 viral load of 3.4-fold during an outbreak, which is sustained for 30 to 45 days after the genital lesions appear [41,42]. Individuals who had acute HIV-1 infection in the Rakai Health Sciences Program study who were HSV-2 seropositive at the time of HIV-1 seroconversion had higher viral loads at 5 and 15 months following their estimated seroconversion date [20]. In addition to the effect on transmission of HIV, treatment of HSV-2/HIV seropositive individuals may have the added benefit of affecting disease progression because of these effects on viral load. This potential benefit, however, remains to be proven in a clinical trial of HSV-2 suppression.

Summary

Antiviral agents aimed at treating HSV-2 chronically infected individuals have proven to be effective in the prevention of symptomatic genital herpes and the reduction of viral shedding. These agents play a key role in current HIV prevention trials that will assess the role of suppression of HSV-2 infection on the risk for HIV acquisition and transmission. An added clinical benefit of treating HSV-2/HIV–coinfected individuals is the potential survival benefit, as suggested by earlier studies and by the recent findings that HSV-2/HIV dually infected individuals have higher viral loads [32]. The results of the current HSV-2 suppression trials may provide additional tools to fight the global spread of HIV infection. Treatment of HSV-2/HIV dually infected individuals may prove to be a low-cost intervention to improve clinical outcomes and delay the need for antiretroviral therapy.

References

[1] Gray RH, Wawer MJ, Brookmeyer R, et al. Probability of HIV-1 transmission per coital act in monogamous, heterosexual, HIV-1-discordant couples in Rakai, Uganda. Lancet 2001; 357(9263):1149–53.
[2] Kreiss JK, Coombs R, Plummer F, et al. Isolation of human immunodeficiency virus from genital ulcers in Nairobi prostitutes. J Infect Dis 1989;160(3):380–4.
[3] Plummer FA, Wainberg MA, Plourde P, et al. Detection of human immunodeficiency virus type 1 (HIV-1) in genital ulcer exudate of HIV-1-infected men by culture and gene amplification. J Infect Dis 1990;161(4):810–1.
[4] Wald A, Link K. Risk of human immunodeficiency virus infection in herpes simplex virus type 2-seropositive persons: a meta-analysis. J Infect Dis 2002;185(1):45–52.
[5] Wasserheit JN. Epidemiological synergy. Interrelationships between human immunodeficiency virus infection and other sexually transmitted diseases. Sex Transm Dis 1992;19(2): 61–77.
[6] Fleming DT, McQuillan GM, Johnson RE, et al. Herpes simplex virus type 2 in the United States, 1976 to 1994. N Engl J Med 1997;337(16):1105–11.
[7] Sanchez J, Volquez C, Totten PA, et al. The etiology and management of genital ulcers in the Dominican Republic and Peru. Sex Transm Dis 2002;29(10):559–67.
[8] Greenblatt RM, Lukehart SA, Plummer FA, et al. Genital ulceration as a risk factor for human immunodeficiency virus infection. AIDS 1988;2(1):47–50.
[9] Mbizvo MT, Mashu A, Chipato T, et al. Trends in HIV-1 and HIV-2 prevalence and risk factors in pregnant women in Harare, Zimbabwe. Cent Afr J Med 1996;42(1):14–21.
[10] del Mar Pujades Rodriguez M, Obasi A, Mosha F, et al. Herpes simplex virus type 2 infection increases HIV incidence: a prospective study in rural Tanzania. AIDS 2002;16(3):451–62.
[11] Reynolds SJ, Risbud AR, Shepherd ME, et al. Recent herpes simplex virus type 2 infection and the risk of human immunodeficiency virus type 1 acquisition in India. J Infect Dis 2003; 187(10):1513–21.
[12] Benedetti JK, Zeh J, Corey L. Clinical reactivation of genital herpes simplex virus infection decreases in frequency over time. Ann Intern Med 1999;131(1):14–20.

[13] Wald A, Zeh J, Selke S, et al. Virologic characteristics of subclinical and symptomatic genital herpes infections. N Engl J Med 1995;333(12):770–5.
[14] Cunningham AL, Turner RR, Miller AC, et al. Evolution of recurrent herpes simplex lesions. An immunohistologic study. J Clin Invest 1985;75(1):226–33.
[15] Koelle DM, Abbo H, Peck A, et al. Direct recovery of herpes simplex virus (HSV)-specific T lymphocyte clones from recurrent genital HSV-2 lesions. J Infect Dis 1994;169(5):956–61.
[16] Moriuchi M, Moriuchi H, Williams R, et al. Herpes simplex virus infection induces replication of human immunodeficiency virus type 1. Virology 2000;278(2):534–40.
[17] Gadkari DA, Quinn TC, Gangakhedkar RR, et al. HIV-1 DNA shedding in genital ulcers and its associated risk factors in Pune, India. J Acquir Immune Defic Syndr Hum Retrovirol 1998;18(3):277–81.
[18] Mbopi-Keou FX, Gresenguet G, Mayaud P, et al. Interactions between herpes simplex virus type 2 and human immunodeficiency virus type 1 infection in African women: opportunities for intervention. J Infect Dis 2000;182(4):1090–6.
[19] Schacker T, Ryncarz AJ, Goddard J, et al. Frequent recovery of HIV-1 from genital herpes simplex virus lesions in HIV-1-infected men. JAMA 1998;280(1):61–6.
[20] Serwadda D, Gray RH, Sewankambo NK, et al. Human Immunodeficiency virus acquisition associated with genital ulcer disease and herpes simplex virus type 2 infection: a nested case-control study in Rakai, Uganda. J Infect Dis 2003;188(10):1492–7.
[21] Grosskurth H, Gray R, Hayes R, et al. Control of sexually transmitted diseases for HIV-1 prevention: understanding the implications of the Mwanza and Rakai trials. Lancet 2000; 355(9219):1981–7.
[22] Hudson CP. Community-based trials of sexually transmitted disease treatment: repercussions for epidemiology and HIV prevention. Bull World Health Organ 2001;79(1):48–58.
[23] Grosskurth H, Mosha F, Todd J, et al. Impact of improved treatment of sexually transmitted diseases on HIV infection in rural Tanzania: randomised controlled trial. Lancet 1995; 346(8974):530–6.
[24] Kamali A, Kinsman J, Nalweyiso N, et al. A community randomized controlled trial to investigate impact of improved STD management and behavioural interventions on HIV incidence in rural Masaka, Uganda: trial design, methods and baseline findings. Trop Med Int Health 2002;7(12):1053–63.
[25] Wawer MJ, Sewankambo NK, Serwadda D, et al. Control of sexually transmitted diseases for AIDS prevention in Uganda: a randomised community trial. Rakai Project Study Group. Lancet 1999;353(9152):525–35.
[26] Kaul R, Kimani J, Nagelkerke NJ, et al. Monthly antibiotic chemoprophylaxis and incidence of sexually transmitted infections and HIV-1 infection in Kenyan sex workers: a randomized controlled trial. JAMA 2004;291(21):2555–62.
[27] White RG, Orroth KK, Korenromp EL, et al. Can population differences explain the contrasting results of the Mwanza, Rakai, and Masaka HIV/sexually transmitted disease intervention trials?: a modeling study. J Acquir Immune Defic Syndr 2004;37(4): 1500–13.
[28] Korenromp EL, White RG, Orroth KK, et al. Determinants of the impact of sexually transmitted infection treatment on prevention of HIV infection: a synthesis of evidence from the Mwanza, Rakai, and Masaka intervention trials. J Infect Dis 2005;191(Suppl 1): S168–78.
[29] Chen CY, Ballard RC, Beck-Sague CM, et al. Human immunodeficiency virus infection and genital ulcer disease in South Africa: the herpetic connection. Sex Transm Dis 2000;27(1): 21–9.
[30] Orroth KK, Korenromp EL, White RG, et al. Higher risk behaviour and rates of sexually transmitted diseases in Mwanza compared to Uganda may help explain HIV prevention trial outcomes. AIDS 2003;17(18):2653–60.

[31] Mertz GJ, Jones CC, Mills J, et al. Long-term acyclovir suppression of frequently recurring genital herpes simplex virus infection. A multicenter double-blind trial. JAMA 1988;260(2): 201–6.
[32] Cooper DA, Pehrson PO, Pedersen C, et al. The efficacy and safety of zidovudine alone or as cotherapy with acyclovir for the treatment of patients with AIDS and AIDS-related complex: a double-blind randomized trial. European-Australian Collaborative Group. AIDS 1993;7(2):197–207.
[33] Schacker T, Hu HL, Koelle DM, et al. Famciclovir for the suppression of symptomatic and asymptomatic herpes simplex virus reactivation in HIV-infected persons. A double-blind, placebo-controlled trial. Ann Intern Med 1998;128(1):21–8.
[34] Youle MS, Gazzard BG, Johnson MA, et al. Effects of high-dose oral acyclovir on herpesvirus disease and survival in patients with advanced HIV disease: a double-blind, placebo-controlled study. European-Australian Acyclovir Study Group. AIDS 1994;8(5): 641–9.
[35] Corey L, Wald A, Patel R, et al. Once-daily valacyclovir to reduce the risk of transmission of genital herpes. N Engl J Med 2004;350(1):11–20.
[36] Celum CL, Robinson NJ, Cohen MS. Potential effect of HIV type 1 antiretroviral and herpes simplex virus type 2 antiviral therapy on transmission and acquisition of HIV type 1 infection. J Infect Dis 2005;191(Suppl 1):S107–14.
[37] Schacker T, Zeh J, Hu HL, et al. Frequency of symptomatic and asymptomatic herpes simplex virus type 2 reactivations among human immunodeficiency virus-infected men. J Infect Dis 1998;178(6):1616–22.
[38] Schacker T, Ryncarz AJ, Goddard J, et al. Frequent recovery of HIV-1 from genital herpes simplex virus lesions in HIV-1-infected men. JAMA 1998;280(1):61–6.
[39] Conant MA, Schacker TW, Murphy RL, et al. Valaciclovir versus aciclovir for herpes simplex virus infection in HIV-infected individuals: two randomized trials. Int J STD AIDS 2002;13(1):12–21.
[40] Romanowski B, Aoki FY, Martel AY, et al. Efficacy and safety of famciclovir for treating mucocutaneous herpes simplex infection in HIV-infected individuals. Collaborative Famciclovir HIV Study Group. AIDS 2000;14(9):1211–7.
[41] Mole L, Ripich S, Margolis D, et al. The impact of active herpes simplex virus infection on human immunodeficiency virus load. J Infect Dis 1997;176(3):766–70.
[42] Schacker T, Zeh J, Hu H, et al. Changes in plasma human immunodeficiency virus type 1 RNA associated with herpes simplex virus reactivation and suppression. J Infect Dis 2002; 186(12):1718–25.

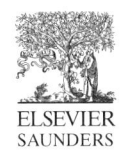

Managing Patients with Genital Herpes and their Sexual Partners

Raj Patel, MD[a], Anne Rompalo, MD[b],*

[a]Department of Genitourinary Medicine, Royal South Hampshire Hospital, Southhampton, Hants, United Kingdom
[b]Johns Hopkins University School of Medicine, Baltimore, MD 21287, USA

There is increasing recognition of the growing size and significance of the genital herpes epidemic. Recent developments in the wide-scale availability of type-specific herpes simplex virus (HSV) serologic assays have meant that many previously undiagnosed mild, atypical, and subclinical infections may now be diagnosed with some degree of confidence without the use of Western blots. The value of such diagnostics is controversial. However, the importance of HSV with its facilitation of HIV transmission and acquisition, the availability of various preventative strategies for limiting vertical HSV transmission, and the growing evidence that condoms, some educational and counseling interventions, and antiviral therapies may limit sexual transmission, have challenged many of the arguments against wider testing of the population.

The alpha herpesviruses herpes simplex virus type 1 (HSV-1) and herpes simplex virus type 2 (HSV-2) can cause various clinical syndromes that are clinically indistinguishable. With the decline of herpes infections in childhood, most first acquisitions of HSV-1 are delayed in many populations until adult life [1,2], when they are equally divided between pharyngeal and genital sites [3]. For some parts of the world, most genital acquisitions in young people involve HSV-1 [4]. When it occurs in adult life, there is a tendency for HSV-1 to be particularly severe [5]. Although the initial acquisition episode may be clinically indistinguishable, the nature and pattern of subsequent recurrence by either HSV-1 or HSV-2 are generally different. HSV-1 infections are rarely troublesome (on average recur approximately once a year or less in the genital area), whereas most individuals who have symptomatic HSV-2 will have significantly more severe disease activities

---

* Corresponding author.
 E-mail address: arompalo@jhmi.edu (A. Rompalo).

(HSV-2 infections recur four to six times per year in the first few years). Therefore, HSV-2 infections cause most severe and recurrent genital infections and consequently contribute to most genital herpes-related morbidity.

Medical importance of genital herpes simplex virus

The consequences of genital infection with HSV are not confined merely to the genital area or necessarily to the individual concerned. Psychosexual morbidity is a frequent and significant problem for many people who have recurrent genital HSV [6]. Genital HSV infection is the most common cause of genital ulceration worldwide, and as such is seen as an important contributor to the transmission and acquisition of HIV not only in the developing world but also among higher-risk groups in the developed world (modeling suggests that HSV-2 contributes more than 50% of the attributable risk for HIV acquisition in many populations) [7]. HSV is a rare cause of serious disseminated infection in the immunocompetent outside of pregnancy. Genital HSV is an important preventable cause of severe neonatal disease and occurs in approximately 1 in 3000 live births in North America. HSV remains an important and significant pathogen in the immunocompromised. Direct and indirect costs of incident genital HSV infection in the United States are currently estimated to be more than $1.8 billion and are projected to exceed $2.7 billion annually by 2015 [8].

The extent of the problem

Serologic surveys in many developed countries show that the rates of these infections continue to rise, although some plateauing of disease may have recently occurred among some population groups. For North America, the levels of HSV-2 prevalence rose by over 30% during the late 1970s, 1980s, and early 1990s.

HSV-2 infection is not seen in children; rates begin to rise with the onset of sexual activity. This rise is particularly steep among some ethnic minorities and has been shown to be associated with markers of social deprivation, partner change, and high-risk sexual behavior [9]. Most HSV-2 infections in any population are undiagnosed. Most people carrying virus will have symptomatic episodes, but these may be mild and atypical. In addition to symptomatic episodes, virtually all individuals will have asymptomatic episodes of viral reactivation when virus will be present on the skin surface in high titre in the absence of signs (subclinical disease) or symptoms (asymptomatic disease) [10]. Clinical (typical and atypical episodes), subclinical, and asymptomatic disease are all potentially infectious [11]. Such infectivity is amenable to interventions that limit transmission. Historically there has been considerable pessimism as to the extent and usefulness of interventions to modify HSV transmission. The results of recent studies question these assumptions. This article focuses on the developments in management aimed at identification of new patients who have HSV and the prevention of onward transmission of infection, in particular the management of serodiscordant couples.

Identification of herpes simplex virus infection

HSV infection can be diagnosed through the identification of herpesviruses using traditional antigen detection tests (culture, enzyme immunoassay [EIA], or polymerase chain reaction tests [PCR]) or by demonstrating herpes antibodies. Antigen detection is widely used for symptomatic patients and has distinct advantages: it is easy to perform, widely available, and inexpensive, and does not require the use of much new technology. In addition, antigen detection tests clearly establish the site of infection and are highly specific. However, tests require the presence of lesions and are often variably sensitive. Culture will only pick up between one half and two thirds of PCR-positive disease [12]. Antigen detection tests cannot be used to exclude infection, which is a particular problem when investigating symptoms that may be atypical for HSV or when screening for infection in asymptomatic patients. Less then 3% of patients shed virus asymptomatically on any one day, making the probability of finding virus through antigen detection on any such day fairly small. Typing is possible with culture and some PCR tests but is not possible with currently available EIAs.

Serologic tests can overcome some of the limitations of antigen detection tests. Because background rates of nongenital HSV infection (essentially HSV-1) are high in many populations, these tests need to differentiate between HSV-1 and HSV-2 infection to be useful. These viruses are closely related (over 50% of the genome is shared) and many epitopes are common. However, enough differences are present to allow identification of immunologic type-specific responses. Serologic tests for HSV infection have been developed that take advantage of the differing immunologic responses to HSV-1 and HSV-2 infection. Most tests rely on the identification of type-specific responses to glycoprotein gG-1 and gG-2 (of HSV-1 and HSV-2, respectively). Glycoprotein G-based tests exploiting a range of technologies have been developed and carefully validated using sera from culture-proven cases and children (HSV-2 negative). These gold standard tests have been used to determine the natural history and seroprevalence of HSV and have shaped the understanding of the range of HSV infection. They remain available in some reference laboratories. More recently, commercial kits have been developed that have been validated against these gold standard tests. These tests are widely available and some have been approved by the Food and Drug Administration.

Characteristics of currently available herpes-specific tests

Three IgG-based type-specific antibody assays are currently licensed and widely used in the United States: POCkit HSV-2 (Diagnology, Belfast, Ireland) and the HerpeSelect-1 and -2 ELISA IgG and HerpeSelect-1 and -2 Immunoblot IgG (Focus Technology, Cypress, California). The POCkit provides point-of-care test results, whereas the HerpeSelect technologies are laboratory-based.

The Focus HerpeSelect-1 and -2 ELISA IgG are sold separately and offer independent HSV-1 and HSV-2 testing. These tests have been validated in antenatal and STD populations where results have been compared with the University of Washington Western blot assay (UW-WB performed in the laboratory of Dr. Rhoda Ashley [13]). For the HSV-1 ELISA, sensitivity was reported as 91% to 96% and specificity 92% to 95%. The HSV-2 ELISA had 96% to 100% sensitivity and 96% to 97% specificity for the same groups [13].

The Focus HerpeSelect Immunoblot (IB) has also been compared with the UW-WB, giving a sensitivity of 99% to 100% and a specificity of 93% to 95% for HSV-1. For HSV-2, sensitivity of 97% to 100% and specificity of 94% to 98% have been reported in clinical trials using the Focus HerpeSelect IB [14].

The Diagnology POCkit HSV-2 test uses capillary blood and offers a rapid point-of-care result. The test generates a result within 10 minutes and has been assessed against the UW-WB. High sensitivity and specificity of 93% to 100% and 94% to 107%, respectively, have been reported with this test [14], although other investigators have suggested that frequent intermediate results make the tests difficult to read and lower the sensitivity and specificity to unacceptable levels [14].

Reliability of herpes simplex virus type 2–positive type-specific serology results

There has been considerable debate as to whether a gG-based test can be positive in a patient who has not been infected with HSV-2. The specificity of these assays has been assessed by testing populations at very low risk for acquiring HSV-2. One such study looking at sera from 100 very low-risk students found no positives with either the POCkit or Focus HerpeSelect ELISA (also negative by UW-WB) [14]. This finding would suggest that the specificity is high for all three tests. Other studies have reported false-positive HerpeSelect ELISA results, finding that most of these seem to occur in those with the low-positive range (index value 1.0–3.0) often in the presence of possible HSV-1 coinfection. If this is the case, then the positive predictive value (PPV) in low-risk populations may be unacceptably low. There may also be significant variability in test performance for samples taken from some racial groups [15]. The consequences of declaring a patient to have HSV-2 who is uninfected are potentially serious, and therefore testing algorithms are being developed to assist clinicians in interpreting results among patients when the PPV is low. Most expert guidelines recommend that an unexpected positive result in a patient who does not have symptoms or a sexual history suggestive of risk for HSV-2 should be followed up with repeat testing for antibodies—ideally with a different test, but if this is not possible, then with the same test at a later time. The recent introduction and wider availability of commercial Western blot may greatly improve the interpretation of positive serology in many regions.

Reliability of a herpes simplex virus type 2–negative type-specific serology test

Serologic tests (both Western blot and type-specific gG-based) are frequently negative during the early stages of infection, and may take a variable time to become positive as the humoral response matures. Having established a measurable antibody response, it may be possible for seroreversion to occur over time especially if recurrences are not frequent. Few longitudinal cohort studies repeating HSV serologies in subjects who have mild or absent clinical disease have been reported. One such study following more than 1100 young male military recruits found that with repeat 6-monthly sampling using a panel of four serology tests, between 6% to 21% of individuals showed a positive to negative shift [16]. Although such patients appear to have lost their type-specific responses, they may continue to be identifiable on tests for HSV-type common antibodies.

Clinical place of serologic assays

Serologic tests can be used diagnostically in symptomatic patients, as an aide to counseling, for assessing the partners of those who have infection, for screening patients who are at high risk for HSV, and for population-based mass screening.

Serologic tests as part of the investigation of symptomatic patients

In a 3-year review of the usefulness of serodetermination in 127 cases attending a sexually transmitted infection (STI) center, the investigators concluded that HSV serology is most useful diagnostically in cases of recurrent genital ulceration [17]. Tests in such cases are inconclusive when only HSV-1 antibody is found. Clinicians found that when tests were performed in conjunction with antigen detection tests, HSV serology in first-episode disease helped stage (primary or initial) and contributed to establishing the diagnosis when antigen tests failed or were inconclusive.

Testing has the potential to confuse; anecdotal cases are reported where the attribution of recurrent genital symptoms to HSV-2 infection (following sero-identification) has delayed a more appropriate and accurate dermatologic diagnosis. Serology was found to be rarely helpful with atypical, nonulcerative symptoms.

Serologic testing of partners of those who have herpes simplex virus

Serologic testing can help with the counseling of couples where one partner has diagnosed HSV infection [18]. Where seroconcordance is found, it may be appropriate to retest the previously undiagnosed partner if they are asymptomatic. Following education and counseling, most such partners will recognize some HSV-related symptoms and signs [18] even if asymptomatic at diagnosis. Usefulness is diminished when partner's HSV type is unknown.

Serodiscordant couples need careful counseling regarding the risks for transmission and possible interventions, as discussed later.

Testing high-risk populations

High rates of HSV-2 infection are reported among STI clinic attendees, and there is some debate as to whether it is appropriate to offer high-risk groups serologic testing for HSV. Proponents of testing develop four arguments:

1. Patients want HSV testing. Surveys of patient views on testing show that most patients would want type-specific HSV testing if it were available to them [19]. However, when serologic identification is made available with counseling (STI clinic patients), fewer patients choose to be tested, suggesting that informed take-up may be far from universal even among higher-risk groups [20,21].
2. Testing will provide for better symptomatic control for patients. Most of the new infections identified serologically will prove to be symptomatic. Most HSV disease is likely to be atypical. Serologic identification will provide for easier and earlier symptom recognition. However, detractors from a screening strategy would argue that much of the disease detected is likely to be mild or trivial in nature.
3. Testing will reduce the risk for onward HSV transmission to sexual partners through education and behavioral change (discussed later) [22] or antiviral therapy. For this group, any benefit remains highly theoretic and assumes that behavioral change can be realized through education and counseling. There is also an assumption that should such a risk reduction strategy be mediated through the introduction of antivirals, funders will be willing to pay for continuous therapy and previously

asymptomatic patients will be happy to comply with such continuous therapy.
4. Testing will reduce HIV transmission and acquisition. There is a close epidemiologic link between HSV-2 and HIV acquisition [7]. Studies suggest that this risk is mediated by visible lesional disease and unrecognized disease. Prospective studies indicate that genital ulcer disease is a strong mediator of HIV acquisition. Couples studies from the developing world show that coinfection of HIV and HSV leads to greater HIV viral loads and greater transmissibility [23]. Trials of HSV control with antivirals in HIV infecteds and susceptibles in an attempt to modify the transmission dynamics of HIV are currently underway [23]. Although results are awaited, some clinicians feel that HSV status should be identified in all patients who have HIV and those at higher risk for HIV acquisition. These patients should be counseled regarding the additional risk their HSV status adds to their risk for HIV acquisition and possible HIV transmission in the hope that this will improve the chances of behavioral modification. In addition, some clinicians are advocating the earlier use of continuous antiviral suppression for HSV therapy in these groups.

Screening in pregnancy

Genital HSV disease in a pregnant woman carries the risk for possible miscarriage, foetal death, and neonatal infection. This risk for neonatal infection is maximal for those women who acquire disease in late pregnancy, although an excess of risk does remain for those who acquire disease before the third trimester [24]. The arguments for screening women and their partners during pregnancy are based on developing strategies that would diminish third-trimester acquisitions of new disease and extend ideal medical management to those already infected to either limit neonatal transmission (eg, antivirals, selective caesarean section) or the early identification of active neonatal infection [25]. The recent demonstration of a lower vertical transmission rate of HSV when women were delivered by caesarian section [26] has fueled the debate as to ideal medical management of women who have established HSV infection.

Although a wide serologic testing strategy involving pregnant women and their partners is superficially extremely attractive, cost–benefit analysis in many countries suggests that unless the local rate of neonatal disease is high, any screening policy is unlikely to be valuable [27,28]. In addition, the potential beneficiaries of such a strategy are often those mothers who are poorly served by health care and currently do not access services. Finally, there is no evidence that behavioral change can be modified in pregnancy and consequently, screening may indirectly deliver a greater level of medical intervention in previous low-risk pregnancies. However, although screening may not be practical or currently advised, many potentially serodiscordant couples will self-identify to the clinician. Management should aim at keeping these pregnant women disease-free during the third trimester. Despite the absence of data supporting interventions for this group, many clinicians would advocate either abstinence or condoms and continuous suppressive therapy with valacyclovir.

Wider screening of the general population

Rates of HSV are in excess of 25% in many developed countries. Modeling suggests that rates will reach 40% in the absence of any practical intervention [8]. For the general population (relatively low-risk), the same limitations to testing exist as for high-risk groups. Limited modeling of counseling interventions that may be based on a general screening strategy suggest a cost of $8200 per case of further HSV transmission averted [8]. These costs may be improved on if testing algorithms can be developed that do not require confirmation for all low-risk positives and if clinicians are happy to use antiviral therapy to manage transmission risk.

Can screening for herpes simplex virus be damaging?

Some clinicians and ethicists argue that in the absence of clear and effective interventions to manage transmission, the identification of herpes infection in those who were previously asymptomatic may be damaging and consequently unethical [29]. The published evidence that screening may identify HSV infection in those who may not be able to cope with the diagnosis is currently based only on reported anecdote [18]. Attempts to produce prospective studies looking at psychologic well-being before and after HSV screening with long-term follow-up to assess adjustment is hampered by the sheer size of numbers needed to produce meaningful follow-up cohorts and by the difficulties of administering long-term psychologic follow-up. Certainly for symptomatic disease, follow-up studies show that most patients appear to cope well with a diagnosis. Poor adjustment may be predicted by severe disease and is occasionally a feature of preexisting underlying psychologic morbidity [30]. Disease identified through screening strategies is unlikely to be clinically severe. A recent screening study looking at adjustment to an HSV diagnosis has shown that those who coped most poorly with genital HSV infection at 3 months after diagnosis were more likely before diagnosis to report unsatisfactory social and intimate relationships (Zimet GD, personal communication) [31]. Outside this group, it seems that a diagnosis of HSV is unlikely to be damaging and may be valuable to the public good if onward transmission can be halted. The benefit of screening is intimately linked to the ability to manage transmission risk.

Managing transmission risk

Much is known about HSV transmission. Transmissions are more frequent from men to women, risk is greatest early in a relationship, and most transmissions are frequently found in couples where the index case is undiagnosed with HSV. When transmissions occur in relationships where serodiscordance has been established, they are most frequently associated with atypical or clinically unapparent disease.

Transmission concern is one of the major anxieties reported by patients who have new and established diagnoses of genital HSV. Factors contributing to transmission are summarized in Box 1 and several of these are potentially modifiable. Four strategies (with varying levels of evidence and success) have been proposed that may limit the transmission risk.

Disclosure of diagnosis

Studies show that when both members of a partnership are aware of their possible serodiscordance, the transmission risk per sexual act is substantially lower than for relationships where one or both partners is unaware of the risk [32,33]. Such data supports the notion that awareness of one's diagnosis with disclosure to one's partner may be helpful in preventing transmission, as this would presumably allow an individual to minimize risk through selective abstinence, condom use, and possible antiviral therapy. In addition, if the partner is also aware of their diagnosis, this may assist

---

Box 1. Risk factors identified as associated with HSV-2 transmission/acquisition

Biologic
- Age
- Gender
- Race
- Duration of partner's infection
- Partner's shedding rates
- Infection with other HSV type in either partner

Behavioural
- Number and choice of sex partners
- Duration of relationships
- Stage of relationship
- Sexual frequency
- Knowledge of partner's serostatus
- Condom use
- Ability to recognize HSV lesions

risk reduction through an understanding of why selective abstinence and condom use may be required. Such a strategy has not been tested in any formal study but is consistent with current medical practice and medicolegal advice regarding disclosure.

Selective abstinence

For most patients, a significantly large proportion of any genital viral shedding occurs concurrently with the presence of some genital lesions or symptoms.

Patients can be taught to recognize some of their symptomatic and clinical disease episodes and may be able to reduce risk through selective abstinence during these times and immediately afterwards [22]. The levels and extent of exposure to their partner will be reduced, but it is important to emphasize to patients that this will not reduce risk in relation to asymptomatic shedding and that risk will still remain in these instances. Some weak natural history data suggests that patients are able to use disease recognition to modify the timing of sex and that for couples aware of their discordance, sexual behavior can be timed to avoid episodes of overt clinical disease [22].

Condom use

Condoms act as mechanical barriers to genital infections. Despite the virtual impermeability that latex presents to herpesviruses, condoms can fail to protect against herpes viral transmission. Three factors are thought to contribute to this: HSV is frequently shed from multiple sites, some of which are not amenable to protection by male condom use; many couples engage in considerable unprotected genital contact before using condoms for penetrative sexual intercourse; and condoms may fail during penetrative sex because of breakage or slippage. Studies of the effectiveness of condom use for preventing HSV transmission are difficult to perform ethically and practically. Indirect evidence for condom effectiveness comes from well-documented natural history studies of transmission in serodiscordant couples where diaries of sexual activity, symptomatology, and condom use were kept. These show that the male condom, when used consistently, will protect men and women from genital HSV acquisition [33,34]. These studies also show that despite an awareness of serodiscordance, and with intensive education and counseling, consistent condom use is difficult to achieve. At present there are only limited data for the effectives of other barriers and no data for microbicides in preventing transmission. Wald [34] has proposed that consistent condom use may diminish transmission risk by 50%.

Antiviral therapy

Suppressive antiviral therapy has an impact on reducing the sexual transmission of HSV from an infected partner [35]. In the valacyclovir transmission study, a once-daily 500-mg dose of valacyclovir prevented between half and three quarters of all transmissions in 1484 monogamous couples over an 8-month period, and had an additive effect over condom use alone. Corey and colleagues [35] concluded that the transmission effects would also be applicable to nonmonogamous heterosexual couples, although more studies are needed in men who have sex with men and in couples where the susceptible partner is immunocompromised. This data may also not be applicable to pregnant women, where the acquisition rate is significantly higher than in the general population.

It would then appear that transmission risk is modifiable to some extent through the use of antiviral therapy, the promotion of condom use, and the promotion of disease awareness and disclosure. Although these strategies may not be acceptable patients at all times, they may become highly relevant to patients at different stages of their infection (early in a relationship or during pregnancy).

Several expert guidelines now recommend that all the options for risk reduction be communicated as part of patient assessment and counseling.

References

[1] Lafferty WE. The changing epidemiology of HSV-1 and HSV-2 and implications for serological testing. Herpes 2002;9(2):51–5.
[2] Nahmias AJ, Lee FK, Beckman-Nahmias S. Sero-epidemiological and -sociological patterns of herpes simplex virus infection in the world. Scand J Infect Dis Suppl 1990;69:19–36.
[3] Langenberg AG, Corey L, Ashley RL, et al. A prospective study of new infections with herpes simplex virus type 1 and type 2. Chiron HSV Vaccine Study Group. N Engl J Med 1999;341(19):1432–8.
[4] Malkin JE. Epidemiology of genital herpes simplex virus infection in developed countries. Herpes 2004;11(Suppl 1):2A–23A.
[5] Lowhagen GB, Tunback P, Andersson K, et al. First episodes of genital herpes in a Swedish STD population: a study of epidemiology and transmission by the use of herpes simplex virus (HSV) typing and specific serology. Sex Transm Infect 2000;76(3):179–82.
[6] Patel R, Boselli F, Cairo I, et al. Patients' perspectives on the burden of recurrent genital herpes. Int J STD AIDS 2001;12(10):640–5.
[7] Wald A, Link K. Risk of human immunodeficiency virus infection in herpes simplex virus type 2-seropositive persons: a meta-analysis. J Infect Dis 2002;185(1):45–52.
[8] Fisman DN, Lipsitch M, Hook EW III, et al. Projection of the future dimensions and costs of the genital herpes simplex type 2 epidemic in the United States. Sex Transm Dis 2002;29(10):608–22.
[9] Fleming DT, McQuillan GM, Johnson RE, et al. Herpes simplex virus type 2 in the United States, 1976 to 1994. N Engl J Med 1997;337(16):1105–11.
[10] Wald A, Zeh J, Selke S, et al. Virologic characteristics of subclinical and symptomatic genital herpes infections. N Engl J Med 1995;333(12):770–5.
[11] Barton SE, Davis JM, Moss VW, et al. Asymptomatic shedding and subsequent transmission of genital herpes simplex virus. Genitourin Med 1987;63(2):102–5.
[12] Wald A, Huang ML, Carrell D, et al. Polymerase chain reaction for detection of herpes simplex virus (HSV) DNA on mucosal surfaces: comparison with HSV isolation in cell culture. J Infect Dis 2003;188(9):1345–51.
[13] Ashley RL. Performance and use of HSV type-specific serology test kits. Herpes 2002;9(2):38–45.

[14] Saville M, Brown D, Burgess C, et al. An evaluation of near patient tests for detecting herpes simplex virus type-2 antibody. Sex Transm Infect 2000;76(5):381–2.
[15] Ashley-Morrow R, Nollkamper J, Robinson NJ, et al. Performance of focus ELISA tests for herpes simplex virus type 1 (HSV-1) and HSV-2 antibodies among women in ten diverse geographical locations. Clin Microbiol Infect 2004;10(6):530–6.
[16] Schmid DS, Brown DR, Nisenbaum R, et al. Limits in reliability of glycoprotein G-based type-specific serologic assays for herpes simplex virus types 1 and 2. J Clin Microbiol 1999; 37(2):376–9.
[17] Munday PE, Vuddamalay J, Slomka MJ, et al. Role of type specific herpes simplex virus serology in the diagnosis and management of genital herpes. Sex Transm Infect 1998;74(3): 175–8.
[18] Oliver L, Wald A, Kim M, et al. Seroprevalence of herpes simplex virus infections in a family medicine clinic. Arch Fam Med 1995;4(3):228–32.
[19] Fairley I, Monteiro EF. Patient attitudes to type specific serological tests in the diagnosis of genital herpes. Genitourin Med 1997;73(4):259–62.
[20] Mullan HM, Munday PE. The acceptability of the introduction of a type specific herpes antibody screening test into a genitourinary medicine clinic in the United Kingdom. Sex Transm Infect 2003;79(2):129–33.
[21] Zimet GD, Rosenthal SL, Fortenberry JD, et al. Factors predicting the acceptance of herpes simplex virus type 2 antibody testing among adolescents and young adults. Sex Transm Dis 2004;31(11):665–9.
[22] Patel R. Educational interventions and the prevention of herpes simplex virus transmission. Herpes 2004;11(Suppl 3):155A–60A.
[23] Celum C, Levine R, Weaver M, et al. Genital herpes and human immunodeficiency virus: double trouble. Bull World Health Organ 2004;82(6):447–53.
[24] Brown ZA, Selke S, Zeh J, et al. The acquisition of herpes simplex virus during pregnancy. N Engl J Med 1997;337(8):509–15.
[25] Kinghorn GR. Debate: the argument for. Should all pregnant women be offered type-specific serological screening for HSV infection? Herpes 2002;9(2):46–7.
[26] Brown ZA, Wald A, Morrow RA, et al. Effect of serologic status and cesarean delivery on transmission rates of herpes simplex virus from mother to infant. JAMA 2003;289(2):203–9.
[27] Barnabas RV, Carabin H, Garnett GP. The potential role of suppressive therapy for sex partners in the prevention of neonatal herpes: a health economic analysis. Sex Transm Infect 2002;78(6):425–9.
[28] Baker D, Brown Z, Hollier LM, et al. Cost-effectiveness of herpes simplex virus type 2 serologic testing and antiviral therapy in pregnancy. Am J Obstet Gynecol 2004;191(6): 2074–84.
[29] Krantz I, Lowhagen GB, Ahlberg BM, et al. Ethics of screening for asymptomatic herpes virus type 2 infection. BMJ 2004;329(7466):618–21.
[30] Miyai T, Turner KR, Kent CK, et al. The psychosocial impact of testing individuals with no history of genital herpes for herpes simplex virus type 2. Sex Transm Dis 2004;31(9): 517–21.
[31] Patel R. Supporting the patient with genial herpes. Herpes, in press.
[32] Wald A, Baseman J, Selke S, et al. Sexual transmission of genital herpes simplex virus (HSV): a time-to-event analysis of risk factors associated with rapid acquisition. Presented at the 2000 National STD Prevention Conference. Milwaukee, Wisconsin, December 4–7, 2000.
[33] Wald A, Langenberg AG, Link K, et al. Effect of condoms on reducing the transmission of herpes simplex virus type 2 from men to women. JAMA 2001;285(24):3100–6.
[34] Wald A, Langenberg A, Kexel E, et al. Condoms protect men and women against herpes simplex virus type 2 (HSV-2) acquisition. Presented at the National STI Prevention Conference. San Diego, CA, March 5–8, 2002.
[35] Corey L, Wald A, Patel R, et al. Once-daily valacyclovir to reduce the risk of transmission of genital herpes. N Engl J Med 2004;350(1):11–20.

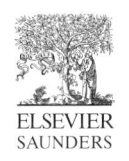

Diagnosis and Management of Oncogenic Cervical Human Papillomavirus Infection

Patti E. Gravitt, PhD[a],*, Roxanne Jamshidi, MD[b]

[a] Johns Hopkins Bloomberg School of Public Health, Department of Epidemiology, 615 North Wolfe Street, Room E6535, Baltimore, MD 21205, USA
[b] Johns Hopkins Bayview Medical Center, 4940 Eastern Avenue, Baltimore, MD 21224, USA

The epidemiology and natural history of cervical human papillomavirus infection

Human papillomaviruses (HPVs) are small, closed circle (episomal), double-stranded DNA viruses. Infectious particles are comprised of the nearly 8000 base pair genome encapsulated by a nonenveloped icosahedral capsid of approximately 55 nm in diameter. The papillomavirus family encompasses an ever-expanding group of hundreds of viruses, all of which are species-specific in their infectivity. Among the HPVs, there are more than 100 viruses that have been fully sequenced and identified. These viruses are characterized based on nucleic acid sequence homology rather than serologic reactivity, resulting in classification of HPVs by genotypes rather than the more traditional serotype nomenclature [1]. Phylogenetic analysis of HPV DNA sequences [2] reveal clusters of related viruses that share tissue tropism (predominantly mucosal versus cutaneous) and oncogenic potential. In particular, the HPV genotypes mapping to phylogenetic clades A5, A6, A7, and A9 (including confirmed high-risk types 16, 18, 31, 33, 35, 39, 45, 51, 52, 56, 58, 59, 68, 73, and 82) have been shown in population-based studies to be associated with a high risk for cancer [3]. Other clades include types that may commonly infect the ano/oral/genital tract, but are not associated with cancer development. Included in this group are HPV types 6

Dr. Gravitt is supported by a Career Development Award (P50 CA98252) from the National Institutes of Health.
* Corresponding author.
 E-mail address: pgravitt@jhsph.edu (P.E. Gravitt).

and 11 (clade A10), which cause anogenital warts in men and women, but are rarely, if ever, found in invasive cancers.

It is now well-established that HPV is sexually transmitted [4]. HPV infection is not systemic, and transmission is thought to occur through mechanical abrasion of an infected epithelial surface with an uninfected epithelium. HPV DNA can be detected in vulvar, vaginal, cervical, oral, and anal samples in women [5,6], and penile shaft, glans, foreskin, scrotum, oral, and anal samples in men [7–9]; however, most cases of HPV are clinically asymptomatic. Primary prevention of transmission by condom use appears to be of limited effectiveness [10], likely because of the broad range of epithelial targets for infection in men and women, absence of detectable symptoms to identify an infected partner, and inconsistent condom use (eg, lack of use during abrasive foreplay). However, evaluation of condom effectiveness in preventing HPV transmission is complicated by the difficulty in obtaining a reliable diagnosis of HPV infection in men to confirm exposure, and in accurately ascertaining proper condom use.

For HPV subtypes with oncogenic potential, the natural history of infection in men is not well understood. Men are almost always clinically asymptomatic and risk for HPV-associated penile cancer is low, even in men who have HIV and other cases of profound immunosuppression. Cross-sectional prevalence estimates of HPV serology are lower for men than for women in the same population [11]. The data to date present conflicting results regarding the epidemiology of male genital HPV infection, with some studies demonstrating a negative age association similar to that observed in women [12,13] and others finding no association with age or number of sexual partners [14,15]. A consistent protective effect of circumcision on the risk of penile HPV has been demonstrated [14,16], and may suggest that HPV infection is more common and has a longer duration when infecting nonkeratinized mucosal epithelial surfaces. Aside from the low-risk genital wart manifestations of HPV 6 and 11, HPV infection in men rarely leads to disease. Because of the low cancer risk and still unknown natural history of HPV in men, virologic testing of this group is not recommended. Furthermore, the method of doing viral testing would not be clear at all. For example, serologic testing has acknowledged sensitivity limitations [9], and sampling site and coverage in men is problematic [14]. A notable exception is the high risk for anal neoplasia resulting from anal HPV infection among men who have sex with men, particular those who have HIV [17]. Screening by anal cytology and anoscopy may be beneficial among this high-risk group [18], though no official recommendations have been issued.

Because of the strong association of HPV with invasive cervical cancer, research on HPV infection has targeted women, and thus the remainder of this article focuses primarily on the natural history and management of cervical HPV infection. A large body of epidemiologic research has allowed the development of a model of the natural history of HPV-associated cervical cancer (Fig. 1) whereby HPV is acquired by sexual transmission and

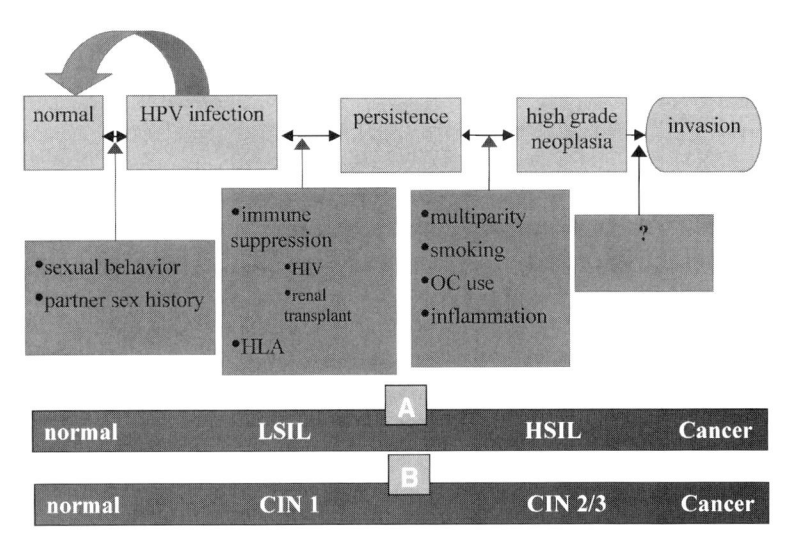

Fig. 1. Natural history of HPV-associated cervical cancer. Bar A refers to cytologic diagnosis as it parallels natural history schema; bar B refers to histologic diagnosis. ?, unknown; CIN, cervical intraepithelial neoplasia; HLA, human leucocyte antigen; HSIL, high-grade squamous intraepithelial lesion; LSIL, low-grade squamous intraepithelial lesion; OC, oral contraceptive.

is largely transient, whereas persistent infection with high-risk HPV confers a high risk for developing high-grade neoplasia and cancer. Data supporting this causal model and factors associated with each transition point are discussed later.

Cervical HPV infection seems to follow one of two patterns. Incident infection is often accompanied by cytologic changes, such as koilocytes, usually within 3 to 6 months. However clearance of the virus and cytologic abnormalities seems to occur in more than 85% of patients. Women whose infection persists for 12 months or more have the highest risk for disease progression.

Prevalent cervical HPV infection is associated with lifetime and recent sexual behavior of the woman or that of her partner [19,20]. Age-stratified HPV incidence reflects the sexual mode of transmission, with incidence peaking around the age of sexual debut and declining to nadir around the third decade of life [21]. In some populations, particularly those in the developing world, a second peak of HPV prevalence occurs around the age of menopause [22–24]. This is unlikely caused by a cohort effect, as a recent population-based cohort study in Colombia reported a similar bimodal age-specific incidence of HPV infection, with recent sexual behavior strongly associated with new infection in older and younger women [21]. Infection with one or more of the more than 50 [genital] HPV genotypes is a common occurrence among sexually active women, but clears rapidly in most cases. A closed cohort of young college women reported up to 60% cumulative infection with genital tract HPV over a 3-year period [25] as estimated by biannual sampling. Recently, Brown and colleagues [26] studied the cumulative prevalence of HPV in a small cohort of 60 adolescent women who had frequent sampling (average two times per week), either by cervical swab during a pelvic examination or by vaginal self-swab. In this cohort, more than 80% of sexually active participants had detectable HPV during the average 2-year follow-up. Among the three women who reported no history of sexual intercourse, HPV was never detected, the prevalence of multiple infection was common (>80% of HPV-positive subjects had more than one HPV type), and the average duration of infection was approximately 6 months. Natural history studies that followed larger cohorts and used less frequent sampling intervals also demonstrate that most (approximately 90%) HPV infections resolve spontaneously, lasting an average of 12 months postinfection [25,27]. Collectively, these data demonstrate that HPV is a nearly ubiquitous, but transient, infection in most sexually active women. As such, HPV infection cannot be managed using direct screening strategies employed for other, less common sexually transmitted infections (STIs), such as screening in adolescent and young adult women, or partner notification.

HPV resolution requires an effective host immune response. The long duration of HPV infection is attributed to the virus' ability to subvert innate immune responses by several mechanisms [28]. The humoral and cellular arms of the adaptive immune response are operational [29], but it is the cytotoxic T-cell response that appears critical to effect viral resolution. Neutralizing immunity based on HPV seroconversion is not thought to play an important role in the resolution of HPV infection for several reasons: (1) less than 70% of incident HPV infections develop serum antibodies after 18 months of initial DNA detection [30]; (2) transient infection is associated with a failure to seroconvert [30], and (3) prevalent seroreactivity does not appear to protect against incident type-specific infection [31,32]. Although antibodies do not appear to play an essential role in the resolution of existing lesions, vaccine-induced antibodies were proved to be effective in prevention of infection, at least in the short-term [33,34]. Alternatively, T-cell immunosuppression has been shown to have a profound effect on the risk for HPV infection and persistence [17], highlighting the significance of the T-cell response. HIV-positive women have at least double the HPV prevalence of HIV-negative women who report similar risk profiles [35], and the risk for persistent HPV is strongly associated with degree of immunosuppression [36]. These data highlight not only the importance of host responses for resolution of natural infection, but also define the HIV-positive population as a high-risk group for HPV-associated malignancies [37].

The initial period after infection is critical. During the 6 to 12 months required for immune recognition, most cervical HPV infections will remain clinically asymptomatic. Manifestations of HPV infection are usually only detected by cervical cytology as part of cervical cancer Papanicolaou screening programs. In these programs, cytologic results are classified according to the Bethesda System, as presented in Box 1 (Fig. 2). Papanicolaou test results can be broadly categorized as low-grade squamous intraepithelial lesions (LSIL), (see Fig. 2) high-grade squamous intraepithelial lesions (HSIL) (Fig. 3), and cancer. In addition to these criteria, the Bethesda system adopts an equivocal category for essentially indeterminate tests not falling precisely into these defined categories, termed *atypical squamous cells* (ASC) and subgrouped as "of undetermined significance" (ASC-US) (Fig. 4) or "cannot exclude HSIL" (ASC-H). Fig. 1 includes a conceptual correlation between the natural history model of HPV-associated cervical cancer and the Bethesda categorization of clinical outcomes. As demonstrated in this model, it is now accepted that most LSIL diagnoses simply reflect the cytologic manifestations of HPV replication. Studies have found that these lesions are commonly detected following an incident HPV infection with cumulative incidence increasing with screening frequency; ranging from 28% 36-month cumulative incidence (95% confidence interval [CI], 25%–32%) in young women seen at 6-month intervals [38] to 47.2% 36-month cumulative incidence (95% CI, 39%–56%) among young women seen at 4-month intervals [39]. However, these low-grade lesions, like asymptomatic HPV infection, are likely to resolve; the average duration of LSIL in one study was estimated at 5.5 months (95% CI, 4.2–7.9), with 85% of lesions clearing during study follow-up [39]. This fact highlights the low risk for and transient nature of LSILs, particularly in women younger than 30 years.

Although the host response to infection is effective in most women, few will develop a persistent infection, defined as detection of the same HPV type for more than 12 months. The presence of persistent infection with the same high-risk genotype has been shown to confer a strong risk for development of subsequent neoplasia [40,41]. The risk for HSIL among older women (mean age of 33 years) was 11.67 (4.1–33.3) if the same oncogenic type was detected at two visits (versus HPV-negative at both visits) 4 months apart [41]. The risks were higher in young women (aged 20–29 years) when examining type-specific persistent oncogenic HPV infection using 2-year sampling intervals (odds ratio of 813, 95% CI 168–3229) [40]. The difference in the magnitude of these risk estimates almost certainly reflects the definition of persistent infection (4 months versus 24 months). A recent prospective cohort study, however, demonstrated that the transit time from incident high-risk HPV infection to development of HSIL averaged 14 months [39], suggesting that long-term persistence is not an absolute requirement for lesion development. A retrospective cohort study of carcinoma in situ, which examined the presence of HPV-16 DNA in prediagnostic Papanicolaou tests, demonstrated that the probably of being HPV 16–positive steadily increased as the time of diagnosis approached, reaching a peak of more than 50% at 2 years before diagnosis, but rising steadily from as much as 14 years before diagnosis [42]. These data can be interpreted as suggesting that although long-term persistence (>2 years) of

Box 1. The 2001 Bethesda System

I. Specimen adequacy
   Satisfactory for evaluation (note presence /absence of endocervical/transformation zone component)
   Unsatisfactory for evaluation...(specify reason)
      Specimen rejected/not processed (specify reason)
      Specimen processed and examined, but unsatisfactory for evaluation of epithelial abnormality because of (specify reason)
II. General categorization (optional)
   Negative for intraepithelial lesion or malignancy
   Epithelial cell abnormality
   Other
III. Interpretation/result
   Negative for intraepithelial lesion or malignancy
      Organisms
            Trichomonas vaginalis
            Fungal organisms morphologically consistent with *Candida* species
            Shift in flora suggestive of bacterial vaginosis
            Bacteria morphologically consistent with *Actinomyces* species
            Cellular changes consistent with herpes simplex virus
      Other non-neoplastic findings (optional to report; list not comprehensive)
            Reactive cellular changes associated with:
               inflammation (includes typical repair)
               radiation
               intrauterine contraceptive device
            Glandular cells status posthysterectomy
            Atrophy
   Epithelial cell abnormalities
      Squamous cell
            Atypical squamous cells (ASC)
               of undetermined significance (ASC-US)
               cannot exclude HSIL (ASC-H)
            Low-grade squamous intraepithelial lesion (LSIL)
               encompassing: human papillomavirus/mild dysplasia/ cervical intraepithelial neoplasia (CIN) 1
            High-grade squamous intraepithelial lesion (HSIL)
               encompassing: moderate and severe dysplasia, carcinoma *in situ*; CIN 2 and CIN 3
            Squamous cell carcinoma

> Glandular cell
>   Atypical glandular cells (AGC) (specify endocervical, endometrial, or not otherwise specified)
>   Atypical glandular cells, favor neoplastic (specify endocervical or not otherwise specified)
>   Endocervical adenocarcinoma in situ (AIS)
>   Adenocarcinoma
> *Other (list not comprehensive)*
>   Endometrial cells in a woman ≥40 years of age
>
> ---
>
> *Adapted from* Solomon D, Davey D, Kurman R, et al. The 2001 Bethesda System: terminology for reporting results of cervical cytology. JAMA 2002;287(16): 2114; with permission.

oncogenic HPV is not necessary for HSIL development, persistent detection of oncogenic HPV of the same type is certainly predictive of HSIL risk, possibly by representing a more sensitive marker for occult disease that is underdiagnosed by conventional methods. Diagnosis of a high-grade lesion requires excisional treatment as part of current successful cervical cancer prevention programs. Therefore, estimates of HSIL duration cannot be ethically derived. However, short-term follow-up studies of biopsy confirmed [high grade lesions indicate] that a significant fraction of high-grade lesions (20%–50%) resolve without intervention [43,44].

The strength of association between high risk (HR)-HPV infection and invasive cervical cancer is unprecedented in cancer epidemiology, with odds ratios exceeding 45 in most cases [3]. However, this association must be considered in the context of the high prevalence of transient HPV infection among sexually active women and the frequent resolution of HPV-associated lesions. It can therefore be concluded that HR-HPV infection is a necessary but insufficient cause of invasive cervical cancer. Besides

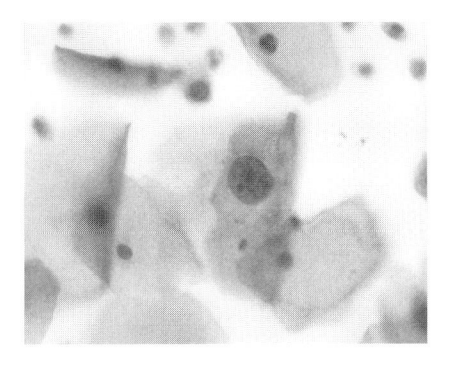

Fig. 2. Example of Pap smear diagnosed as LSIL.

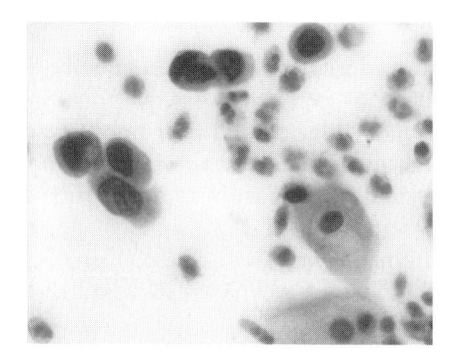

Fig. 3. Example of Pap smear diagnosed as HSIL.

infection with HR-HPV, the other factors influencing risk for progression to invasive cervical cancer are less well-defined. To date, multiparity [45,46] and cigarette smoking [46–48] have been consistently found to be increased among cervical cancer cases relative to HPV-positive controls. In addition, long-term use of oral contraceptives (>5 years) [46,49–52], co-infection with other sexually transmitted infections (eg, *Chlamydia trachomatis* and herpes simplex virus) [52–56], and inflammation [57,58] have been found to increase the risk for HPV-associated cervical cancer, although these observations are generally less consistent than those demonstrated for parity and smoking. Identification of these cofactors that interact with HR-HPV to cause cancer remain the focus of intensive research efforts.

HPV infection is a common result of sexual activity, easily transmitted, and frequently self-limiting with no clinical manifestation. However, in rare circumstances, HR-HPV infection can result in development of invasive cervical cancer. Reduction in morbidity and mortality resulting from cervical HPV infections is therefore best achieved by the appropriate detection and treatment of premalignant sequelae of infection. The

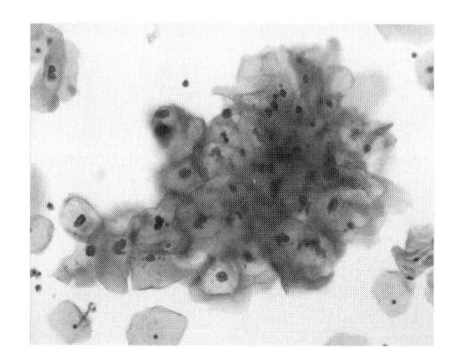

Fig. 4. Example of Pap smear diagnosed as ASC-US.

following sections of this article discuss the current recommendations for management of cervical HPV infections, with an emphasis on detection and treatment of high-grade lesions (histopathologic diagnosis of cervical intraepithelial neoplasia [CIN] grade 2 or more severe) through cervical cancer screening programs.

Although traditional approaches over the past 50 years have centered on Papanicolaou screening, the development and availability of newer testing methods that allow direct detection of HPV DNA have revolutionized the field, leading to a reevaluation of optimal cervical cancer screening strategies. Of utmost importance in the consideration of how and when to use an HPV DNA diagnostic test is the positive and negative predictive value of HPV DNA testing in populations of high HPV prevalence (eg, women younger than 30 years and women who have HIV) versus populations of low HPV prevalence (eg, women older than 30 years).

Cervical cancer screening: current management guidelines and role of human papillomavirus testing

Screening and treatment of cancer precursor lesions have led to a dramatic reduction in cervical cancer incidence in the developed world [59]. Successful programs are based on the Papanicolaou test, which uses microscopy to detect cytologic changes consistent with neoplasia from an exfoliated cervical cell sample. This section reviews the current cervical cancer screening guidelines, the management of abnormal screening results (including the management of atypical results using HPV testing), and the future of HPV DNA testing in cervical cancer screening programs.

Multiple professional organizations (including the American Cancer Society [ACS], US Preventive Services Task Force [USPSTF], American College of Obstetrics and Gynecology, and the American Society for Colposcopy and Cervical Pathology) have recently evaluated the evidence-based literature regarding cervical cancer natural history, screening, and prevention, and have issued revised guidelines [60–62]. These guidelines recommend ages to begin and end screening, screening intervals, screening of hysterectomized women, and the use of new technologies (eg, liquid-based smears) and HPV DNA testing. A sample of the guidelines from the USPSTF is presented in Box 2. These screening guidelines were developed for the general population, and may require modification for unique subgroups, including HIV-positive women, women who have in utero diethylstilbestrol (DES) exposure, and women who are immunocompromised because of organ transplant, chemotherapy, or chronic corticosteroid treatment. Management for these subgroups are detailed in the ACS guidelines [60], and are not discussed in this article.

The success of Papanicolaou screening is dependent on several factors: adequate sampling of the cervix, trained cytopathologists for accurate

> **Box 2. Screening recommendations from the US Preventive Services Task Force**
>
> - The USPSTF strongly recommends screening for cervical cancer in women who have been sexually active and have a cervix.
> - The USPSTF recommends against routinely screening women older than age 65 for cervical cancer if they have had adequate recent screening with normal Papanicolaou tests and are not otherwise at high risk for cervical cancer.
> - The USPSTF recommends against routine Papanicolaou screening in women who have had a total hysterectomy for benign disease.
> - The USPSTF concludes that the evidence is insufficient to recommend for or against the routine use of new technologies to screen for cervical cancer.
> - The USPSTF concludes that the evidence is insufficient to recommend for or against the routine use of HPV testing as a primary screen for cervical cancer.
>
> ---
>
> Screening for cervical cancer, recommendations and rationale, US Preventive Services Task Force. Available at: http://www.ahrq.gov/clinic/3rduspstf/cervcan/cervcanrr.pdf. Accessed April 28, 2005.

interpretation, ability to follow-up abnormal smears, treatment of confirmed precursor lesions, and frequent screening.

The smear quality is determined by the adequate representation of endocervical and ectocervical cells. The standard for cervical cell collection is the use of an extended-tip Ayre's spatula directed to the cervical os for collection of a sample of ectocervical cells, followed by a sample of the endocervix using an endocervical brush. Both samples are smeared onto the same glass slide and fixed using 95% ethanol or commercial spray fixatives. Alternative collection devices have recently become available in the market, including the "broom" sampling device, which simultaneously samples the ectocervix and endocervix. In addition, various brands of liquid fixatives have been brought to the market. These fixatives are used as a "liquid Pap," where the sampled cervical cells are rinsed into a fixative vial, an aliquot of which is used in an automated procedure in a pathology laboratory to create a monolayer of cells on a slide, that is stained and interpreted using standard methods. The value of the liquid Pap is twofold: it avoids the potentially obscuring features of cellular clumping, blood, and inflammatory cells and it allows for "reflex" HPV testing as discussed in detail later. Although some studies have reported improved performance using the liquid Pap compared with conventional smears, the performance has not been considered sufficiently different to recommend a preferred method [60]. An important practical consideration in choosing conventional versus liquid Pap is cost: liquid Paps are currently more costly than conventional smears. Saslow et al [60] provide a detailed review of the evidence regarding the use of the liquid-based technologies. Whether or not the liquid Pap is cost-effective remains the subject of some controversy.

Conventional and thin-layer smears are fixed and stained, and interpreted by certified cytopathologists according to the Bethesda System (see Box 1). First proposed in 1988, the Bethesda System has been revised twice, most recently in 2001 [63]. This system categorizes the observed cytologic changes into multiple groups; this article focuses on the broad categories of ASC-US, LSIL, HSIL, and cancer.

Two criteria should be considered when evaluating a Papanicolaou screening result: the adequacy and grade of abnormality. Generally, unsatisfactory smears should be repeated within 2 to 4 months. Satisfactory smears may be annotated to indicate absence or endocervical or transformation zone component on the slide. This occurs if the transformation zone was not well-sampled, a common occurrence in pregnant women and postmenopausal women in whom the transformation zone has receded into the endocervical canal. The clinical significance of this absence on cytological screening is unknown. If a woman has normal recent cervical cytology without results of ASC-US or worse, repeat cervical cytology screening can be continued annually. However, if a woman has had a recent abnormal Papanicolaou test result without three subsequent negative smears, an incompletely visualized cervix, an immunocompromised state, or poor prior screening, a repeat cytologic sampling should be done within 6 months [64].

The current guidelines incorporate use of standard Papanicolaou test cytology and newer HPV DNA diagnostic tests. There is a single diagnostic assay that is approved by the US Food and Drug Administration for the specific detection of high-risk HPV infection. The Hybrid Capture 2 Test (Digene Diagnostics, Gaithersburg, Maryland) is designed to detect one or more of the 13 HPV genotypes that has confirmed association with cervical cancer development (HPV 16, 18, 31, 33, 35, 39, 45, 51, 52, 56, 58, 59, and 68). The test uses a signal amplification technology and approaches the sensitivity of consensus polymerase chain reaction–based methods [65]. Clinically, there is no value in determining the presence of a low-risk HPV infection, as most are self-limiting with no risk for significant disease. Therefore, HPV DNA testing should be used to clarify equivocal results (ASC-US triage) or in combination with Papanicolaou tests as a potentially more sensitive but similarly specific screen among populations that have lower overall HPV prevalence (eg, women older than 30 years).

Figure 5 outlines the basic recommended algorithm for follow-up based on the results of the Pap smear. It should be reiterated that Papanicolaou

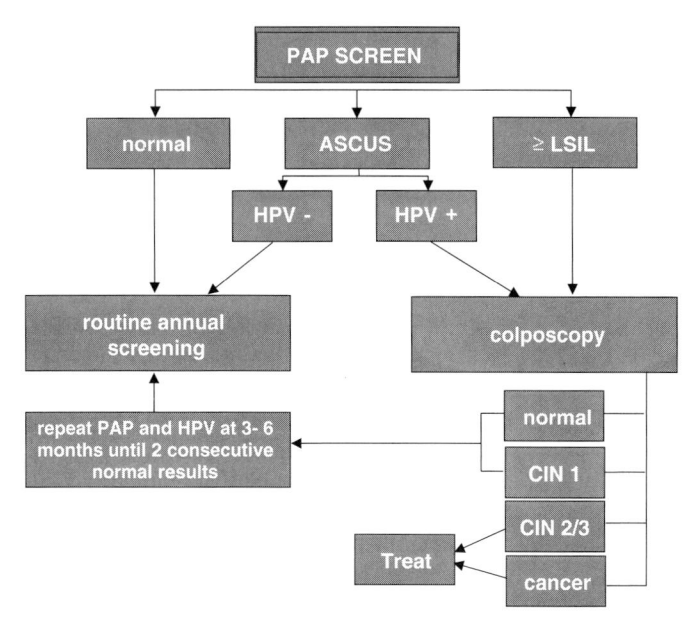

Fig. 5. Pap smear management algorithm. ≥LSIL – includes LSIL, HSIL and carcinoma in situ. ASCUS, atypical cells of undetermined significance; CIN, cervical intraepithelial neoplasia; LSIL, low-grade squamous intraepithelial lesion.

test cytology is a screening test, the results of which are used to triage only the highest-risk patients for diagnostic testing or colposcopy. The colposcopic examination involves a more rigorous visualization of the cervix with the aid of magnification following application of a 3% to 5% acetic acid solution. The acetic acid will cause lesions to become white and visible. Biopsies are taken from suspicious acetowhite lesions and used for histologic diagnosis, which is considered the gold standard for detection of cervical neoplasia.

When using the Papanicolaou test as the sole screening method, the goal is to identify women who are at risk for harboring a CIN 2 or more severe lesion (CIN 2+) for referral to diagnostic colposcopy. Currently, all Papanicolaou test diagnoses of ASC-H, LSIL, HSIL, or cancer are referred for colposcopy. In the past, the management of the ASC-US result was variable across centers, but now can include either follow-up by repeat Papanicolaou test in 3 to 6 months, or triage based on HR-HPV testing. HPV triage of ASC-US Papanicolaou test results is especially attractive when used with the liquid cytology option, as the residual material from the liquid Pap can be used for reflex HPV testing if the Papanicolaou test comes back as ASC-US, without the need to see the patient again. In this option, women who have ASC-US results that are found to be HR-HPV negative are asked to return for routine screening, as the risk for occult disease is low in these women. Women who have an ASC-US Papanicolaou test and a positive HR-HPV test are referred for colposcopy. The rationale for these colposcopy referral recommendations based on smear results has been confirmed in multiple studies, including a large randomized trial of management strategies for ASC-US/LSIL diagnoses [66,67]. The ASCUS/LSIL Triage Study (ALTS) trial enrolled 3488 women who had a referral ASC-US Papanicolaou test result, and 1572 women who had a referral LSIL. Each referral group was randomized to one of three management strategy arms: (1) immediate colposcopy, where all ASCUS and LSIL Papanicolaou tests are referred; (2) HPV triage, where women who have either a positive HPV DNA test or HSIL on enrollment cytology were referred; and (3) conservative management, where women were referred if the Papanicolaou test result was more than the HSIL. The HPV triage arm for the LSIL group was closed early because more than 80% of these women were found to be HR-HPV–positive. The results of this trial demonstrated that referral using a threshold diagnosis of HSIL is highly specific (eg, many HSIL positive Papanicolaou tests will be confirmed on histopathology as CIN 2+) but insensitive (eg, only 30% of confirmed CIN 2+ will have been detected by Papanicolaou test as HSIL), whereas referral using a threshold of ASC-US is highly sensitive (correctly identifying 70% to 80% of CIN 2+) but nonspecific (most positive Papanicolaou test will be normal or CIN 1 on biopsy). The specificity of ASC-US referral with HPV triage was significantly better without a sacrifice in sensitivity, as only 50% of ASC-US Papanicolaou tests were determined to be HR-HPV–positive, and all high-grade disease was detected in this group. Therefore, most current recommendations refer all women who have a Papanicolaou test diagnosis of ASC-US or more severe (or HPV-positive ASC-US) for colposcopic evaluation. An exception to this may be in the management of LSIL in adolescent women, for whom continued close cytologic screening without immediate referral to colposcopy may be warranted [68]. The consequence of this recommendation, one that favors sensitivity above specificity, is an increased cost because of expensive follow-up and testing of a large number of women, most of whom will be found to have normal cervices on colposcopic evaluation.

During follow-up, if the colposcopist suspects a lesion during this examination, a biopsy is taken and the histopathologic diagnosis is used to confirm the final diagnosis. Unfortunately, although the terminology for grading cytopathologic and histopathologic results has been standardized over time, it has not converged. Histopathologic grading of cervical biopsies uses the CIN terminology. This classification can be viewed as loosely analogous to the Bethesda System of squamous intraepithelial lesion categorization, where LSIL is inclusive of CIN 1 and HSIL is inclusive of CIN 2, CIN 3, and carcinoma in situ. Treatment is triggered after a confirmed diagnosis of CIN 2+. The interpretation of the CIN classification scheme in the context of the natural history of HPV and cervical cancer must be emphasized. It is now largely recognized that CIN 1 likely reflects nothing more than cytologic changes caused by HPV infection, and as such harbors a high probability of spontaneous resolution. Therefore, the management of CIN 1 diagnoses usually involves repeat Papanicolaou (or HPV) testing at 3 to 6 months to ensure lesion regression. A CIN 2 diagnosis is thought to represent an amalgam of "heightened" CIN 1 and true CIN 3 lesions. Because a significant fraction of CIN 2 will progress if untreated, however, this diagnosis triggers management by excisional therapy (usually loop electroexcision procedure or cold knife cone). CIN 3 is considered a truer cancer precursor, with additional viral and genetic changes that significantly increase the risk for lesion persistence or progression and should always be treated.

Role of new human papillomavirus virus–specific tests

The indication for HPV DNA testing has been evaluated by many studies. Testing for the presence of even HR-HPV outside of the context of cervical cancer screening is not indicated, because of the lack of treatment options and the high probability of detecting an insignificant, self-limiting infection. However, there are two clear indications for HPV DNA testing in the context of cervical cancer screening: ASC-US triage and primary cervical cancer screening in women older than 30 years of age.

It is estimated that more than 2 million of the 55 million Papanicolaou tests performed annually in the United States (3.6%) are interpreted as ASC-US. The 2001 revised Bethesda classification has dichotomized the ASC category to ASC-US and ASC-H, the latter representing approximately 10% of the ASC interpretations; all of these diagnoses should trigger colposcopic referral. The remaining ASC-US diagnoses actually represent a conglomerate of benign changes, low-grade lesions, and high-grade lesions. Because a significant fraction of CIN 2+ will be diagnosed as a result of an ASC-US referral, observational follow-up management of these patients is not recommended. As described above, the results of the ALTS trial indicated that triage of only HR-HPV DNA–positive ASC-US results to colposcopy reduces the rate of referral by approximately 50% while maintaining a high sensitivity (at least as sensitive as immediate colposcopy and more sensitive than repeat Papanicolaou testing) [67]. However, HPV DNA testing was not found to be an effective triage strategy for the referral of LSIL-positive Papanicolaou tests, as most (approximately 80%) were HR-HPV–positive [66]. Cost-effectiveness analyses show that liquid-based cytology with reflex HPV DNA testing is the most cost-effective strategy while maintaining same or greater life expectancy benefits when compared with other strategies for the management of ASC-US [69].

Since the discovery that HPV infection with one of about 13 viral genotypes is a necessary cause of invasive cervical cancer, researchers have explored the possibility of replacing Papanicolaou screening with a more objective test for patients who are at risk for cervical cancer and those who have prevalent HR-HPV infection. The rationale and implication of HPV testing as a primary screening strategy has been reviewed in detail by Franco [70]. The clinical relevance of a positive cervical HPV DNA test will be strongly age-dependent. Women younger than 30 years are significantly more likely to harbor a transient, self-limiting HR-HPV infection and intensive management of these women would result in a tremendous burden on the health care system, and an HPV–positive diagnosis would result in an unacceptable increase in undue patient anxiety. Therefore, the population most amenable to an HPV DNA primary screening application is women older than age 30. A positive HPV result in these women is much more likely to represent clinically relevant, persistent HR-HPV infection as a marker of prevalent CIN 2+. In such a primary screening algorithm, only women who have a positive HPV test would be referred for a Papanicolaou test or colposcopic examination. The value of this strategy is the result of the complementation of two factors: the low prevalence of HR-HPV infection in this age group, and the significantly increased probability of false-positive Papanicolaou test results caused by misinterpretation of menopausal changes. An additional benefit of HPV testing in this group is the value added from the high negative predictive value (NPV) of HPV DNA testing (eg, the likelihood of the absence of disease among HPV-negative patients). The high NPV assures that women who test negative are unlikely to have prevalent high-grade neoplasia at the time of testing. Because of the long latency of cervical cancer progression, this information can be safely used to increase the screening intervals among the older women who have had at least three preceding normal Papanicolaou tests and are currently HPV-negative [71].

The multicenter HPV in Addition to Routine Testing study conducted in the United Kingdom demonstrated the feasibility of primary screening in women aged 30 to 60 years. The results of this study confirmed an increased sensitivity of HPV testing versus Papanicolaou testing using a borderline change threshold (97.1% versus 76.6%, respectively) [71]. Though less specific, HPV-positive women who have negative or borderline cytologic results could be safely monitored by repeat testing at 12 months, thereby reducing total colposcopy referral while maintaining improved CIN 2+ detection.

Summary

Cervical HPV infection should be managed less as a typical STI and more as a strong risk factor predisposing to cervical cancer development. HPV infection is undeniably transmitted predominantly through sexual contact. However, the fact that more than 80% of women followed over time will acquire at least one HR-HPV infection reflects the ubiquitous nature of the infection and the ease of transmission. Although the behavioral profiles typically associated with an increased risk for STI (including lifetime partner number, age at first intercourse, and so forth) will certainly lead to an increased risk for HPV detection, there is a high absolute prevalence of HPV even among women who have few lifetime sex partners. It could be argued that to counsel patients for an HPV infection as an STI would be counterproductive, as short of absolute abstinence, the prevention of infection is difficult and treatment options, short of excisional procedures for neoplasia, are limited.

The real promise held in this area is the availability of an apparently highly effective prophylactic HPV vaccine, targeting at least HPV 16, 18, 6, and 11 [33,34]. This vaccine cocktail, if it achieved 100% coverage, could theoretically prevent 50% to 70% of invasive cervical cancers and most genital warts. Vaccination will be required among women before initiation of sexual contact, presumably among girls 10 to 13 years of age. Many programmatic issues remain regarding the implementation of HPV vaccine programs, including the marketing of the vaccine as STI or cancer prevention, as reviewed in detail by Gravitt and Shah [72]. Even in the era of potentially effective vaccines, screening for cervical cancer is likely to remain a priority in cervical cancer prevention programs for at least several decades. Vaccine trials have proven high short-term efficacy; however, these effects were clearly type-specific and antibody titers gradually decrease postvaccination. It is unclear whether the protection will remain over an individual's lifetime without vaccine booster, and oncogenic HPV infections not targeted by vaccination will continue to contribute to risk for development of cervical intraepithelial neoplasia and cancer. Therefore, although the public health success of HPV vaccination is undoubtedly promising, the role of cervical cancer screening as a secondary prevention effort should not be trivialized. In fact, the nature of screening programs should continue to be reevaluated in the context of effective but limited spectrum vaccines.

Acknowledgment

The authors are grateful to Dorothy Rosenthal, MD for providing the cytologic photographs.

References

[1] de Villiers EM. Human pathogenic papillomavirus types: an update. Curr Top Microbiol Immunol 1994;186:1–12.
[2] Chan SY, Delius H, Halpern AL, et al. Analysis of genomic sequences of 95 papillomavirus types: uniting typing, phylogeny, and taxonomy. J Virol 1995;69(5):3074–83.
[3] Munoz N, Bosch F, de Sanjose S, et al. Epidemiologic classification of human papillomavirus types associated with cervical cancer. N Engl J Med 2003;348(6):518–27.
[4] Bosch F, Lorincz A, Munoz N, et al. The causal relation between human papillomavirus and cervical cancer. J Clin Pathol 2002;55:244–65.

[5] Bauer HM, Ting Y, Greer CE, et al. Genital human papillomavirus infection in female university students as determined by a PCR-based method. JAMA 1991;265(4):472–7.
[6] Palefsky JM, Holly EA, Ralston ML, et al. Prevalence and risk factors for anal human papillomavirus infection in human immunodeficiency virus (HIV)-positive and high-risk HIV-negative women. J Infect Dis 2001;183(3):383–91.
[7] Weaver BA, Feng Q, Holmes KK, et al. Evaluation of genital sites and sampling techniques for detection of human papillomavirus DNA in men. J Infect Dis 2004;189(4):677–85.
[8] Palefsky JM, Shiboski S, Moss A. Risk factors for anal human papillomavirus infection and anal cytologic abnormalities in HIV-positive and HIV-negative homosexual men. J Acquir Immune Defic Syndr 1994;7(6):599–606.
[9] Kreimer AR, Alberg AJ, Daniel R, et al. Oral human papillomavirus infection in adults is associated with sexual behavior and HIV serostatus. J Infect Dis 2004;189(4):686–98.
[10] Manhart LE, Koutsky LA. Do condoms prevent genital HPV infection, external genital warts, or cervical neoplasia? A meta-analysis. Sex Transm Dis 2002;29(11):725–35.
[11] Stone KM, Karem KL, Sternberg MR, et al. Seroprevalence of human papillomavirus type 16 infection in the United States. J Infect Dis 2002;186(10):1396–402.
[12] Franceschi S, Castellsague X, Dal Maso L, et al. Prevalence and determinants of human papillomavirus genital infection in men. Br J Cancer 2002;86(5):705–11.
[13] Svare EI, Kjaer SK, Worm AM, et al. Risk factors for genital HPV DNA in men resemble those found in women: a study of male attendees at a Danish STD clinic. Sex Transm Infect 2002;78(3):215–8.
[14] Baldwin SB, Wallace DR, Papenfuss MR, et al. Human papillomavirus infection in men attending a sexually transmitted disease clinic. J Infect Dis 2003;187(7):1064–70.
[15] Lazcano-Ponce E, Herrero R, Munoz N, et al. High prevalence of human papillomavirus infection in Mexican males: comparative study of penile-urethral swabs and urine samples. Sex Transm Dis 2001;28(5):277–80.
[16] Castellsague X, Bosch FX, Munoz N, et al. Male circumcision, penile human papillomavirus infection, and cervical cancer in female partners. N Engl J Med 2002;346(15):1105–12.
[17] Palefsky J, Holly E. Immunosuppression and co-infection with HIV. J Natl Cancer Inst Monogr 2003;31:41–6.
[18] Aberg JA, Gallant JE, Anderson J, et al. Primary care guidelines for the management of persons infected with human immunodeficiency virus: recommendations of the HIV Medicine Association of the Infectious Diseases Society of America. Clin Infect Dis 2004;39(5):609–29.
[19] Smith JS, Bosetti C, Munoz N, et al. Chlamydia trachomatis and invasive cervical cancer: a pooled analysis of the IARC multicentric case-control study. Int J Cancer 2004;111(3):431–9.
[20] Bosch FX, Castellsague X, Munoz N, et al. Male sexual behavior and human papillomavirus DNA: key risk factors for cervical cancer in Spain. J Natl Cancer Inst 1996;88(15):1060–7.
[21] Munoz N, Mendez F, Posso H, et al. Incidence, duration, and determinants of cervical human papillomavirus infection in a cohort of Colombian women with normal cytological results. J Infect Dis 2004;190(12):2077–87.
[22] Molano M, Posso H, Weiderpass E, et al. Prevalence and determinants of HPV infection among Colombian women with normal cytology. Br J Cancer 2002;87(3):324–33.
[23] Herrero R, Hildesheim A, Bratti C, et al. Population-based study of human papillomavirus infection and cervical neoplasia in rural Costa Rica. J Natl Cancer Inst 2000;92(6):464–74.
[24] Lazcano-Ponce E, Herrero R, Munoz N, et al. Epidemiology of HPV infection among Mexican women with normal cervical cytology. Int J Cancer 2001;91(3):412–20.
[25] Ho GY, Bierman R, Beardsley L, et al. Natural history of cervicovaginal papillomavirus infection in young women. N Engl J Med 1998;338(7):423–8.
[26] Brown DR, Shew ML, Qadadri B, et al. A longitudinal study of genital human papillomavirus infection in a cohort of closely followed adolescent women. J Infect Dis 2005;191(2):182–92.

[27] Franco EL, Villa LL, Sobrinho JP, et al. Epidemiology of acquisition and clearance of cervical human papillomavirus infection in women from a high-risk area for cervical cancer. J Infect Dis 1999;180(5):1415–23.
[28] Tindle RW. Immune evasion in human papillomavirus-associated cervical cancer. Nat Rev Cancer 2002;2(1):59–65.
[29] Stanley MA. Immunobiology of papillomavirus infections. J Reprod Immunol 2001; 52(1–2):45–59.
[30] Carter JJ, Koutsky LA, Hughes JP, et al. Comparison of human papillomavirus types 16, 18, and 6 capsid antibody responses following incident infection. J Infect Dis 2000;181(6): 1911–9.
[31] Viscidi RP, Schiffman M, Hildesheim A, et al. Seroreactivity to human papillomavirus (HPV) types 16, 18, or 31 and risk of subsequent HPV infection: results from a population-based study in Costa Rica. Cancer Epidemiol Biomarkers Prev 2004;13(2):324–7.
[32] Viscidi R, Snyder B, Cu-Uvin S, et al. Human papillomavirus capsid antibody response to natural infection and risk of subsequent HPV infection in HIV-positive and HIV-negative women. Cancer Epidemiol Biomarkers Prev 2005;14(1):283–8.
[33] Koutsky LA, Ault KA, Wheeler CM, et al. A controlled trial of a human papillomavirus type 16 vaccine. N Engl J Med 2002;347(21):1645–51.
[34] Harper DM, Franco EL, Wheeler C, et al. Efficacy of a bivalent L1 virus-like particle vaccine in prevention of infection with human papillomavirus types 16 and 18 in young women: a randomised controlled trial. Lancet 2004;364(9447):1757–65.
[35] Palefsky JM, Minkoff H, Kalish LA, et al. Cervicovaginal human papillomavirus infection in human immunodeficiency virus-1 (HIV)-positive and high-risk HIV-negative women. J Natl Cancer Inst 1999;91(3):226–36.
[36] Ahdieh L, Klein R, Burk RD, et al. Prevalence, incidence and type-specific persistence of human papillomavirus in human immunodeficiency virus (HIV)-positive and HIV-negative women. J Infect Dis 2001;184(6):682–90.
[37] Frisch M, Biggar R, Engels E, et al. AIDS-Cancer match registry study group. Association of cancer with AIDS-related immunosuppression in adults. JAMA 2001;285(13):1736–45.
[38] Woodman CB, Collins S, Winter H, et al. Natural history of cervical human papillomavirus infection in young women: a longitudinal cohort study. Lancet 2001;357(9271):1831–6.
[39] Winer RL, Kiviat NB, Hughes JP, et al. Development and duration of human papillomavirus lesions, after initial infection. J Infect Dis 2005;191(5):731–8.
[40] Kjaer SK, van den Brule AJ, Paull G, et al. Type specific persistence of high risk human papillomavirus (HPV) as indicator of high grade cervical squamous intraepithelial lesions in young women: population based prospective follow up study. BMJ 2002;325(7364): 572.
[41] Schlecht NF, Kulaga S, Robitaille J, et al. Persistent human papillomavirus infection as a predictor of cervical intraepithelial neoplasia. JAMA 2001;286(24):3106–14.
[42] Ylitalo N, Josefsson A, Melbye M, et al. A prospective study showing long-term infection with human papillomavirus 16 before the development of cervical carcinoma in situ. Cancer Res 2000;60(21):6027–32.
[43] Alvarez R, Conner M, Weiss H, et al. The efficacy of 9-cis-retinoic acid (aliretinoin) as a chemopreventive agent for cervical dysplasia: results of a randomized double-blind clinical trial. Cancer Epidemiol Biomarkers Prev 2003;12(2):114–9.
[44] Follen M, Atkinson EN, Schottenfeld D, et al. A randomized clinical trial of 4-hydroxyphenylretinamide for high-grade squamous intraepithelial lesions of the cervix. Clin Cancer Res 2001;7(11):3356–65.
[45] Munoz N, Franceschi S, Bosetti C, et al. Role of parity and human papillomavirus in cervical cancer: the IARC multicentric case-control study. Lancet 2002;359(9312):1093–101.
[46] Castellsague X, Munoz N. Cofactors in human papillomavirus carcinogenesis—role of parity, oral contraceptives, and tobacco smoking. J Natl Cancer Inst Monogr 2003;(31): 20–8.

[47] Plummer M, Herrero R, Franceschi S, et al. Smoking and cervical cancer: pooled analysis of the IARC multi-centric case–control study. Cancer Causes Control 2003;14(9):805–14.
[48] Castle PE, Wacholder S, Lorincz AT, et al. A prospective study of high-grade cervical neoplasia risk among human papillomavirus-infected women. J Natl Cancer Inst 2002; 94(18):1406–14.
[49] Moreno V, Bosch FX, Munoz N, et al. Effect of oral contraceptives on risk of cervical cancer in women with human papillomavirus infection: the IARC multicentric case-control study. Lancet 2002;359(9312):1085–92.
[50] Green J, Berrington de Gonzalez A, Smith JS, et al. Human papillomavirus infection and use of oral contraceptives. Br J Cancer 2003;88(11):1713–20.
[51] Shapiro S, Rosenberg L, Hoffman M, et al. Risk of invasive cancer of the cervix in relation to the use of injectable progestogen contraceptives and combined estrogen/progestogen oral contraceptives (South Africa). Cancer Causes Control 2003;14(5):485–95.
[52] Smith JS, Green J, Berrington de Gonzalez A, et al. Cervical cancer and use of hormonal contraceptives: a systematic review. Lancet 2003;361(9364):1159–67.
[53] Smith JS, Herrero R, Bosetti C, et al. Herpes simplex virus-2 as a human papillomavirus cofactor in the etiology of invasive cervical cancer. J Natl Cancer Inst 2002;94(21): 1604–13.
[54] Tran-Thanh D, Provencher D, Koushik A, et al. Herpes simplex virus type II is not a cofactor to human papillomavirus in cancer of the uterine cervix. Am J Obstet Gynecol 2003;188(1):129–34.
[55] Lehtinen M, Koskela P, Jellum E, et al. Herpes simplex virus and risk of cervical cancer: a longitudinal, nested case-control study in the Nordic countries. Am J Epidemiol 2002; 156(8):687–92.
[56] Wallin KL, Wiklund F, Luostarinen T, et al. A population-based prospective study of Chlamydia trachomatis infection and cervical carcinoma. Int J Cancer 2002;101(4):371–4.
[57] Castle PE, Hillier SL, Rabe LK, et al. An association of cervical inflammation with high-grade cervical neoplasia in women infected with oncogenic human papillomavirus (HPV). Cancer Epidemiol Biomarkers Prev 2001;10(10):1021–7.
[58] Yang YC, Chang CL, Huang YW, et al. Possible cofactor in cervical carcinogenesis: proliferation index of the transformation zone in cervicitis. Chang Gung Med J 2001;24(10): 615–20.
[59] Peto J, Gilham C, Fletcher O, et al. The cervical cancer epidemic that screening has prevented in the UK. Lancet 2004;364(9430):249–56.
[60] Saslow D, Runowicz CD, Solomon D, et al. American Cancer Society guideline for the early detection of cervical neoplasia and cancer. CA Cancer J Clin 2002;52(6):342–62.
[61] Cox JT. The clinician's view: role of human papillomavirus testing in the American Society for Colposcopy and Cervical Pathology Guidelines for the management of abnormal cervical cytology and cervical cancer precursors. Arch Pathol Lab Med 2003;127(8):950–8.
[62] Screening for cervical cancer: recommendations and rationale. Available at: http://www.ahrq.gov/clinic/3rduspstf/cervcan/cervcanrr.pdf. Accessed January 15, 2003.
[63] Solomon D, Davey D, Kurman R, et al. The 2001 Bethesda System: terminology for reporting results of cervical cytology. JAMA 2002;287(16):2114–9.
[64] Davey DD, Austin RM, Birdsong G, et al. ASCCP patient management guidelines: Pap test specimen adequacy and quality indicators. Am J Clin Pathol 2002;118(5):714–8.
[65] Peyton CL, Schiffman M, Lorincz AT, et al. Comparison of PCR- and hybrid capture-based human papillomavirus detection systems using multiple cervical specimen collection strategies. J Clin Microbiol 1998;36(11):3248–54.
[66] ALTS. A randomized trial on the management of low-grade squamous intraepithelial lesion cytology interpretations. Am J Obstet Gynecol 2003;188(6):1393–400.
[67] ALTS. Results of a randomized trial on the management of cytology interpretations of atypical squamous cells of undetermined significance. Am J Obstet Gynecol 2003;188(6): 1383–92.

[68] Moscicki AB, Shiboski S, Hills NK, et al. Regression of low-grade squamous intra-epithelial lesions in young women. Lancet 2004;364(9446):1678–83.
[69] Kim JJ, Wright TC, Goldie SJ. Cost-effectiveness of alternative triage strategies for atypical squamous cells of undetermined significance. JAMA 2002;287(18):2382–90.
[70] Franco EL. Primary screening of cervical cancer with human papillomavirus tests. J Natl Cancer Inst Monogr 2003;31:89–96.
[71] Cuzick J, Szarewski A, Cubie H, et al. Management of women who test positive for high-risk types of human papillomavirus: the HART study. Lancet 2003;362(9399):1871–6.
[72] Gravitt P, Shah K. A virus-based vaccine may prevent cervical cancer. Curr Infect Dis Rep 2005;7:125–31.

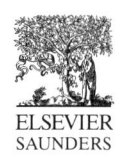

Counseling the Patient who has Genital Herpes or Genital Human Papillomavirus Infection

Terri Warren, RN, ANP[a],*, Charles Ebel, BA[b]

[a]Westover Heights Clinic, 2330 NW Flanders Street, Suite 207,
P.O. Box 13827, Portland, OR 97210, USA
[b]American Social Health Association, P.O. Box 13827,
Research Triangle Park, NC 27709, USA

The most common viral sexually transmitted infections (STIs), herpes simplex virus (HSV) and human papillomavirus (HPV), present special challenges for clinicians and their patients. The potential difficulty stems from several factors, including the time restraints placed on clinicians; the complexity of the infections; and the emotional distress that is felt by some patients, especially at the time of diagnosis. Yet, clinicians can make a significant difference in how patients adjust to diagnosis of these STIs. This article provides clinicians with counseling messages, both medical and psychosocial, for patients who have HSV or HPV.

Genital herpes simplex virus infection

How do patients view having genital herpes? In a telephone survey that was conducted by the American Social Health Association in 1999, 96% of respondents queried said that a diagnosis of HIV infection would be "very traumatic." Sixty-eight percent said the same about having genital herpes. To put this in better perspective, 54% found breaking up with a significant other "very traumatic" and 51% said the same about getting fired from their job. This infection, although not usually a severe problem medically, can have a remarkable impact on the lives of those who are diagnosed. At this writing, approximately one in four people older than age 18 in the United States are infected with HSV-2; of those infected, almost 90% are unaware

* Corresponding author.
 E-mail address: twestover@aol.com (T. Warren).

[1,2]. HSV-2 is common, and with improved diagnostics and more societal awareness, cases will come to the attention of clinicians more often than in the past. In this section, we discuss how best to counsel patients who have genital herpes.

Two kinds of counseling are needed after a diagnosis of genital HSV. The first is what might be called medical counseling. This deals with clinical issues—facts about the disease and its physical impact on the patients. The second kind of counseling deals with the emotional aspects of having herpes—its impact on sexuality, self-esteem, and social interactions with others. Both kinds of counseling are important, and one without the other leaves gaps that may block patients from having a full understanding of their infection.

Barriers to dialogue about herpes simplex virus

Before talking about specific counseling topics, it is useful to think about barriers to honest dialog about herpes from both clinician and patient perspectives. In a study of patients' perceptions of the adequacy of counseling, Gilbert et al [3] found some common barriers that patients cited relative to herpes counseling with their clinician. The most common (57%) was embarrassment. Discussing herpes necessarily means discussing sex—both past and future behavior. Discussing sex with people you know well is hard enough, but discussing it with a clinician you may not know well or who, in the past, has dealt only with nonsexual issues, is not easy. For example, people who have sex partners of the same gender never may have raised this topic with a clinician, but discussing what kinds of behaviors put the patient at risk for contracting herpes may require this disclosure. An additional topic that may be difficult to discuss is specific sexual behaviors that could transmit infection in the future, such as oral and anal sex, and who can do what with whom involving various body parts.

Another obstacle that was identified in the Gilbert et al [3] study, cited by 24% of respondents, was time constraints. Particularly in these days of managed care, patients may sense the clinician being rushed to see another patient, and may feel awkward or uncomfortable about asking questions that take up too much time. Lastly, because herpes can be a complex issue, patients often feel unprepared in an office visit to deal with all of the issues that are raised by this infection, particularly if they are having a first episode. They may be too surprised or distressed by the diagnosis to be able to think about which questions to ask. In the Gilbert et al study [3], 25% of patients described the complexity of herpes infection as a barrier to discussion.

Barriers are perceived by clinicians as well. The clinician who has patients waiting to be seen in other examination rooms may feel the time constraint issue even more acutely. What was initially scheduled as a simple urinary tract infection may prove to be a first episode of genital herpes and throw off an entire day's schedule. Although the clinician may wish to take the time to address all of the patient's questions, he or she also needs to respect the time of other patients in the office. Keeping abreast of all of the latest information about herpes can be challenging, especially when there are so many disease states on which to stay current, and clinicians are reluctant to provide answers to questions unless they are certain they are correct. The emotional aspect of the disease cuts both ways. Although patients may be distressed by this diagnosis, clinicians also are frustrated by the lack of a cure, and find the emotionally charged response to this infection difficult to tackle.

In some cases, barriers may be significant, but for purposes of this article we will assume the clinician has adequate time, is up to date on HSV, and has a patient who is eager to understand his or her infection. What do patients want to learn about and discuss?

Herpes simplex virus talking points with patients

1. The medical counseling discussion might well start with the common nature of the infection—the information that one in four adults has this but most do not know that they are infected [1,2]. Fleming et al's [1] study also found that women are 45% more likely to be infected than men; this probably is due, in large part, to anatomy. People in all settings are vulnerable to herpes; individuals of all colors and ethnicities can be infected, regardless of educational level, including city-dwelling and suburban residents. This is not a disease of one particular group. Having more partners does put one at greater risk for HSV, but a person can be infected after having only one partner or even only oral sex [2].

2. Herpes is likely to recur, in the form of symptomatic recurrences and periods of asymptomatic viral shedding. Patients need to know that there is no cure for herpes and it most likely will recur; however, it is better to avoid the use of the word "incurable." Typically, genital HSV-2 will recur four to six times per year, significantly more often than genital HSV-1, which recurs less than once per year on average [4,5]. If someone acquires HSV-2 orally, it rarely recurs in the healthy adult [6]. The good news is that outbreaks of genital HSV-2 decrease in frequency over time in most people [5,7].

In addition to recognized recurrences, patients must be told that herpes virus can be active and infectious to others when there are no apparent symptoms. This concept of asymptomatic shedding may be the most challenging topic for herpes education. Although patients are not contagious at all times, they cannot be assured that the risk of infectiousness is zero on any given day (see "Special considerations for HSV"). A study by Mertz et al [8] looked at heterosexual couples where one was infected with HSV-2 and the other was not. Seventy percent of new cases of herpes in this trial were transmitted when the infected person had no apparent symptoms. This study, along with known rates of asymptomatic viral shedding, tells us that the patient's comprehension and acceptance of this concept is important in reducing transmission.

3. Antiviral medication can have a dramatic impact on the course of the infection and psychosocial sequelae, including social concerns. Although shedding and recurrences are not good news for patients, there are effective treatments for herpes. An appropriate part of the medical counseling discussion is choosing a treatment that fits the needs of a particular patient. Treatments can change the frequency of recurrences, duration of outbreaks, and risk of transmission to others. Daily antiviral therapy reduces the frequency of recurrences by approximately 75% [9,10]. Medication that is taken at the beginning of a recurrent outbreak reduces the duration of pain, viral shedding, and the lesion by one to two days, although patients—given the choice—prefer daily therapy over episodic outbreak therapy [11]. In discordant couples, where one is infected with HSV-2 and the other is not, transmission can be reduced by 48% when the infected person takes antiviral therapy daily [12]. For couples in which one partner has HSV-2 infection and the other does not, suppressive antiviral therapy should be recommended for the partner who has HSV-2 to reduce the rate of transmission [13]. Adding regular condom use can cut the risk of transmission even more [14,15].

In addition to the medical benefit, treatment also can provide a psychologic benefit. Because transmission of this infection is a major concern among those who have herpes, having a good method to reduce transmission is important. People who have recurrent genital herpes who were started on daily suppression had significantly reduced illness concern and anxiety [16–18].

Patients may have specific questions about treatments, especially about safety. There are three antiviral medications for genital herpes to choose from; most often these are covered by health insurance plans. These nucleoside analogs were shown to be safe when taken daily over long periods of time, up to 20 years [19]. Generally, it is not necessary to draw safety labs or put patients on drug holidays; however, in patients who have kidney impairment, it may be necessary to check a creatinine clearance and reduce the dose of antiviral medication, based on the value obtained.

4. Women who have herpes can bear children safely. Transmission rates to newborns from women who are antibody positive and have no symptoms at the time of delivery are less than 1% [20]. Women who acquire genital HSV-1 or -2 in the third trimester are at high risk for infecting their newborns (30%–50%) [20]; susceptible women of infected partners should be counseled carefully about abstinence or condom use to avoid this problem. Infected men who are concerned about passing HSV to their partner while trying to impregnate them should be offered suppressive therapy during this time to reduce the risk of transmission.

5. Virus typing and the testing of partners often are valuable in proper management. It is useful to offer testing to partners of patients who are infected [13,21,22]. Because almost 90% of persons who are infected with HSV-2 do not know it [1], many couples who think they are discordant (one infected and the other not) when tested, find that both are infected [12].

Couples who are infected with the same type of virus do not need to be concerned about viral activity causing problems within the sexual relationship, and can feel free to enjoy their sexual relationship without concerns about transmission or triggering new outbreaks.

The issue of testing to determine discordancy necessarily raises the topic of typing of the virus. HSV-1 and -2 have different recurrence rates in the genital area. In addition, patients who have genital HSV-1 should be told that they are susceptible to getting HSV-2 infection in the genital area [23]. The person who already has HSV-2 is highly unlikely to acquire HSV-1 [24].

Couples who believe that they always have been monogamous may be greatly upset when a diagnosis of genital herpes is made in one or both partners, causing suspicions that one of them may have been unfaithful. About one third of new genital herpes cases is caused by HSV-1; in college students, that number is significantly higher [25,26]. Many of these cases of genital HSV-1 are transmitted by oral to genital contact during oral sex [25,26]. Therefore, if the viral isolate is typed as HSV-1, and the couple participates in oral sex, transmission within the relationship is a plausible explanation. HSV-1 also can be shed from the mouth in the absence of symptoms, just as HSV-2 can be shed from the genitals asymptomatically [27]. A cold sore need not be present for oral to genital transmission to occur. Education about viral type may help partners to clarify a source of infection and future risk—or absence of risk.

6. *Patients should be made aware that herpes infections usually have no long-term impact on their general health.* Exceptions include increased HIV acquisition risk and neonatal herpes infection. The person who has HSV-2 genital infection has twice the risk of acquiring HIV, should they be exposed [28–30]. In addition, recent data suggest that transmission of HIV is more likely in the person who has HSV-2 infection [31,32]. Neonatal herpes likely can be avoided with proper identification of women who are infected and with appropriate interventions at the time of labor and delivery to decrease the risk of transmission to the neonate [33].

Counseling related to psychosocial adjustment of herpes simplex virus

Although the medical counseling issues often are straightforward and sometimes easier to handle, the psychosocial issues that surround a herpes diagnosis are more complicated and present more long-term problems. Counseling for these kinds of issues can be broken down into topics that should be discussed at the diagnostic visit and topics that might be discussed better at a follow-up visit.

Initial visit

People who are being newly diagnosed with genital herpes cannot listen well. They often are surprised—even stunned—and may be processing internally while you are trying to share information. Other emotions that are experienced by patients may include guilt, fear, and denial ("the blood test must be wrong") [34]. Questions from newly diagnosed patients often relate to concrete, immediate concerns, such as "Who gave this to me?" and "How long have I had it?" It is wise to suggest strongly that you believe that their diagnosis is herpes but withhold a definitive statement until you have laboratory confirmation. It also is best not to make medical statements like "this is your first infection" based on clinical appearance alone because many cases are recurrences from infection years ago [35]. Remember that pronouncements about first infections have medical and psychosocial implications because relationships may be involved intimately in the medical diagnosis. Although you cannot say with certainty from whom a patient acquired the infection, you may be able to help with how long they have had it (see "Special Considerations for HSV").

Anger often is present at the initial visit [34], and questions about fidelity may come up quickly. Patients should be reassured that they could have had this for a long time, or their partner could have been infected for a long time and recently infected them; a third party need not be involved. Encourage patients not to jump to conclusions. If you strongly suspect herpes, transmission should be discussed, at least briefly, at this visit. Patients need to know that they could be infectious between the visit and the time you get the laboratory tests back.

Sometimes patients are so overwhelmed by the diagnosis that they just do not know which questions to ask first. It may be helpful to say: "I know there are so many questions on your mind right now. We can get together again in a few weeks for a follow-up visit, but right now, can you tell me what your biggest concern is?" This will allow a patient to focus and allow you to help them, even in a time-pressured situation. Medicines should be prescribed if new herpes is suspected, without waiting for laboratory results. Waiting for results of a positive culture (an insensitive test) before treatment could prolong a bad outbreak unnecessarily. Because the medicines are activated only by the presence of virus, patients will excrete it if there is no HSV infection.

It is helpful to provide reading materials and a list of good websites. Patients will be hungry for information that you may not have time to give right away. Resources allow them to pursue this learning on their own. Finally, at the first visit, it is worth stating in clear terms that having herpes does not change the core of the patient. It does not make them less worthwhile or "damaged goods." It is a virus, not a judgment. Allow this to sink in and be absorbed between the first visit and the follow-up.

Follow-up visit

Follow-up visits allow you to talk with patients in more depth. Typical topics that come up for discussion include transmission reduction, shedding, how to tell partners about the herpes, self-esteem issues, sexual dysfunction related to transmission concerns, and general anxiety and depression related to the diagnosis of HSV. Dibble and Swanson [36] and Levenson et al [37] found that there were differences in how men and women adjust to herpes and what attitudes predict more depression related to a herpes diagnosis [36,37]. In women, increased anger, decreased vigor, increased confusion, a negative attitude toward herpes, self-concealment, somatization, lack of feeling desirable, and stress symptoms from genital herpes predicted more depression. In men, increased depression was predicted by increased anger, a negative attitude toward herpes, and a decreased willingness to share personal information with a stranger. Patients should be encouraged to share their diagnosis with at least one other person to avoid the isolation that is felt so often with this diagnosis. They often will discover that people that they already know also have herpes, which will provide reassurance that they are not alone with this infection.

Patients often worry that stress is a trigger for recurrences. This can become a vicious cycle because people who worry that having stress will cause outbreaks, potentially produce stress about stress! Rein [38] found that intermittent stress was not a factor in increased recurrences, although persistent stress showed a tendency to precipitate an increased frequency of outbreaks. Two other studies found no relationship between emotional stress and HSV recurrence rates [39,40].

Reinforcement should be given to the concept of continuing self-esteem and self-acceptance [41]. Remind patients that the virus does not do a personality inventory or check the number of past sexual partners that a person has had before it invades a cell. It just invades a cell. Making this concept clear repeatedly may be one of the most effective tools we have for helping people to accept themselves with this infection.

It may be useful to identify a therapist in the community who will talk to patients who have herpes, should the need arise. In addition, herpes support groups are available around the country, with technical support from the American Social Health Association. Locations can be found on their website, www.ashastd.org.

Special considerations for herpes simplex virus

Determining length of infection

Laboratory assays can help to determine how recently an HSV infection was acquired. If a swab is gathered from a lesion (polymerase chain reaction [PCR] or culture) and typed, it can be compared with an antibody result from serum that is drawn on the same day. For example, if a patient has a positive PCR for HSV-2 and a negative antibody test for HSV-2, this is likely (but not absolutely) a first infection—the patient has not had an opportunity to make antibody because the infection is so new [42]. Any other combination of swab and antibody test will not give such clear results about how long someone might have been infected. Questions about source partner may be approached by offering to test sexual partners by serology. If the partner is negative, he or she is an unlikely source of the infection; if the partner is positive, it is possible—although not certain—that the infection came from him or her.

Asymptomatic patients who test positive

What about patients who get a positive blood test for HSV-2 but cannot recall ever having symptoms of genital herpes? For a patient who has subtle symptoms, testing and counseling can be especially complicated. Research shows that people who simply test positive by type-specific IgG blood test but never have had recognized symptoms shed at the same rate, on their asymptomatic days, as those who have recognized infection and up to 12 outbreaks per year [43]. This makes a strong case for testing and identifying those who are infected but do not know it. In this same study, after careful instruction about the subtleties of herpes symptoms, 87% of those who were infected—but identified as asymptomatic—learned to identify a symptom that was consistent with herpes by the end of approximately 3 months of daily home swabbing. Part of the medical counseling that may be most valuable is teaching patients the fine points about how and where herpes symptoms can present. This can turn an asymptomatic, antibody-positive patient into one who recognizes outbreaks or symptoms and can avoid sex during times of high viral shedding. It also can give patients a feeling of power over an infection that previously lived in their body without ever being noticed or recognized.

Asymptomatic shedding

Clinicians may find some patients ask, "How do you know about asymptomatic shedding?" Through a process called daily home swabbing, patients in research studies are taught to swab their genitalia for some extended period of time [43,44]. Early studies used culture to look for viral shedding but newer studies use PCR, a much more sensitive test [45]. People who are newly diagnosed will shed virus often, approximately 40% of the days sampled [46]. Patients, including those who have newer and more established infections, will shed, on average, approximately 11% to 28% of the days swabbed [12,43,47].

Importance of herpes simplex virus counseling

Clinicians can make a significant difference in how people adjust to having this life-long, highly stigmatized STI. When given repeatedly to several different patients, the herpes counseling messages—medical and psychosocial—can be made concise, kind, and fit into a busy day. Patients who have HSV will benefit greatly when time is taken to address these challenging issues.

Genital human papillomavirus infection

Although it is a new field of inquiry by comparison with genital herpes, behavioral and educational aspects of genital HPV infection are now acknowledged as increasingly important, given the emergence of HPV DNA testing as a frequent adjunct to Pap testing and likely development of successful vaccines against several HPV types. The use of HPV tests along with cytology creates an increasing need for clinicians to explain the term "human papillomavirus" in the context of Pap testing. This conversation, in turn, raises questions of how best to manage perceptions of HPV as a "cancer virus" and to manage patient attitudes toward the concept of a chronic, if silent, STI.

The numbers of people who potentially are affected by these considerations are large. Annual prevalence of genital HPV infection in the United States, including high- and low-risk types, is estimated at 6.2 million among 15- to 44-year-olds [48]. Current prevalence is estimated at 20 million, and it is believed that up to 50% to 80% of sexually active adults are exposed to, and infected with, genital HPV at some point [49,50]. Although only a small proportion of these infections become persistent and progress to cervical cancer, in 2002 there were an estimated 13,000 cases of invasive cervical cancer in the United States and 4100 deaths among women older than 20 [51]. Meanwhile, external genital warts (EGWs), which usually are associated with low-risk HPV types 6 and 11, remain one of the leading lesion-causing STIs. The National Disease and Therapeutic Index estimated 264,000 office visits for EGWs in 2003 [52]; an estimated 1% of all HPV infections is believed to result in EGWs [49].

Psychosocial aspects of genital human papillomavirus infection

Several published papers have focused on the psychosocial sequelae of genital HPV, and the topic seems to be one of increasing interest, with several studies ongoing. Historically, behavioral researchers have established that abnormal Pap tests are associated with distress because of anxiety about cancer and the fear that an abnormal test in some way suggests promiscuous or deviant behavior [53,54]. Against this backdrop, the introduction of HPV testing potentially deepens some of these patient concerns about test results. In general, some of the same factors that can complicate a genital herpes diagnosis contribute to potential psychosocial stressors with genital HPV—lack of curative treatment for underlying viral infection, the sexually transmitted nature of the infection and ongoing potential for transmission, and the lack of a highly effective strategy for protecting sexual partners.

Investigators in this field generally find common ground in characterizing an HPV diagnosis as having the potential to provoke emotional reactions, such as anger, shame, or concerns about social isolation [54–56]. One recent article suggests that anxiety, concern, and distress were higher in women who tested positive for HPV than in women who had abnormal Pap test results and that women who had HPV perceived themselves to be at high risk for cancer [57].

A 1996 survey of patients who had genital warts or cervical lesions, by Clarke et al [55], showed that significant percentages of persons with a history of genital HPV had high levels of anxiety about disclosing the information to sexual partners and feared rejection and social isolation as a result of having a potentially chronic viral infection. More than half of respondents expressed worry about being judged negatively by others, and nearly three quarters cited fear of transmitting genital HPV to a sexual partner.

Other investigators also made reference to the potential social stigma of HPV and the potential difficulty of disclosing an HPV diagnosis to partners. In a 2000 study by Keller et al [58], 51% of HPV-positive subjects believed that they should disclose this information to future sexual partners, whereas only 31% actually reported doing so. Similar to a herpes diagnosis, an HPV diagnosis often raises questions about fidelity in established relationships and creates mutual suspicions; a person who tests positive for HPV may consider his or her current partner as the source of infection, whereas the partner may suspect infidelity [59].

Although there is strong suggestion that HPV, like other STIs, carries some degree of social stigma, establishing whether it has a significant impact on sexual behavior and sexual satisfaction has been elusive. In one study, more than two thirds of respondents reported that HPV had a negative initial impact on feelings of sexual desirability and spontaneity [55]. A subsequent study by Reed et al [60] showed no significant effect on sexual impulses or physical intimacy among a group of women who were diagnosed with subclinical HPV based on DNA testing. In addition, Keller et al's [58] disclosure study observed that instances of rejection as a result of disclosure and negative impact on sexual relations are rare.

Linnehan and Groce [56] surveyed college health settings and report that clinicians generally characterize psychosocial issues as the most difficult aspect of management for those who test positive for HPV. These observations are consistent with the reported experience of clinicians in a recent study that focused on the interactions between health care providers and a group of women who were diagnosed with HPV based on DNA testing [61]. Clinicians characterized the patient responses with reference to anger, fear, and a desire to lay blame. Patients frequently raised questions about the source of their HPV infection; wanted more information about the long-term health effects of HPV and required follow-up; and in particular sought clear guidance on HPV's impact on future sexual activity. The health care professionals who were surveyed for the study cited an urgent need for quality educational materials and access to referrals, such as toll-free helplines and other free resources for patients.

Several experts have urged caution in the use of HPV DNA tests because positive test results can have a negative psychosocial impact on patients [57,62,63]. Some specify that clinicians should deliver pretest counseling about HPV as a first step in gaining consent for the use of HPV DNA tests, so that patients are not blind-sided by the issue of sexual transmission [63].

The educational challenge of human papillomavirus

Educational counseling for patients who have HPV poses several challenges to clinicians. The first of these is the comparatively steep learning curve for most patients. In contrast to genital herpes, for which the first barrier to counseling arguably might be patient misperceptions about herpes, for HPV there is likely to be a major gap in awareness. Studies among college students suggest that two thirds of young adults have not heard of HPV, and that many of those who are aware of HPV have low knowledge scores [64,65]. In yet another indication that HPV historically has been low on the radar screen of sex education curricula, a 2003 study that involved several large family planning and university health clinics in south Florida found that only 22% of women who participated in a screening survey had any knowledge of HPV [66]. An additional study by Naoom et al [67] focused on adolescent women and documented, in focus group interviews, that the vast majority had no recall of having learned about HPV in high school sex education or reproductive health classes.

Although HPV may not be a familiar term to most women, increasing press coverage in recent years is making its mark on a segment of the patient population. Here, misperceptions and anxiety come into play as additional challenges. Anhang et al [68] performed a content analysis on 111 news media reports on HPV and found that most took a cervical cancer angle on the story: 36% reported on HPV in a context of new tests for cervical cancer (HPV DNA tests); 30% focused on the HPV–cervical cancer link; and 27% characterized HPV as a STI—the cause of EGWs. Generally, the media reports were not comprehensive in their explanation of genital HPV and frequently left out salient points. Only 26% of the stories, for example, made clear that most HPV-positive women do not get cervical cancer, and only 14% explained that HPV often causes no symptoms. Additionally, the stories on new HPV screening tests omitted content on transmission risk and prevention. Stories that took the sexual transmission angle tended to omit content on cervical cancer screening.

In a parallel study, the same research group conducted focus groups with 48 women to discover how women react to a standard educational brochure on the topic and identify their most pressing educational needs [69]. In general, women tended to overestimate their risk of cancer, and younger women differentiated themselves by focusing on the sexually transmitted nature of HPV, the potential for embarrassing symptoms, and the possible need for disclosure to partners.

Key counseling messages for patients who have human papillomavirus

Several experts and leading reproductive health organizations have developed messages to address the educational needs of patients who are HPV-positive in a variety of clinical scenarios. These include a paper that reflects the top 10 questions of persons who contact the National HPV and Cervical Cancer Prevention Resource Center, operated by the American Social Health Association, along with consensus message points as developed by a national advisory committee of HPV experts [70]. The American Society for Colposcopy and Cervical Pathology also developed a set of educational messages that include HPV testing as an integral part of cervical cancer screening, and the American Cancer Society has tested and published a consumer educational brochure [71,72]. Finally, several journal articles have offered observations on facts that need emphasis to address major areas of confusion and misinformation among women on the topic of genital HPV and cancer risk [59,69].

Taken together, this literature suggests several key points to emphasize in HPV-related counseling:

1. *HPV is a common virus among sexually active adults and can cause various kinds of skin warts.* Among the more than 100 types of HPV, some types affect the genital area. HPV often is present without causing signs or symptoms. Genital HPV is so common that anyone who has had a sexual partner is likely to have been exposed. It is transmitted through skin-to-skin contact, including intercourse.
2. *A healthy immune system almost always suppresses or eliminates HPV infection over a period of time.* It may take some time, but it is important for patients to know that it is still possible to have a normal, healthy life, even with HPV.
3. *Understanding the difference between low-risk and high-risk types of HPV is key.* Among the many types of genital HPV, some may cause minor cells changes, such as warts. These are called "low-risk types." If warts are present, they can be treated in several ways. Other types of HPV can cause the kinds of cell changes on the cervix that usually are detected by Pap tests. These are called "high-risk types" because they increase the risk of cervical cancer. It is important to remember that the overwhelming majority of women who have high-risk types do not develop cervical cancer—or even have abnormal Pap results.
4. *The importance of screening cannot be overlooked.* Cervical cancer can be prevented with regular screening tests and with treatment if abnormal cells become a problem. The Pap test gives important protection by detecting early signs of cervical cancer.
5. *HPV tests play a new role.* Today, to supplement Pap tests, there also are specific tests for common genital HPV types, and it can be helpful to have this information about HPV status. HPV tests are added to Pap

screening in some cases to clarify Pap results and to determine what kind of follow-up is needed. In women who are 30 and older, HPV tests are approved as a routine test to be done along with Pap tests.
6. *Determining the source of infection is not straightforward.* Most sexually active persons acquire genital HPV at some point, and the virus may be present for long periods of time without causing signs or symptoms. Most individuals who have HPV do not know that they are infected. Therefore, it is impossible, in most cases, to know when and from whom a person became infected. It should not be assumed that a current partner is the source of infection.
7. *Address issues of risk reduction among partners.* Transmission to partners is difficult to prevent, short of abstinence. When HPV is diagnosed in persons who are in long-term relationships, the odds are good that the current partner already has the same HPV types and has developed immunity to those types. Condoms do not offer complete protection, but they can reduce the risk of EGWs and cervical abnormalities.
8. *Genital HPV infection rarely affects fertility.* When cervical lesions require treatment, most often the treatment leaves the cervix sufficiently intact to preserve fertility. During pregnancy, warts and HPV lesions may grow faster, and warts may require removal. Only in rare cases is HPV passed from mother to child, and a history of HPV does not indicate the need for a Cesarean section or other special procedures.

Special considerations for human papillomavirus

The underlying challenge of providing HPV-related educational counseling is one of balancing the need to provide key information with the potential for creating unwarranted feelings of distress. Several of the studies that were mentioned here emphasize the tendency for persons who test positive for HPV to overestimate their risk of cancer. In addition, the focus group study by Anhang et al [68] emphasized the desire of female subjects to receive educational counseling that is tailored to their specific risks. The suggestion that is implicit here is that even the best educational materials likely will leave the individual with the specific question of "What does this mean for me?"

Clinicians also are cautioned to review carefully the content of educational materials that are provided to patients. A review of such resources by Brandt et al in 2003 [73] revealed that most were deficient, either in providing adequate content on HPV or in delivering information effectively at an appropriate reading level. Several publishers, including those cited here [70–72], have developed or updated their materials since the U.S. Food and Drug Administration approval of the combination DNA-Pap as a primary screen in women who are 30 and older. The latest generation of educational tools attempts to explain HPV testing to readers as a routine part of cervical cancer screening and provide a basic explanation of HPV without using emotional or stigmatizing language.

External genital warts

Patient concerns with EGWs often are similar to those with cervical HPV infection. Important messages to impart to patients who have EGWs include the following:

Genital warts almost always are associated with "low-risk," non-oncogenic HPV types. Warts do not increase cancer risk, and need not change the frequency of Pap testing [74].

A current partner is likely to have HPV infection already, even if he or she does not exhibit symptoms. It is not necessary for the partner to be seen by the clinician, although this may have educational or clinical value in some cases [74].

Treatment alone may not eliminate all risk of transmission. Duration of infectivity is not known; however, the use of latex condoms may help to reduce the risk of HPV-associated disease, including genital warts in men and cervical cancer in women [74,75].

Partners

With reference to the questions of infidelity that were cited earlier in this article, patients will benefit from understanding that the incubation period of HPV is uncertain and an HPV diagnosis does not necessarily mean that either partner has been unfaithful. Disclosure to partners can be challenging, and patients who are well-informed and able to put HPV in perspective are likely to feel more competent to communicate well with partners [76].

Pregnancy

Women often have questions about the potential impact of HPV infection on pregnancy, and it is important to provide reassurance about EGWs and cervical HPV infection. Cesarean section is not recommended for women who have genital warts unless the warts threaten to obstruct the birth canal or cause excessive bleeding at the time of labor [74]. As with EGWs, transmission to the newborn is rare. Cesarean section is not recommended for a woman because of cervical cell changes.

Summary

Educational counseling has an important role in managing patients who have viral STIs, such as genital herpes and genital HPV infections. Given the lack of a curative therapy for both, patients may require long-term management and may need to be attentive to recurring symptoms. In addition, both diagnoses may raise issues of persisting infectiousness along with a need for patient counseling about the potential risk to partners and risk reduction strategies. Lastly, dozens of published papers over the years describe potential psychosocial sequelae for patients who have genital herpes, and there is a growing psychosocial literature on genital HPV as well. Clinicians can make a significant difference in patient adjustment to the diagnosis of an STI, and addressing these challenging issues will benefit patients greatly.

References

[1] Fleming DT, McQuillan GM, Johnson RE, et al. Herpes simplex virus type 2 in the United States, 1976 to 1994. N Engl J Med 1997;337(16):1105–11.
[2] Leone P, Fleming DT, Gilsenan AW, et al. Seroprevalence of herpes simplex virus-2 in suburban primary care offices in the United States. Sex Transm Dis 2004;31(5):311–6.
[3] Gilbert LP, Schulz SL, Ebel C. Education and counselling for genital herpes: perspectives from patients. Herpes 2002;9(3):78–82.
[4] Engelberg R, Carrell D, Krantz E, et al. Natural history of genital herpes simplex virus type 1 infection. Sex Transm Dis 2003;30(2):174–7.
[5] Wald A, Zeh J, Selke S, et al. Virologic characteristics of subclinical and symptomatic genital herpes infections. N Engl J Med 1995;333:770–5.
[6] Wald A, Ericsson M, Krantz E, et al. Oral shedding of herpes simplex virus type 2. Sex Transm Infect 2004;80(4):272–6.
[7] Benedetti J, Zeh J, Corey L. Clinical reactivation of genital herpes simplex virus infection decreases in frequency over time. Ann Intern Med 1999;131(1):14–20.
[8] Mertz GJ, Benedetti J, Ashley R, et al. Risk factors for the sexual transmission of genital herpes. Ann Intern Med 1992;116(3):197–202.
[9] Reitano M, Tyring S, Lang W, et al. Valaciclovir for the suppression of recurrent genital herpes simplex virus infection: a large-scale dose range-finding study. J Infect Dis 1998; 178(3):603–10.
[10] Sacks SL. Famciclovir suppression of asymptomatic and symptomatic recurrent anogenital herpes simplex virus shedding in women: a randomized, double-blind, double-dummy, placebo-controlled, parallel-group, single-center trial. J Infect Dis 2004;189(8):1341–7.
[11] Romanowski B, Marina RB, Roberts JN. Valtrex HS230017 Study Group. Patients' preference of valacyclovir once-daily suppressive therapy versus twice-daily episodic therapy for recurrent genital herpes: a randomized study. Sex Transm Dis 2003;30(3):226–31.
[12] Corey L, Wald A, Patel R, et al. Valacyclovir HSV Transmission Study Group. Once-daily valacyclovir to reduce the risk of transmission of genital herpes. N Engl J Med 2004;350(1): 11–20.
[13] ACOG Practice Bulletin. Clinical management guidelines for obstetrician-gynecologists, number 57, November 2004. Gynecologic herpes simplex virus infections. Obstet Gynecol 2004;104(5 Pt 1):1111–8.
[14] Wald A, Langenberg A, Link K, et al. Effect of condoms on reducing the transmission of herpes simplex virus type 2 from men to women. JAMA 2001;285(24):3100–6.
[15] Casper C, Wald A. Condom use and the prevention of genital herpes acquisition. Herpes 2002;9(1):10–4.
[16] Brentjens M, Yeung-Yue K, Lee PC, et al. Recurrent genital herpes treatments and their impact on quality of life. Pharmacoeconomics 2003;21(12):853–63.

[17] Carney O, Ross E, Bunker C, et al. A prospective study of the psychological impact on patients with a first episode of genital herpes. Genitourin Med 1994;70(1):40–5.
[18] Carney O, Ross E, Ikkos G, et al. The effect of suppressive oral acyclovir on the psychological morbidity associated with recurrent genital herpes. Genitourin Med 1993; 69(6):457–9.
[19] Tyring SK, Baker D, Snowden W. Valacyclovir for herpes simplex virus infection: long-term safety and sustained efficacy after 20 years' experience with acyclovir. J Infect Dis 2002; 186(Suppl 1):S40–6.
[20] Brown ZA, Wald A, Morrow RA, et al. Effect of serologic status and cesarean delivery on transmission rates of herpes simplex virus from mother to infant. JAMA 2003;289(2): 203–9.
[21] Song B, Dwyer DE, Mindel A. HSV type specific serology in sexual health clinics: use, benefits, and who gets tested. Sex Transm Infect 2004;80(2):113–7.
[22] Ashley RL. Sorting out the new HSV type specific antibody tests. Sex Transm Infect 2001; 77(4):232–7.
[23] Sucato G, Wald A, Wakabayashi E, et al. Evidence of latency and reactivation of both herpes simplex virus (HSV)-1 and HSV-2 in the genital region. J Infect Dis 1998;177(4): 1069–72.
[24] Brown Z, Selke S, Zeh J, et al. The acquisition of herpes simplex virus during pregnancy. N Engl J Med 1997;337(8):509–15.
[25] Roberts CM, Pfister JR, Spear SJ. Increasing proportion of herpes simplex virus type 1 as a cause of genital herpes infection in college students. Sex Transm Dis 2003;30(10): 797–800.
[26] Lafferty WE, Downey L, Celum C, et al. Herpes simplex virus type 1 as a cause of genital herpes: impact on surveillance and prevention. J Infect Dis 2000;181(4):1454–7.
[27] da Silva L, Guimaraes A, Victoria J, et al. Herpes simplex virus type 1 shedding in the oral cavity of seropositive patients. Oral Dis 2005;11(1):13–6.
[28] Blower S, Ma L. Calculating the contribution of herpes simplex virus type 2 epidemics to increasing HIV incidence: treatment implications. Clin Infect Dis 2004;39(Suppl 5): S240–7.
[29] Freedman E, Mindel A. Epidemiology of herpes and HIV co-infection. J HIV Ther 2004; 9(1):4–8.
[30] Celum C, Levine R, Weaver M, et al. Genital herpes and human immunodeficiency virus: double trouble. Bull World Health Organ 2004;82(6):447–53.
[31] Celum CL, Robinson NJ, Cohen MS. Potential effect of HIV type 1 antiretroviral and herpes simplex virus type 2 antiviral therapy on transmission and acquisition of HIV type 1 infection. J Infect Dis 2005;191(Suppl 1):S107–14.
[32] Corey L, Wald A, Celum CL, et al. The effects of herpes simplex virus-2 on HIV-1 acquisition and transmission: a review of two overlapping epidemics. J Acquir Immune Defic Syndr 2004;35(5):435–45.
[33] Watts D, Brown Z, Money D, et al. A double-blind, randomized, placebo-controlled trial of acyclovir in late pregnancy for the reduction of herpes simplex virus shedding and cesarean delivery. Am J Obstet Gynecol 2003;188(3):836–43.
[34] Melville J, Sniffen S, Crosby R, et al. Psychosocial impact of serological diagnosis of herpes simplex virus type 2: a qualitative assessment. Sex Transm Infect 2003;79(4):280–5.
[35] Diamond C, Selke S, Ashley R, et al. Clinical course of patients with serologic evidence of recurrent genital herpes presenting with signs and symptoms of first episode disease. Sex Transm Dis 1999;26(4):221–5.
[36] Dibble SL, Swanson JM. Gender differences for the predictors of depression in young adults with genital herpes. Public Health Nurs 2000;17(3):187–94.
[37] Levenson JL, Hamer RM, Myers T, et al. Psychological factors predict symptoms of severe recurrent genital herpes infection. Psychosom Res 1987;31(2):153–9.
[38] Rein M. Stress and genital herpes recurrences in women. JAMA 2000;283(11):1394.

[39] Rand KH, Hoon EF, Massey JK, et al. Daily stress and recurrence of genital herpes simplex. Arch Intern Med 1990;150(9):1889–93.
[40] Hoon EF, Hoon PW, Rand KH, et al. A psycho-behavioral model of genital herpes recurrence. Psychosom Res 1991;35(1):25–36.
[41] Nack A. Damaged goods: women managing the stigma of STDs. Deviant Behav 2000;21(2): 95–121.
[42] Langenberg AG, Corey L, Ashley RL, et al. A prospective study of new infections with herpes simplex virus type 1 and type 2. Chiron HSV Vaccine Study Group. N Engl J Med 1999;341(19):1432–8.
[43] Wald A, Zeh J, Selke S, et al. Reactivation of genital herpes simplex virus type 2 infections in asymptomatic seropositive persons. N Engl J Med 2000;342(12):844–50.
[44] Sacks S, Griffiths P, Corey L, et al. HSV shedding. Antiviral Res 2004;63(Suppl 1):S19–26.
[45] Wald A, Huang M, Carrell D, et al. Polymerase chain reaction for detection of herpes simplex virus (HSV) DNA on mucosal surfaces: comparison with HSV isolation in cell culture. J Infect Dis 2003;188(9):1345–51.
[46] Gupta R, Wald A, Krantz E, et al. Valacyclovir and acyclovir for suppression of shedding of herpes simplex virus in the genital tract. J Infect Dis 2004;190(8):1374–81.
[47] Wald A, Corey L, Cone R, et al. Frequent genital herpes simplex virus 2 shedding in immunocompetent women: effect of acyclovir treatment. J Clin Invest 1997;99(5):1092–5.
[48] Weinstock H, Berman S, Cates W Jr. Sexually transmitted diseases among American youth: incidence and prevalence estimates, 2000. Perspect Sex Reprod Health 2004;36(1):6–10.
[49] Koutsky L. Epidemiology of genital human papillomavirus infection. Am J Med 1997; 102(5A):3–8.
[50] Jenkins D, Sherlaw-Johnson C, Gallivan S. Can papilloma virus testing be used to improve cervical cancer screening? Int J Cancer 1996;65(6):763–73.
[51] Wright TC Jr, Schiffman M, Solomon D, et al. Interim guidance for the use of human papillomavirus DNA testing as an adjunct to cervical cytology for screening. Obstet Gynecol 2004;103(2):304–9.
[52] Centers for Disease Control and Prevention. Sexually transmitted disease surveillance 2003. Atlanta (GA): U.S. Department of Health and Human Services; 2003.
[53] Campion MJ, Brown JR, McCance DJ, et al. Psychosexual trauma of an abnormal pap smear. Br J Obstet Gynaecol 1988;95(2):175–81.
[54] Waller J, McCaffery KJ, Forrest S, et al. Human papillomavirus and cervical cancer: issues for biobehavioral and psychosocial research. Ann Behav Med 2004;27(1):68–79.
[55] Clarke P, Ebel C, Catotti DN, et al. The psychosocial impact of human papillomavirus infection: implications for health care providers. Int J STD AIDS 1996;7:197–200.
[56] Linnehan M, Groce NE. Psychosocial and educational services for female college students with genital human papillomavirus infection. Fam Plann Perspect 1999;31(3):137–41.
[57] Maissi E, Marteau TM, Hankins M, et al. Psychological impact of human papillomavirus testing in women with borderline or mildly dyskaryotic cervical smear test results: cross sectional questionnaire study. BMJ 2004;328(7451):1293–9.
[58] Keller M, von Sadovszky V, Pankratz B, et al. Self-disclosure of HPV infection to sexual partners. West J Nurs Res 2000;22(3):285–302.
[59] Monk B, Wiley DJ. Human papillomavirus infections: truth or consequences. Cancer 2004; 100(2):225–7.
[60] Reed B, Ruffin MT IV, Gorenflo DW, et al. The psychosexual impact of human papillomavirus cervical infections. J Fam Pract 1999;48(2):110–6.
[61] Brandt H, Sharpe PA, Abbott JM, et al. Health care providers' interactions with women who have human papillomavirus (HPV). Presented at the 131st Annual Meeting of the American Public Health Association. San Francisco, November 15–19, 2003.
[62] Helmerhorst TJM, Meijer CJLM. Cervical cancer should be considered as a rare complication of oncogenic HPV infection rather than a STD. Int J Gynecol Cancer 2002; 12:235–6.

[63] Harper D. Why am I scared of HPV? CA Cancer J Clin 2004;54(5):245–7.
[64] Baer H, Allen S, Braun L. Knowledge of human papillomavirus infection among young adult men and women: implications for health education and research. J Community Health 2000;25(1):67–78.
[65] Yacobi E, Tennant C, Ferrante J, et al. University students' knowledge and awareness of HPV. Prev Med 1999;28(6):535–41.
[66] Packing-Ebuen J, Rayko H, Wallace F, et al. Lack of HPV knowledge: what women don't know could hurt them... Presented at the 131st Annual Meeting of the American Public Health Association. San Francisco, November 15–19, 2003.
[67] Naoom S, Buie ME, Daley E, et al. HPV: adolescents at risk for a potentially life threatening disease. Presented at the 131st Annual Meeting of the American Public Health Association. San Francisco, November 15–19, 2003.
[68] Anhang R, Stryker JE, Wright TC Jr, et al. News media coverage of human papillomavirus. Cancer 2004;100(2):308–14.
[69] Anhang R, Wright TC Jr, Smock L, et al. Women's desired information about human papillomavirus. Cancer 2004;100(2):315–20.
[70] Gilbert L, Alexander L, Grosshans JF, et al. Answering frequently asked questions about HPV. Sex Transm Dis 2003;30(3):193–4.
[71] American Cancer Society. What women should know about HPV and cervical health. 2003. Available at: http://www.cancer.org/docroot/NWS/content/NWS_2_1x_What_Women_Should_Know_about_HPV_and_Cervical_Health.asp. Accessed December 14, 2004.
[72] American Society for Colposcopy and Cervical Pathology. What women should know about HPV and cervical health. 2004. Available at: http://www.asccp.org/pdfs/patient_edu/women_should_know.pdf. Accessed December 2, 2004.
[73] Brandt H, McCree DH, Lindley LL, et al. A formal evaluation of existing printed HPV educational materials. Presented at the 131st Annual Meeting of the American Public Health Association, San Francisco, CA, November 15–19, 2003.
[74] Centers for Disease Control and Prevention. Sexually transmitted diseases treatment guidelines 2002. MMWR 2002;51(No. RR-6):53–9.
[75] National Institutes of Health. Workshop summary: scientific evidence on condom effectiveness for sexually transmitted disease (STD) prevention. Bethesda (MD): U.S. Department of Health and Human Services; 2001.
[76] Reitano M. Counseling patients with genital warts. Am J Med 1997;102(5A):38–43.

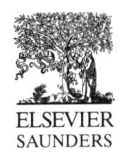

Progress in Vaccines for Sexually Transmitted Diseases

Lawrence R. Stanberry, MD, PhD*, Susan L. Rosenthal, PhD

Department of Pediatrics and the Sealy Center for Vaccine Development, University of Texas Medical Branch, Children's Hospital, 301 University Boulevard, Galveston, TX 77555, USA

Although treatment affords some control of the ongoing sexually transmitted infection (STI) epidemic, the high prevalence of asymptomatic STIs and the chronic/persistent nature of some STIs (eg, human immunodeficiency virus, herpes simplex virus, human papillomavirus) point to the need for prevention. Bacterial STIs can cause end-organ damage, such as pelvic inflammatory disease, without significant symptoms, further supporting the need for primary prevention. Potential prevention strategies include abstinence or delaying sexual initiation, conscientious partner selection, use of condoms, antiviral suppression, and the use of microbicides and vaccines. Vaccines are attractive because durable protection would be expected following completion of the immunization regimen, whereas other strategies require consistent use or implementation. Furthermore, vaccines have the potential to afford indirect protection to those who are unimmunized through community immunity, but widespread uptake will be needed to impact the epidemic spread of STIs. This review discusses the progress toward vaccine development for *Chlamydia trachomatis, Neisseria gonorrhoeae*, human papillomavirus, and herpes simplex virus.

Financial support: National Institute of Health Grants #HD40151; # AI52372.

Conflicts of interest: L.R. Stanberry—recent research funding, GlaxoSmithKline; consultant, GlaxoSmithKline, Novartis, NanoBio; speakers' bureau, Novartis. S.L. Rosenthal—recent research funding, GlaxoSmithKline, Novartis, Merck; consultant, GlaxoSmithKline, Merck.

* Corresponding author.
E-mail address: l.stanberry@utmb.edu (L.R. Stanberry).

Chlamydia trachomatis

Chlamydia vaccine development began in the 1950s with research on inactivated whole cell preparations intended for the control of ocular trachoma. These trials established that the protection afforded by the vaccine was specific for the strain of chlamydia used in preparing the product, and antigens contained in the whole cell preparations induced immunopathologic responses when breakthrough infection occurred. Human trials of the whole cell vaccines were discontinued because of limited protection and significant safety concerns. Experience with the whole cell vaccines led to the concept that a safe and effective chlamydia vaccine would need to contain protective antigens but be free of antigens that engendered immunopathologic responses [1]. Therefore, the focus shifted to the development of subunit vaccines.

A few subunit candidates have been proposed that parallel the increased knowledge of the organism. Most work has centered on the major outer membrane protein (MOMP), but animal model studies indicate that MOMP vaccines do not afford sufficient protection [2,3]. Various other known and putative outer membrane proteins (OMP), including cysteine-rich OMP2 and OMP3, are being evaluated as subunit antigens [1,4]. Other subunits have also been proposed, including chlamydia heat shock proteins (HSPs) [5], the cytidine triphosphate synthetase [6], *crpA* [7], and an exoglycolipid [8]. Immune responses to chlamydial HSP-60 antigen have been detected in patients who have chlamydial pelvic inflammatory disease. Because the protein is similar to the human homolog, it has been hypothesized that molecular mimicry may result in autoimmune inflammatory damage that contributes to chlamydial pathogenesis [9]. The chlamydia trachomatis genome encodes over 900 proteins, thus it is likely that many new candidate antigens will be identified in the future.

In addition to the search for new antigens, some research has also explored new means of delivering subunits, including DNA vaccines [6] and vector systems such as Vibrio cholerae ghosts and lactobacillus mutants [4,10].

No reported clinical trials of Chlamydia vaccines are currently ongoing. Of the big four vaccine companies (GlaxoSmithKline, Wyeth, Merck, and Sanofi Pasteur) only Sanofi Pasteur has publicly identified chlamydia as one of their long-term targets for vaccine development.

Neisseria gonorrhoeae

The development of a vaccine against gonorrhea has been hampered by a limited understanding of what constitutes protective immunity and the lack of an animal model [11,12]. A human male urethral gonococcal challenge model has been developed and used to examine protection against mucosal infection. However, this model is not useful in assessing the ability of a vaccine to protect against upper genital tract infection and disease such as pelvic inflammatory disease [13]. Multistrain variability and the potential for gonococcal infection to cause immunosuppression that result in a weak pathogen-specific immune response of short duration may contribute to the capability of the gonococcus to cause repeated infections. Multistrain variability must be considered in vaccine development to ensure that the proteins selected will afford protection against diverse gonococcal strains [14]. One immune evasion strategy may be the induction of antibodies to the reduction-modifiable protein (Rmp) that blocks the function of bactericidal antiporin antibodies [15]. Currently, research is focused on transferrin binding; pilin and porin proteins; the discovery of new antigens; and development of strategies for delivering subunits that are free of contaminating Rmp protein [16–18]. There are no candidates currently in clinical trials, although Sanofi-Pasteur has identified gonococcal vaccines as a target for long-term vaccine development.

Human papillomavirus

There are over 30 human papillomaviruses (HPVs) known to infect the human genital tract. HPVs are responsible for anogenital warts, cervical and anal dysplasia, and associated cervical, anal, and penile cancers. The greatest public health burden of HPV infection is cervical cancer, which is a leading cause of mortality among women in developing countries. The annual cost of Papanicolaou testing and treatment for cervical dysplasia is in excess of $3.5 billion in the United States [19]. Because HPVs can establish persistent infections, there are efforts to develop vaccines to treat chronically infected patients (therapeutic vaccines) and vaccines to protect individuals from becoming infected or establishing a persistent infection (prophylactic vaccines). Antibody-mediated immunity seems to be important in affording protection against initial infection (prophylaxis); however, robust cell-mediated immunity is probably required to ensure long-term protection and is critical for therapeutic vaccines [20].

Only limited amounts of some HPVs can be grown using specialized tissue culture systems, making it difficult to develop vaccines using traditional methods. The advent of molecular biologic techniques has made the development of HPV-subunit and -vectored vaccines feasible. HPVs contain a small circular DNA genome that encodes only six early (E) and two late (L) proteins. E1 and E2 proteins are involved in viral DNA replication; E4 and E5 proteins are involved in amplification of the viral genome in the upper layers of the epithelium; E6 and E7 proteins of high-risk HPV types are involved in oncogenic transformation; and L1 and L2 proteins form the viral capsid. The L proteins are capable of self-assembly into empty capsids referred to as virus-like particles (VLPs) that lack the HPV viral genome and hence are incapable of causing infection. The VLPs are immunogenic, which makes them attractive vaccine candidates; however, because they are type-specific vaccines, they must include various strain-specific VLPs to provide broad protection. The E6 and E7 genes are expressed in high-grade dysplastic lesions and cancer, making their gene products likely therapeutic vaccine antigens.

There is much current interest in developing therapeutic vaccines that target the treatment of dysplasia, HPV-associated cancers, and anogenital warts. Because of their role in malignant transformation, HPV E6 and E7 gene products have been the primary candidates in therapeutic vaccines targeting dysplasia and cancer. Strategies discussed later include subunit vaccines containing potent adjuvants, live vaccinia virus engineered to express HPV gene products, and novel approaches such as HSP–HPV peptide vaccines and autologous dendritic cell vaccines.

Most therapeutic vaccine trials have focused on dysplasia and neoplasia. A therapeutic vaccine consisting of a mutated HPV-16 E7 protein expressed as a fusion product with a portion of the *Haemophilus influenzae* B protein D, and combined with an adjuvant system containing monophosphoryl lipid A (MPL) plus the saponin extract QS21, was evaluated in a few women who had HPV-16–positive cervical intraepithelial neoplastic (CIN) lesions. The vaccine, developed by GlaxoSmithKline, enhanced humoral and cell-mediated immunity, but there was no clinical response [21,22]. A live vectored vaccine consisting of modified vaccinia Ankara (MVA)–HPV E2 was evaluated in 36 women who had CIN lesions. The vaccine, administered by direct intrauterine injection weekly for 6 weeks, was immunogenic and the presence of cytotoxic T-lymphocyte activity correlated with regression of precancerous lesions [23]. Xenova has developed two products focused on neoplasia, TA-HPV, a vaccinia construct expressing HPV-16 and -18 E6/E7, and TA-CIN, a recombinant fusion protein consisting of HPV-16 L2/E6/E7. Studies of TA-HPV in women who had vulvar and vaginal intraepithelial neoplasia showed the vaccine induced humoral and T-cell immunity and a reduction in lesion size [24,25]. Twenty-nine women who had high-grade anogenital intraepithelial neoplasia were treated with a regimen consisting of three injections of TA-CIN at 4-week intervals followed by a single administration of TA-HPV by dermal scarification. The regimen increased TA-CIN–specific T-cell proliferative responses and γ-interferon–producing lymphocytes, but no clear clinical benefit was noted. Although six patients demonstrated some clinical response, there was no relationship between observed immunologic responses and clinical outcome [26]. Stressgen Biotechnologies has developed a vaccine consisting of HPV E7 covalently linked to a HSP. The company announced in November 2004 that a trial of its candidate vaccine HspE7 produced a 40% response rate among 21 women who had high grade cervical dysplasia [27]. German investigators evaluated a vaccine consisting of autologous monocyte-derived dendritic cells pulsed with recombinant HPV-16 or HPV-18 E7 in 15 stage IV patients who had cervical cancer [28]. The vaccine induced T-cell responses in 4 of 11 subjects, but no objective clinical response was observed. Another phase 1/2 trial by Kaufmann and colleagues evaluated an HPV-16 L1E7 chimeric VLP vaccine in patients who had CIN II/III [29]. Histologic responses were seen in 50% of the vaccine recipients and 15% of the placebo recipients. The current surgical approach to the management of early-stage HPV-associated CIN has high cure rates. To be an acceptable alternative to surgery, therapeutic vaccines will need to produce higher rates of cure than clinical trials have. Therefore, further development of this approach will be necessary before these vaccines become available to clinicians.

There has only been one reported study of a therapeutic vaccine targeting the treatment of anogenital warts. Xenova developed TA-GW, an HPV-6 L2/E7 fusion protein, which was investigated in an open-label study of 27 men who had genital warts. The study showed that the vaccine induced humoral responses in all subjects and lymphoproliferative responses in 19 of 25. Only five subjects cleared their warts within 8 weeks of completing the immunization regimen [30].

Prophylactic HPV vaccines are another matter. Three groups have advanced studies of prophylactic HPV vaccines. A vaccine consisting of HPV-16 L1 VLPs developed by Merck is being evaluated in a double-blind trial involving nearly 2400 women randomized to receive either placebo or 40 μg of HPV-16 VLPs given at day 0, month 2, and month 6. The outcome measures include the incidence of persistent HPV-16 infection, the incidence of acute HPV-16 infection, and the incidence of cervical intraepithelial neoplasia. The incidence of persistent HPV-16 infection was 3.8 per 100 woman-years at risk in the placebo group and 0 per 100 woman-years at risk in the vaccine group during a mean follow-up of 17.4 months [31]. There were 111 cases of incident HPV-16 infection in placebo recipients and seven cases in subjects who were vaccinated during the 48 month follow-up period (vaccine efficacy 94%, 95% CI, 88%–98%). There were 12 cases of HPV-16–related CIN II/III (6 CIN II and 6 CIN III) among the placebo recipients and none among the vaccinated subjects (vaccine efficacy 100%, 95% CI, 65%–100%) [32]. HPV-16 antibody titers were greatest at month 7 (geometric mean titer [GMT] 1519 mMu/mL), fell during month 18 (GMT 202 mMu/mL), and then stabilized during the remainder of the study (GMTs at months 30 and 48 ranged from 28–150 milli Merck units (mMu)/mL) [31,32]. The initial trial investigated a monovalent HPV-16 vaccine, but Merck is currently developing a quadrivalent vaccine containing HPV-6, -11, -16, and -18 VLPs.

GlaxoSmithKline has evaluated a bivalent HPV-16/18 VLP vaccine in a trial involving 1113 women. The vaccine was highly efficacious in preventing incident and persistent infections in fully immunized volunteers. The vaccine was also efficacious in preventing HPV-16– or -18–associated cytologic abnormalities with a vaccine efficacy of 93.5% (95% CI, 51.3%–99.1%). The vaccine was immunogenic and peak antibody titers were over 80 and 100 times greater than those seen in natural HPV-18 and -16 infections, respectively, and even at month 18, the titers were still 10 and 16 times greater than seen with natural HPV-16 and -18 infections, respectively [33].

A recombinant HPV-16 L1 VLP vaccine developed by the National Cancer Institute has been evaluated in phase 1/2 trials. The vaccine was evaluated most recently in a placebo-controlled phase 2 trial involving 220 healthy female volunteers in which the vaccine was shown to induce robust B- and T-cell responses, including strong proliferative and cytokine responses [34,35].

There have been important advances in the development of therapeutic and prophylactic HPV vaccines. Although highly effective therapeutic vaccines may be many years off, recent trials have provided evidence demonstrating proof of the concept. The results of the prophylactic HPV vaccine trials are exciting and provide evidence that vaccines can protect against mucosal infection by STIs. Given the accelerated pace of development, it is likely that Merck and GlaxoSmithKline will have licensed multivalent HPV vaccines within the next few years. It is likely that these vaccines will reduce the need for colposcopy, biopsy, and treatment, but probably will not reduce the need for Papanicolaou testing programs [19]. Trials are also underway to assess the prophylactic efficacy of HPV vaccines in men. Widespread use by both sexes will be important for maximum public health impact.

Herpes simplex virus

Genital herpes may be caused by either herpes simplex virus type 1 (HSV-1) or type 2 (HSV-2). These viruses differ in their genetic and antigenic make-up, but both viruses have a 152-kilobase double-stranded DNA genome that encodes at least 80 gene products, and because of the extensive conservation of B-cell and T-cell epitopes between the two viruses, it is believed that immune responses engendered by proteins from either virus will likely protect against infection or disease caused by the other virus. Antibody responses are predominantly directed at the major envelope glycoproteins B, D, and H/L, and these responses tend to have cross-reactivity with the heterologous virus. However, type-specific B-cell epitopes have been defined on glycoproteins B, D, C, and G, and type-specific T-cell epitopes have been defined on several structural and regulatory proteins, including VP16 and ICP27 [36].

Because HSV establishes latent infection, and periodically reactivates to cause recurrent infections, there have been attempts to make prophylactic and therapeutic vaccines. As HSV-1 is a common cause of genital infection, prophylactic vaccines will need to protect against HSV-1 and HSV-2 infections. However, HSV-1 does not have the same capacity to reactivate from sacral ganglia, as HSV-2 recurrent genital HSV-1 infections are uncommon; therefore, therapeutic HSV vaccines mainly target recurrent HSV-2 genital infections. During the past 15 years, commercial development has focused on the following strategies: subunit glycoprotein vaccines; genetically modified live virus; replication-impaired mutants; DNA-based products; and vectored vaccines. Two HSV glycoproteins, gB and gD, were selected as vaccine antigens. These proteins were known to induce neutralizing antibody responses [37] and to have prophylactic and therapeutic activity in animal models [38–41].

Two subunit vaccines developed by Chiron have been evaluated as therapeutic products. The first vaccine, containing recombinant truncated HSV-2 gD (gD2) adsorbed to alum, was tested in volunteers who had frequently recurring genital herpes. Although the vaccine was only modestly effective in reducing the number of episodes of recurrent disease, this study was the first to provide objective evidence supporting the concept of therapeutic vaccination for controlling persistent viral infections [42]. The second vaccine contained recombinant HSV-2 gD2 and gB2 with MF59, an adjuvant consisting of squalene, polysorbate 80, and sorbitan trioleate. Unfortunately, this vaccine was shown to be ineffective in the treatment of recurrent genital herpes [43].

Cantab (Xenova) developed a replication-impaired viral vaccine by deleting the gene that encodes for a protein (gH) that is essential for viral replication [44]. When the modified virus infects a host cell, the replication cycle of a modified virus proceeds to a point where the missing gene product is required. The vaccine TA-HSV-2 was immunogenic in phase 1 studies, but failed in a phase 2 trial involving 483 patients who had frequently recurring genital herpes [45]. The further development of TA-HSV-2 as a therapeutic vaccine is not planned.

The Theraherp vaccine developed by AuRx consists of a replication-competent HSV-2 virus stripped of the ICP10 protein kinase domain. This virus is capable of replicating, but is less virulent because of the deletion. The vaccine was evaluated in a clinical trial in Mexico involving subjects who had a minimum of five documented herpetic recurrences in the previous year. The vaccine reportedly reduced the number and durations of recurrences [46].

PowderMed has a DNA-based therapeutic HSV vaccine containing a plasmid (pPJV7630) that encodes the HSV-2 ICP0, ICP4, ICP22 and ICP27 antigens. The plasmid is precipitated onto the surface of gold particles 1 to 3 μm in diameter and is administered by ballistic delivery. The vaccine has been shown to be immunogenic in mice, and a phase 1 safety and immunogenicity trial involving 36 volunteers was initiated in October 2004 [47].

Antigenics is developing HSP–based therapeutic vaccines. Cellular HSPs have numerous chaperone functions, including antigen delivery to antigen-presenting cells. The Antigenics AG-702 vaccine consists of HSP complexed to a single immunogenic HSV-2 peptide. AG-702 is being evaluated in a dose-escalation phase 1 trial involving 40 subjects. The evaluation of a second generation vaccine, AG-707, which contains multiple synthetic peptides representing numerous immunogenic HSV-2 proteins, will proceed following the AG-702 proof of principle trial [48].

In the area of prophylactic vaccines, only two recombinant subunit vaccines have advanced to phase 3 clinical evaluation. The first, developed by

Chiron, consisted of recombinant truncated HSV-2 gB and gD with MF59. Two phase 3 studies were conducted: the first enrolled 531 HSV-2 seronegative cohorts who had HSV-2 genital herpes (ie, discordant couples), and the second recruited 1862 volunteers from sexually transmitted disease clinics (ie, high-risk persons). The primary outcome measure of the trials was prevention of infection, an outcome that had not been demonstrated in preclinical animal studies [49]. The vaccine was shown to be ineffective, although post-hoc analysis suggested differences owing to gender (efficacy in women 26%, 95% CI, −29%–58% compared with efficacy in men −4%, 95% CI, −64%–34%) [50]. Work on the vaccine was halted because of failure to demonstrate efficacy.

The second vaccine, developed by GlaxoSmithKline Biologicals, contained recombinant truncated HSV-2 gD and alum combined with the adjuvant 3-de-0-acylated monophosphoryl lipid A (MPL). The vaccine was evaluated in two phase 3 trials. The primary outcome measure of these trials was the prevention of symptomatic genital herpes, with prevention of infection being a secondary outcome measure. The first enrolled 847 HSV-1 and HSV-2 seronegative cohorts who were infected with HSV-2, and the second enrolled 1867 HSV-2 seronegative cohorts who were infected with HSV-2. Both studies demonstrated that the vaccine had an efficacy of 73% to 74% against acquisition of genital HSV-2 disease in HSV seronegative women, but afforded no protection in men or HSV-1–seropositive women [51]. The reasons why the GlaxoSmithKline vaccine worked and the Chiron vaccine did not are uncertain, but might relate to differences in the adjuvant.

Prevention of disease was selected as the primary outcome measure based on preclinical animal studies that showed the vaccine could prevent disease but not mucosal infection [41], and the fact that vaccines in general typically prevent disease not infection. The problem with preventing disease but not HSV infection is that HSV can establish a latent infection and periodically reactivate with potential for transmission to a susceptible contact. From a public health perspective, if an HSV vaccine does not prevent infection, it should reduce the burden of the latent infection and the frequency and magnitude with which individuals shed virus [52].

The GlaxoSmithKline vaccine is being further evaluated in a double-blind, randomized, controlled trial (Herpevac) cosponsored by the National Institutes of Health and GlaxoSmithKline [53]. Modeling of the results of the initial two efficacy trials suggest that universal immunization of young girls can result in decreased spread of HSV-2 among the general population, including men [19]. The mechanism of the gender-specific protection seen with the Chiron and GlaxoSmithKline vaccines is unclear. Two possible, nonexclusive explanations have been suggested. The first is that there are differences in how men and women respond immunologically to these vaccines (eg, women may make a more robust T-cell response to the HSV vaccine). This possibility is easily investigated. The second possibility is that differences in male and female genital anatomy lead to differences in the pathogenesis of the infection. Stratified squamous epithelium covers the circumcised male genitalia, whereas much of the female genital tract is largely comprised of mucosal epithelium that is covered with secretions containing antibodies and T cells. It may be that the vaccine-induced immunity affords greater protection to infection that is initiated at a mucosal site (eg, the vagina) than one where virus entry is through abrasions in keratinized epithelia (eg, the circumcised penis).

Prophylactic vaccine acceptability

Once prophylactic vaccines are developed and available, they will need to be accepted to impact the rates of STIs. To be maximally effective, these vaccines should be given to adolescents before they become sexually experienced. For common STIs, such as HPV and HSV, it is through universal vaccination of all individuals rather than targeting high-risk individuals that the greatest impact will occur [19,54]. Strategies to enhance uptake will need to foster widespread acceptance by health care providers, parents, and adolescents. Research suggests that recommendations from professional organizations will be influential in health care providers' acceptance of STI vaccines [55,56].

There are two common misperceptions that are presented as barriers to recommending STI vaccines to adolescents. The first is that parents will not be supportive of STI vaccination. Contrary to this popular belief, research indicates that the sexual transmission of the disease targeted does not influence parental vaccine acceptability and that parents are likely to be supportive of STI vaccination [56–60]. Although research has indicated that parents will be supportive, there remains the issue of obtaining consent/ assent from the parent and the adolescent. If adolescents are vaccinated in settings where they are unaccompanied by parents (eg, school-based clinics), then obtaining an actual signed consent form may be difficult [61]. Studies of adolescents and young adults also have found high rates of acceptability [62–65], although even these individuals may seek parental opinion. The other popular belief is that individuals will increase sexual risk-taking behaviors following STI vaccination. Participants in one study that queried this belief as it related to an HPV vaccine denied it would change their behavior [58]. It will be important to educate policy-makers about the public health significance of these diseases and the potential of vaccines to improve personal health, protect the unborn and newborn from vertical transmission, and reduce health care costs associated with these ongoing epidemics.

Summary and future directions

The development of effective STI vaccines has been tough. Unlike infections for which bacteremia or viremia are critical elements in the disease pathogenesis (eg, pneumococcal sepsis, measles), STIs are typically mucosal infections and the pathogenesis generally involves local cutaneous spread or dissemination through nonhematogenous routes (eg, intraneuronal spread of HSV). The development of vaccines that provide durable protection against mucosal infection has been problematic. Mucosal infections themselves often do not induce durable protection against re-infection, unlike what is seen with diseases that cause bacteremia or viremia. Hence, analysis of immunity resulting from natural infection may not provide direction in the development of effective vaccines. It is likely that each pathogen has developed strategies through which it evades host immune responses, and it will be important to identify these strategies to improve on nature. Improving the somewhat rudimentary knowledge of mucosal immunology and immune correlates to protection will facilitate the development of STI vaccines. Another problem that has complicated the development of effective STI vaccines has been clinical trial design. Selection of the primary outcome measure can be controversial (eg, prevention of HSV infection versus HSV disease) or imprecise (eg, prevention of pelvic inflammatory disease). Use of discordant couples versus "at risk" populations versus the general public raises other issues including the generalizability of the findings.

The possibility of developing vaccines to control STIs is more promising than ever before. Advances in microbial genetics and understanding of the immunobiology of bacterial STIs make the prospect for the development of chlamydia and gonococcal vaccines optimistic. The exciting results of recent clinical trials have shown that vaccines can be developed that protect against the genital herpes and cervical human papillomavirus infections. To impact the STI epidemic, recommendations for universal rather than high-risk vaccination will be necessary, and behavioral research suggests that these vaccines will be acceptable to health care providers and consumers. Although effective vaccines against bacterial STIs are still many years away, it is likely that vaccines for HSV and HPV infections will be available in the near future. It may not be too soon to start considering the development of combination STI vaccines for adolescents similar to the combination pediatric vaccines commonly used today in infants.

Acknowledgments

The authors would like to acknowledge Laura Hardy for assistance in manuscript preparation.

References

[1] Brunham RC, McClarity G. Chlamydia. In: Stanberry LR, Bernstein DI, editors. Sexually transmitted disease: vaccines, prevention and control. San Diego (CA): Academic Press; 2000. p. 339–68.

[2] Batteiger BE, Rank RG, Bavoil PM, et al. Partial protection against genital reinfection by immunization of guinea-pigs with isolated outer-membrane proteins of the chlamydial agent of guinea-pig inclusion conjunctivitis. J Gen Microbiol 1993;139:2965–72.
[3] Moore T, Ekworomadu CO, Eko FO, et al. Fc receptor-mediated antibody regulation of T cell immunity against intracellular pathogens. J Infect Dis 2003;188:617–24.
[4] Eko FO, He Q, Brown T, et al. A novel recombinant multisubunit vaccine against Chlamydia. J Immunol 2004;173:3375–82.
[5] Hechard C, Grepinet O, Rodolakis A. Molecular cloning of the Chlamydophila abortus groEL gene and evaluation of its protective efficacy in a murine model by genetic vaccination. J Med Microbiol 2004;53:861–8.
[6] Zhang D, Yang X, Berry J, et al. DNA vaccination with the major outer-membrane protein gene induces acquired immunity to Chlamydia trachomatis (mouse pneumonitis) infection. J Infect Dis 1997;176:1035–40.
[7] Starnbach MN, Loomis WP, Ovendale P, et al. An inclusion membrane protein from Chlamydia trachomatis enters the MHC class I pathway and stimulates a CD8 + T cell response. J Immunol 2003;171:4742–9.
[8] Whittum-Hudson JA, Rudy D, Gerard H, et al. The anti-idiotypic antibody to chlamydial glycolipid exoantigen (GLXA) protects mice against genital infection with a human biovar of Chlamydia trachomatis. Vaccine 2001;19:4061–71.
[9] Beagley KW, Timms P. Chlamydia trachomatis infection: incidence, health costs and prospects for vaccine development. J Reprod Immunol 2000;48:47–68.
[10] Turner MS, Giffard PM. Expression of Chlamydia psittaci- and human immunodeficiency virus-derived antigens on the cell surface of Lactobacillus fermentum BR11 as fusions to bspA. Infect Immun 1999;67:5486–9.
[11] Zenilman JM, Deal CD. Gonorrhea: epidemiology, control and prevention. In: Stanberry LR, Bernstein DI, editors. Sexually transmitted disease: vaccines, prevention and control. San Diego (CA): Academic Press; 2000. p. 369–86.
[12] Sparling PF, Thomas CE, Zhu W. A vaccine for gonorrhea. In: Ellis RW, Brodeur BR, editors. Bacterial vaccines. Georgetown (TX): Landes Bioscience; 2003. p. 127–53.
[13] Schmidt KA, Schneider H, Lindstrom JA, et al. Experimental gonococcal urethritis and reinfection with homologous gonococci in male volunteers. Sex Transm Dis 2001;28:555–64.
[14] McKnew DL, Lynn F, Zenilman JM, et al. Porin variation among clinical isolates of Neisseria gonorrhoeae over a 10-year period, as determined by Por variable region typing. J Infect Dis 2003;187:1213–22.
[15] Rice PA, Vayo HE, Tam MR, et al. Immunoglobulin G antibodies directed against protein III block killing of serum-resistant Neisseria gonorrhoeae by immune serum. J Exp Med 1986;164:1735–48.
[16] Rokbi B, Renauld-Mongenie G, Mignon M, et al. Allelic diversity of the two transferrin binding protein B gene isotypes among a collection of Neisseria meningitidis strains representative of serogroup B disease: implication for the composition of a recombinant TbpB-based vaccine. Infect Immun 2000;68:4938–47.
[17] Gulati S, Ngampasutadol J, Yamasaki R, et al. Strategies for mimicking Neisserial saccharide epitopes as vaccines. Int Rev Immunol 2001;20:229–50.
[18] Zhu W, Thomas CE, Sparling PF. DNA immunization of mice with a plasmid encoding Neisseria gonorrhea PorB protein by intramuscular injection and epidermal particle bombardment. Vaccine 2004;22:660–9.
[19] Hughes JP, Garnett GP, Koutsky L. The theoretical population-level impact of a prophylactic human papilloma virus vaccine. Epidemiology 2002;13:631–9.
[20] Stanley MA. Human papillomavirus (HPV) vaccines: prospects for eradicating cervical cancer. J Fam Plann Reprod Health Care 2004;30:213–5.
[21] Simon P, Buxant F, Hallez S, et al. Cervical response to vaccination against HPV16 E7 in case of severe dysplasia. Eur J Obstet Gynecol Reprod Biol 2003;109:219–23.

[22] Hallez S, Simon P, Maudoux F, et al. Phase I/II trial of immunogenicity of a human papillomavirus (HPV) type 16 E7 protein-based vaccine in women with oncogenic HPV-positive cervical intraepithelial neoplasia. Cancer Immunol Immunother 2004;53:642–50.
[23] Corona Gutierrez CM, Tinoco A, Navarro T, et al. Therapeutic vaccination with MVA E2 can eliminate precancerous lesions (CIN 1, CIN 2, and CIN 3) associated with infection by oncogenic human papillomavirus. Hum Gene Ther 2004;5:421–31.
[24] Davidson EJ, Boswell CM, Sehr P, et al. Immunological and clinical responses in women with vulval intraepithelial neoplasia vaccinated with a vaccinia virus encoding human papillomavirus 16/18 oncoproteins. Cancer Res 2003;63:6032–41.
[25] Baldwin PJ, van der Burg SH, Boswell CM, et al. Vaccinia-expressed human papillomavirus 16 and 18 E6 and E7 as a therapeutic vaccination for vulval and vaginal intraepithelial neoplasia. Clin Cancer Res 2003;9:5205–13.
[26] Smyth LJ, Van Poelgeest MI, Davidson EJ, et al. Immunological responses in women with human papillomavirus type 16 (HPV-16)-associated anogenital intraepithelial neoplasia induced by heterologous prime-boost HPV-16 oncogene vaccination. Clin Cancer Res 2004; 10:2954–61.
[27] Stressgen Biotechnologies. Stressgen announces positive phase II data in high grade cervical dysplasia. Available at: http://www.stressgen.com. Accessed December 4, 2004.
[28] Ferrara A, Nonn M, Sehr P, et al. Dendritic cell-based tumor vaccine for cervical cancer II: results of a clinical pilot study in 15 individual patients. J Cancer Res Clin Oncol 2003;129: 521–30.
[29] Schreckenberger C, Kaufmann AM. Vaccination strategies for the treatment and prevention of cervical cancer. Curr Opin Oncol 2004;16:485–91.
[30] Lacey CJ, Thompson HS, Monteiro EF, et al. Phase IIa safety and immunogenicity of a therapeutic vaccine, TA-GW, in persons with genital warts. J Infect Dis 1999;179:612–8.
[31] Koutsky LA, Ault KA, Wheeler CM, et al. A controlled trial of a human papillomavirus type 16 vaccine. N Engl J Med 2002;347:1645–51.
[32] Mao C, Koutsky L, Ault K, et al. Prophylactic human papillomavirus (HPV) 16 virus-like particle (VLP) vaccine prevents HPV16-related cervical intraepithelial neoplasia (CIN) 2–3 [abstract G-3741]. In: Programs and abstracts from the 44th Annual Interscience Conference on Antimicrobial Agents and Chemotherapy. Washington (DC): 2004. p. 72.
[33] Harper DM, Franco EL, Wheeler C, et al. Efficacy of a bivalent L1 virus-like particle vaccine in prevention of infection with human papillomavirus types 16 and 18 in young women: a randomised controlled trial. Lancet 2004;364:1757–65.
[34] Harro CD, Pang YY, Roden RB, et al. Safety and immunogenicity trial in adult volunteers of a human papillomavirus 16 L1 virus-like particle vaccine. J Natl Cancer Inst 2001;93:284–92.
[35] Pinto LA, Edwards J, Castle PE, et al. Cellular immune response to human papillomavirus (HPV)-16 L1 in healthy volunteers immunized with recombinant HPV-16 L1 virus-like particles. J Infect Dis 2003;188:327–38.
[36] Cunningham AL, Mikloska Z. The Holy Grail: immune control of human herpes simplex virus infection and disease. Herpes 2001;8(Suppl 1):6A–10A.
[37] Vestergaard BF. Herpes simplex virus antigens and antibodies: a survey of studies based on quantitative immunoelectrophoresis. Rev Infect Dis 1980;2:899–913.
[38] Berman PW, Gregory T, Crase D, et al. Protection from genital herpes simplex virus type 2 infection by vaccination with cloned type 1 glycoprotein D. Science 1985;227:1490–2.
[39] Dix RD, Mills J. Acute and latent herpes simplex virus neurological disease in mice immunized with purified virus-specific glycoproteins gB or gD. J Med Virol 1985;17:9–18.
[40] Stanberry LR, Bernstein DI, Burke RL, et al. Vaccination with recombinant herpes simplex virus glycoproteins: protection against initial and recurrent genital herpes. J Infect Dis 1987; 155:914–20.
[41] Bourne N, Bravo FJ, Francotte M, et al. Herpes simplex virus (HSV) type 2 glycoprotein D subunit vaccines and protection against genital HSV-1 or HSV-2 disease in guinea pigs. J Infect Dis 2003;187:542–9.

[42] Straus SE, Corey L, Burke RL, et al. Placebo-controlled trial of vaccination with glycoprotein D of herpes simplex virus type 2 immunotherapy of genital herpes. Lancet 1994;343: 1460–3.
[43] Straus SE, Wald A, Kost RG, et al. Immunotherapy of recurrent genital herpes with recombinant herpes simplex virus type 2 glycoproteins D and B: results of a placebo-controlled trial. J Infect Dis 1997;176:1129–34.
[44] McLean CS, Erturk M, Jennings R, et al. Protective vaccination against primary and recurrent disease caused by herpes simplex virus (HSV) type 2 using a genetically disabled HSV-1. J Infect Dis 1994;170:1100–9.
[45] Stanberry LR. Clinical trials of prophylactic and therapeutic herpes simplex virus vaccines. Herpes 2004;11(Suppl 3):161A–9A.
[46] Casanova G, Cancela R, Alonzo L, et al. A double-blind study of the efficacy and safety of the ICP10DPK vaccine against recurrent genital HSV-2 infections. Cutis 2002;70: 235–9.
[47] PowderMed Ltd. PowderMed initiates a phase I clinical trial for a novel therapeutic herpes simplex type 2 (HSV2) DNA vaccine. Available at: http://www.powdermed.com/. Accessed December 5, 2004.
[48] Antigenics Inc. Genital herpes (HSV-2) trial. Available at: http://www.antigenics.com/trials/open/gh/info_gh.html. Accessed December 5, 2004.
[49] Stanberry LR, Myers MG, Stephanopoulos DI, et al. Preinfection prophylaxis with herpes simplex virus glycoprotein immunogens: Factors influencing efficacy. J Med Virol 1989;70: 3177–85.
[50] Corey L, Langenberg AG, Ashley R, et al. Recombinant glycoprotein vaccine for the prevention of genital HSV-2 infection: two randomized controlled trials. Chiron HSV Vaccine Study Group. JAMA 1999;282:331–40.
[51] Stanberry LR, Spruance SL, Cunningham AL, et al. Glycoprotein-D-adjuvant vaccine to prevent genital herpes. N Engl J Med 2002;347:1652–61.
[52] Stanberry L, Cunningham A, Mindel A, et al. Prospects for control of herpes simplex virus disease through immunization. Clin Infect Dis 2000;30:549–66.
[53] National Institute of Allergy and Infectious Diseases. Herpevac trial for women. Available at: http://www.niaid.nih.gov/dmid/stds/herpevac/default.htm. Accessed December 5, 2004.
[54] Garnett GP, Dubin G, Slaoui M, et al. The potential epidemiological impact of a genital herpes vaccine for women. Sex Transm Infect 2004;80:24–9.
[55] Mays RM, Zimet GD. Recommending STI vaccination to parents of adolescents: the attitudes of nurse practitioners. Sex Transm Dis 2004;31:428–32.
[56] Raley J, Followwill K, Zimet GD, et al. Gynecologists' attitudes regarding human papillomavirus vaccination: a survey of Fellows of the American College of Obstetricians and Gynecologists. Infect Dis Obstet Gynecol 2004;12(3–4):127–33.
[57] Mays RM, Sturm LA, Zimet GD. Parental perspectives on vaccinating children against sexually transmitted infections. Soc Sci Med 2004;58:1405–13.
[58] Kahn JA, Rosenthal SL, Hamann T, et al. Attitudes about human papillomavirus vaccine in young women. Int J STD AIDS 2003;14:300–6.
[59] Zimet GD, Mays RM, Strum LA, et al. Parental attitudes about sexually transmitted infection vaccination for their adolescent children. Arch Pediatr Adolesc Med 2005;15: 132–7.
[60] Rosenthal SL, Stanberry LR. Editorial response: parental acceptability of vaccines for sexually transmitted infections. Arch Pediatr Adolesc Med 2005;159:190–2.
[61] Deeks SL, Johnson IL. Vaccine coverage during a school-based hepatitis B immunization program. Can J Public Health 1998;89:98–101.
[62] Boehner CW, Howe SR, Bernstein DI, et al. Viral sexually transmitted disease vaccine acceptability among college students. Sex Transm Dis 2003;30:774–8.

[63] Hoover DR, Carfioli B, Moench EA. Attitudes of adolescent/young adult women toward human papillomavirus vaccination and clinical trials. Health Care Women Int 2000;21: 375–91.
[64] Rosenthal SL, Lewis LM, Succop PA, et al. College students' attitudes regarding vaccination to prevent genital herpes. Sex Trans Dis 1999;26:438–43.
[65] Zimet GD, Mays RM, Winston Y, et al. Acceptability of human papillomavirus immunization. J Womens Health Gend Based Med 2000;9:47–50.

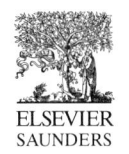

Sexually Transmitted Disease Care in Managed Care Organizations

Zsakeba Henderson, MD*, Guoyu Tao, PhD, Kathleen Irwin, MD, MPH

Division of STD Prevention, Centers for Disease Control and Prevention, 1600 Clifton Road, Mailstop E-80, Atlanta, GA 30333, USA

More than 15 million new cases of bacterial and viral sexually transmitted diseases (STDs) occur annually in the United States [1,2], with over two thirds occurring in people between the ages of 15 and 24 years [2]. Most STD infections are asymptomatic and can cause serious and costly complications if undetected and untreated. These complications include pelvic inflammatory disease (PID), infertility, chronic pelvic pain, and ectopic pregnancy in women; epididymitis and infertility in men; painful genital herpes lesions and human papillomavirus (HPV)-related anogenital warts; dysplasia; and cancer [3,4]. Bacterial and viral STD may facilitate human immunodeficiency virus (HIV) transmission and cause adverse neonatal outcomes [4]. Because these adverse outcomes have substantial short-term and long-term costs, STD prevention is cost-effective. Despite the substantial disease burden and attendant costs, STD prevention and control efforts compete for a position on the nation's health agenda [5].

Until the 1980s, most STD services were provided in public health department STD clinics, community health clinics, private physician's offices, hospital emergency departments, and health maintenance organizations (HMO) [6]. By the late 1990s, about 70% of STD care was provided by private providers or to privately insured persons [7], and the number and hours of dedicated STD clinics had declined substantially [8]. Meanwhile, enrollment in commercial and Medicaid managed care organizations (MCOs) rose dramatically, especially in the South [9] where bacterial STD rates are highest [10]. MCOs are now the principal source of private health care [11] and about two thirds of Medicaid enrollees are enrolled in an MCO

---

* Corresponding author.
  E-mail address: bwc5@cdc.gov (Z. Henderson).

[12]. This major shift of services to MCOs underscores their critical role in STD control [5,13,14].

MCOs have theoretical advantages for STD prevention and control when compared with traditional indemnity coverage, although these advantages may differ by MCO type (Table 1). Compared with network models, staff and group models provide more direct oversight of clinical practice and more centralization of quality assurance and administration, such as independent practice associations, point-of-service plans, and preferred provider organizations. In some MCOs, especially those that directly provide prevention, ambulatory, and hospital care, the financial structure may favor a greater commitment to prevention that might support (1) routine sexual risk assessment and screening, (2) a population-based approach to the provision of services that might support services for STD-exposed sex partners, and (3) the ability to train and guide a large panel of clinicians that would facilitate dissemination of new treatment guidelines. Large MCO administrative databases facilitate tracking of STD services and process outcomes (eg, *Chlamydia trachomatis* screening rates).

The contracts that MCOs negotiate with health care purchasers hold them accountable for delivering specific services and for meeting certain performance standards, such as the MCO performance measure for

Table 1
Types of managed care organizations

Managed care organizations	Service
HMO	Provides, offers, or arranges for coverage of designated health services for a fixed prepaid premium. Three basic models: group, staff, and individual practice association.
Group model HMO	Contracts with one or more independent group practices to provide services to its members in one or more locations.
Staff model HMO	Employs physicians to provide health care to its members. All premiums and other revenues accrue to the HMO, which compensates physicians by salary.
Individual practice association	Contracts with individual practitioners or an association of individual practices in return for a negotiated fee. The IPA then compensates its physicians on a per capita, fee schedule, or other agreed basis.
Preferred provider organization	Contracts with providers of medical care to provide services at discounted fees to members.
Point-of-service plan	Offers the option to its members to choose to receive a service from participating or nonparticipating providers, usually with reduced coverage for services associated with nonparticipating providers.

Data from United States Department of Health and Human Services. Managed care issue forum, glossary of managed care terms. Available at: http://aspe.os.dhhs.gov/progsys/forum/mcobib.htm. Accessed April 18, 2005.

C trachomatis screening [9,13–16]. To determine whether the potential of MCOs to promote STD control has been realized, this article summarizes the quality of STD care available in commercial and Medicaid MCOs over the last decade, barriers to STD control, and interventions that have been used to improve STD care in these settings.

Literature review methods

We reviewed the English language medical literature from North American sources published from January 1990 through June 2004 by searching MEDLINE. We cross referenced the terms *sexually transmitted diseases, prevention, risk assessment, patient education, health education, counseling, screening, testing, treatment, contact tracing, costs,* and *managed care* as MeSH headings and text words. We reviewed articles in which the title, abstracts, or body indicated that the study took place in an MCO or in a population that was largely privately insured or served by private-sector providers. We also accessed project reports, published guidelines, textbooks, and personal communication available in files of the Division of STD Prevention at the Centers for Disease Control and Prevention (CDC) [17]. We restricted our review to *C trachomatis, Neisseria gonorrhoea,* and syphilis. Data on other STDs were sparse, and HIV, hepatitis, and HPV-related conditions were beyond the scope of the review. We summarized information on STD prevalence, guideline use, and quality of six clinical domains: (1) sexual risk assessment, (2) screening, (3) treatment, (4) counseling and patient education, (5) case reporting, and (6) sex partner management. For each domain, we assessed the extent of and barriers to service delivery and interventions that have attempted to improve delivery.

Results

Sexually transmitted disease burden in managed care organization settings

Few studies have specifically addressed STD prevalence or incidence in MCO enrollees. National surveillance data provide an incomplete picture of the burden of the three universally reportable STDs (*C trachomatis, N gonorrhoea* , and syphilis) because most cases represent positive test results reported by laboratories and STDs diagnosed without laboratory tests remain unreported [10], and because case reporting outside of public STD clinics is incomplete [14,15]. Despite these challenges, the proportion of disease reported from the private sector is increasing. In 2003, clinicians practicing outside public STD clinics reported approximately 77% of *C trachomatis* cases, 64% of *N gonorrhoea* cases, and 67% of primary and secondary syphilis cases [10].

General population prevalence studies roughly approximate the burden in MCO populations because so many Americans are enrolled in MCOs. Among the bacterial STDs, *C trachomatis* is the most common, with an estimated annual incidence of 2.8 million cases [2]. Two nationally representative STD prevalence surveys in which most of the sample was privately insured used highly sensitive nucleic acid amplification tests (NAATS). For persons aged 14 to 39 years, *C trachomatis* prevalence was 2.6% in 1999 to 2000 [18]. For adults aged 18 to 26 years, prevalence was 4.2% in 2001 to 2002 [19]. Studies in routinely screened female populations, most of whom were privately insured, show prevalences of 5% to 14% in 15- to 19-year-olds and 3% to 12% in 20- to 25-year-olds [20]. Studies of routinely screened female MCO enrollees show prevalences from 4.2% to 14% among adolescents under 20 years of age and 3% to 4% among women aged 20 to 25 years [21–25].

An estimated 718,000 new cases of *N gonorrhoea* occurred in 2000 [2]. The two national STD prevalence surveys found occurrences of 0.25% among persons aged 14 to 39 years [18] and 0.43% among young adults aged 18 to 26 years [19]. *N gonorrhoea* prevalence in various private sector settings has ranged from 0.1% to 5.0% among asymptomatic patients, from 3.5% to 7% among mixed populations of asymptomatic and symptomatic patients, and from 6% to 11% among patients classified as at risk for STD. *N gonorrhoea* prevalence in private sector settings (other than emergency departments) and commercial MCOs tends to be lower than in public sector settings and Medicaid MCO (Tao et al, submitted for publication, 2004) [26]. Prevalence of *N gonorrhoea* in commercial MCOs may be lower than in public sector settings because commercial MCOs tend to enroll a lower proportion of persons who are at risk for acquiring gonorrhea or have not received screening or treatment for gonorrhea because of low socioeconomic status and limited health care access [10].

Syphilis is much less common than *C trachomatis* or *N gonorrhoea* overall, especially in privately insured populations. About 34,000 cases were reported to CDC in 2003 [2,10]. Although syphilis rates have declined dramatically over the last decade, rates remain high among low-income heterosexual populations in the South, some of whom may be enrolled in Medicaid MCOs, and among men (many of whom have commercial health insurance) who have sex with men (MSM) and have multiple partners [10]. This helps explain why most syphilis cases reported to CDC in 2003 were diagnosed in the private sector [10,27].

Use of sexually transmitted disease clinical practice guidelines

Clinical practice guidelines are widely used tools in many MCOs. The CDC STD treatment guidelines [4] are among those most commonly used by providers in MCOs [28–32]. Evaluations of the relevance of various STD prevention and treatment guidelines to MCOs concluded that the guidelines were generally current and complete, but needed more emphasis on STD risk assessment, STD screening, patient education, risk-reduction counseling, the cost-effectiveness of services, how STD prevention services compare with other prevention services given limited time and resources, and how to integrate STD services into typical MCO practice [30,32].

The few MCOs that have issued formal STD guidelines have used or adapted CDC treatment guidelines or the US Preventive Services Task Force (USPSTF) Guide to Clinical Preventive Services [28]. In a 1998–1999 study of Medicaid MCOs in seven large cities with a high penetration of Medicaid managed care and high bacterial STD rates, the MCOs did not consistently recommend STD practice guidelines to their primary care clinicians [29]. STD services that were explicitly recommended only by some MCOs included prenatal syphilis screening (71%), treating minors without parental/guardian consent (75%), providing preventive counseling while taking a sexual history (57%), alerting public departments to notify sex partners of infected patients (57%), presumptively treating *C trachomatis* in the presence of *N gonorrhoea* (14%), using single-dose *C trachomatis* therapy (40%), advising infected patients to notify sex partners (33%), annually screening sexually active adolescents (15%) and women ages 20 to 24 years (10%) for *C trachomatis*, or testing and treating exposed sex partners regardless of MCO membership or reimbursement (10%) [29]. A 2002 study of Medicaid MCOs in California found that only 9% of contracted primary care physicians reported having STD guidelines from their affiliated MCO or medical group [28].

However, in both studies, most of the affiliated medical group directors and physicians reported that they usually followed recommended STD practices despite the absence of MCO guidelines [28,29].

Quality of sexually transmitted disease care

Underuse, overuse, and misuse of health care can compromise desired health outcomes. In our review, underuse appeared to best characterize STD care in MCOs, especially regarding missed opportunities for risk assessment, screening, counseling and patient education, and sex partner management.

Risk assessment

Several national organizations, including CDC and USPSTF, recommend periodic sexual risk assessment to prompt risk-reduction counseling and patient education or to determine which patients are most likely to benefit from STD screening [30]. Two national population surveys indicated that only 28% of adults in the United States aged 18 to 64 years reported being asked about STD during routine checkups [33], and only 15% of women of reproductive age said they discussed STD with a health

Box 1. Commonly cited barriers to high quality sexually transmitted disease care in managed care organizations

Patient
- Concerns about confidentiality of medical information, medical records, or billing information that would reveal sexual activity
- Discomfort with discussing sexual issues with health care providers
- Stigma associated with STD limits demand for STD services
- Limited understanding of high prevalence and asymptomatic nature of many STDs and serious and long-term consequences of untreated STDs limit demand for routine risk assessment and screening of asymptomatic patients

Provider
- Brief patient encounters and competing clinical priorities discourage sensitive, labor intensive tasks such as sexual risk assessment, patient counseling and education, and sex partner management
- Discomfort discussing sexual issues with patients and doing pelvic examinations (especially on adolescent patients)
- Lack of training in sexual risk assessment and sexual risk-reduction counseling and educating, and sex partner management
- Difficulty keeping up with revised recommendations on STD screening and treatment
- Insufficient or nonconfidential reimbursement methods for routine risk assessment, screening, risk-reduction counseling, patient education, sex partner management, and case reporting
- Lack of awareness of noninvasive STD screening tests

Health system
- Lack of explicit policies/protocols for STD care
- Lack of decision-support tools
- Lack of provider feedback and reminder systems
- Cost-containment pressures that discourage STD prevention services, routine risk assessment, screening, counseling, education, and sex partner management
- Limited support staff to assist with risk assessment, counseling, education, sex partner services, and case reporting
- Medicolegal/liability concerns about potential confidentiality breaches or legal requirements to report evidence of sexual activity of minors (eg, reporting statutory rape, sexual abuse)

- Nonavailability/reimbursement of noninvasive STD screening tests (eg, urine)
- Lack of centralized systems, dedicated staff, or electronic data systems that facilitate case reporting
- Limited organizational commitment and "internal champions" because of stigma and perception that STDs are low-volume, low-cost conditions
- Limited demand by health care purchasers and MCO enrollees for STD quality improvement

professional at their first gynecologic or obstetric visit [34]. Two studies suggested that routine STD risk assessment was less commonly reported by private sector providers than by public sector providers [35,36]. A multicity survey of MCO providers found that 57% reported taking sexual histories and that only 8% used a standard risk assessment form [37]. In a 1998 survey of private providers in Colorado, only 72% reported taking sexual histories [38]. In Medicaid MCOs in the state of Washington, less than half of the adolescent patients had sexual histories documented in medical records for primary care or well-care visits [39]. Among patients diagnosed with STD in a private, nonprofit clinic in the state of Washington, risk information such as past STD, condom use, and partner's gender was documented in less than two thirds of the encounters [40]. Among publicly-funded MCOs in Minnesota, sexual histories were documented in 93% of women diagnosed with STD, but only 66% of women were classified as sexually active by administrative data [26].

Barriers to routine risk assessment in MCOs, such as those listed in Box 1, include lack of policies, protocols, reimbursement, standard forms, and decision-support tools that support risk assessment; competing clinical priorities during brief visits; lack of provider or patient comfort when discussing sexual issues; and concerns about breaches of confidentiality [26,37,41,42]. In a 1999 survey of primary care providers in two commercial MCOs, more than 30% of the providers reported lack of time to elicit sexual histories or to address STD [41].

Interventions that have attempted to promote risk assessment in MCOs include developing policies to promote confidentiality for MCO members, routinely excusing parents from adolescent encounters to allow for risk assessment [21], adopting standard self-administered or provider-administered risk assessment tools [37,43], or using patient-administered computer programs that elicit a sexual history and provide counseling messages tailored to that patient's risks [44]. Other methods include clinician training on risk assessment methods, using nonphysician staff to collect risk information [21], making risk assessment a covered service [45], and increasing reimbursement [46].

Screening of asymptomatic persons and diagnostic testing of symptomatic persons

Screening of asymptomatic patients for STD is recommended for specific population groups to detect the high proportion of patients infected with *C trachomatis*, *N gonorrhoea*, and syphilis who lack symptoms or signs and to prompt early treatment [4]. Guidelines recommend prenatal syphilis screening; *C trachomatis* screening in sexually active female adolescents and young women under the age of 25 years, older women at high risk, and pregnant women; and *N gonorrhoea* screening of high-risk persons and pregnant women [4,30].

In a national sample of commercial MCO claims data during 1998 and 1999, 63% of the pregnant women had claims for syphilis tests, mostly during the first prenatal visit [47]. In publicly-funded MCOs in Minnesota, 88% of the pregnant women had documented syphilis testing [26]. A 1998 national survey of primary care providers, most of whom practiced in private sector settings, found that 3% to 98% reported routine prenatal syphilis testing, with most estimates exceeding 50% [48]. In Medicaid MCOs, 94% of the physicians reported routine prenatal screening for syphilis, as advised by most of their MCOs (71%) [29].

In contrast, screening rates of sexually active women for *C trachomatis*, which has a much higher prevalence than syphilis, are low to moderate in most MCOs. Annual *C trachomatis* screening was reported by 45% of the physicians surveyed in Medicaid MCOs [29], by 32% of the primary care physicians surveyed in Pennsylvania [49], and 54% of the primary care providers surveyed in Colorado [38]. Of the providers who treat adolescents in a commercial MCO, only 67% reported willingness to screen female adolescents for *C trachomatis* [50]. In the 1998 national primary care provider survey, only one third of the physicians reported routinely screening women for *C trachomatis*, although obstetrician/gynecologists reported higher screening rates [48]. Studies of MCO medical records and administrative data have shown that 2% to 55% of the sexually active adolescents and young women are screened annually [21,23,25,26,50,51]. Since the annual *C trachomatis* screening of sexually active female MCO enrollees under 26 years of age was introduced in 1999 as an MCO performance measure, average screening rates have increased slightly in commercial MCOs (from 20% in 1999 to 26% in 2001) and Medicaid MCOs (from 28% in 1999 to 38% in 2001) [52]. Other studies report higher screening rates in MCOs that have high Medicaid enrollment (Table 2) [26].

Although *N gonorrhoea* screening is currently recommended only for high-risk persons because its prevalence varies substantially by geographic, demographic, and sexual characteristics of patients, screening rates vary considerably, reflecting over- and underuse. A 1992 study of *N gonorrhoea* screening of 15- to 21-year-old female patients enrolled in an HMO found that 3% to 10% had evidence of screening or diagnostic tests [51]. In a 1998

Table 2
Percentage[a] of sexually active female enrollees aged 16 to 26 years who were screened for chlamydia by health plan type[b]

	Year	16–20 y (%)	21–26 y (%)	16–26 y (%)
Commercial MCOs	2001	28	25	26
	2000	27	24	25
	1999	22	19	20
Medicaid MCOs	2001	38	38	38
	2000	35	36	36
	1999	27	28	28

Data from Centers for Disease Control and Prevention. Chlamydia screening among sexually active young female enrollees of health plans—United States, 1999–2001. MMWR Morb Mortal Wkly Rep 2004;53(42):983–4.

[a] Average *Chlamydia trachomatis* screening rates were weighted for size of health plan.

[b] Health plan employer data and information set (HEDIS) performance measure, 1999–2001.

national survey of primary care providers, less than one third reported routinely screening asymptomatic men (13%), nonpregnant asymptomatic women (30%), and pregnant women (31%) [48]. In addition, a study of patients in a private, nonprofit clinic system in the state of Washington found that some clinics selectively screened patients for *N gonorrhoea* [40]. In various private sector settings, medical records document *N gonorrhoea* screening or diagnostic testing in up to 71% of female teens or young adults, up to 97% of pregnant women (Tao et al, submitted for publication, 2004), and 34% of sexually active women in Minnesota MCOs [26]. Active marketing of *N gonorrhoea–C trachomatis* combination tests has resulted in their increased use for screening. When these tests are used to screen for *C trachomatis* in populations with low *N gonorrhoea* prevalence, they may yield few positive *N gonorrhoea* cases, low *N gonorrhoea* test predictive value, and poor cost-effectiveness [53].

Provider, health system, and patient-level factors may discourage routine STD screening in MCOs [5,15] (see Box 1). Provider-level barriers include clinician misperception that prevalences of STD and STD risk behaviors in commercial MCOs are low or are correlated with insurance status and race, and the belief that screening is not cost-effective [13,49,50]. Lack of provider comfort with assessing sexual activity and competing clinical priorities during brief visits are other challenges [28,50]. Screening practices vary by provider specialty and the importance of STD to a given practice. For example, in several Medicaid MCOs, obstetrician/gynecologists and family and general practitioners were more likely to report screening young women for *C trachomatis* than were internists or pediatricians [28]. Policy-level factors that discourage screening include lack of reimbursement, screening policies, decision support tools, non-invasive urine screening tests, and performance feedback and reminder systems. Also, few MCOs use generic codes to mask STD tests on billing records [28,49,50,52,54]. Cost-containment pressures favor diagnostic testing of the few symptomatic patients over routine screening of large numbers of asymptomatic patients. This is especially true in capitated MCOs and in MCOs concerned that investing in screening may make them less financially competitive than other MCOs [9]. *C trachomatis* screening is cost-effective from a societal perspective and is ranked among the top ten preventive services in terms of disease averted and cost-effectiveness [55]. However, rapid MCO enrollee turnover, especially in Medicaid MCOs, makes it difficult for a given MCO to reap benefits of prevention in the short term because many sequelae of undetected, untreated infection occur years later [29]. For patients, especially adolescents, the stigma of STD and concerns about maintaining confidentiality of their sexual activity or infection status discourages demand for or acceptance of screening [56].

MCOs have introduced several interventions to increase routine STD screening. Syphilis testing in standard prenatal testing panels, longstanding national screening guidelines, and state regulations mandating syphilis screening have supported high screening rates for decades [47]. Simple interventions to increase *C trachomatis* screening include development, dissemination, and championing of print- and Web-based practice or MCO-specific screening guidelines and protocols [21,25]; posting aggregate HMO STD case counts in provider newsletters to highlight enrollee incidence [57,58]; introducing urine tests [21,54,59]; pooling specimens from numerous patients and retesting only individual specimens from positive pools [53]; using generic STD service billing codes to protect confidentiality [26]; and collecting *C trachomatis* screening tests with every pelvic examination [9]. At one commercial MCO, a protocol to collect *C trachomatis* specimens with routine Pap tests increased screening rates from 61% to 83% in 24 months [25]. A multifaceted intervention involving the use of multimedia educational materials and an intensive office-based "academic detailing" approach increased *C trachomatis* screening rates by 16.9% and 30.4% for Medicaid and commercial enrollees respectively [60]. It has also been shown that new parent rooming-in policies that gave teens time alone with their clinicians to discuss STD screening helped to increase *C trachomatis* screening rates [21].

More complex interventions that have increased screening include Web instruction using clinical cases relevant to MCOs [61] and sending personalized letters inviting MCO enrollees who are classified as high risk through administrative data to undergo *C trachomatis* screening [62]. A system-level practice improvement approach used in adolescent clinics involved forming a quality improvement team, selecting clinic-specific improvement measures, and screening performance feedback. This approach increased *C trachomatis* screening by nearly 40% within 18 months [21,22]. In contrast, no appreciable increase in *C trachomatis* screening was observed in three different MCOs that sent young adult enrollees newsletters with information about *C trachomatis* infection and how to get access to *C trachomatis* screening [63].

Treatment practices

The benefits of screening asymptomatic persons and diagnostic testing of symptomatic persons can be achieved only if infected patients are appropriately treated. MCO databases afford opportunities to assess compliance with treatment guideline recommendations. Studies using such databases document adherence to CDC-recommended treatment regimens for laboratory-confirmed *C trachomatis* in pregnant women, with adherence rates ranging from 89% to 98% [64,65]. The same holds true for treatment of *C trachomatis* in men and nonpregnant women, with compliance ranging from 91% to 97% [26,64]. Several studies have also shown widespread adherence to guidelines that indicate use of single-dose Azithromycin for treating *C trachomatis* in patients whose compliance to longer regimens might be questioned [29,65]. Widespread adherence to CDC-recommended treatment regimens have also been documented for *N gonorrhoea*, despite challenges presented by changes in treatment guidance as a result of emerging drug resistance [4,26,66,67].

CDC recommends presumptive treatment of patients who have a clinical diagnosis of *N gonorrhoea*, *C trachomatis*, or syphilis before laboratory results are available because recommended antibiotics are safe and have few adverse effects, and immediate treatment may prevent serious, costly sequelae and transmission to others [4]. In the 1998 national primary-care provider survey, more than one third of the physicians surveyed reported they presumptively treat patients who have *N gonorrhoea* (56.7%), *C trachomatis* (54.2%), and syphilis (40%) [48]. Of primary care clinicians surveyed in two large commercial MCOs in 1999, 87% reported they would choose antibiotics that would cover *C trachomatis* in a nonpregnant patient who has signs of cervicitis [64]. Most primary care physicians affiliated with Medicaid MCOs in two studies reported they would presumptively treat *C trachomatis* in the presence of *N gonorrhoea* as recommended by CDC [28,29]. In a Massachusetts HMO, all men who had symptomatic urethritis and tested positive for *N gonorrhoea*, and 88% of those who tested positive for *C trachomatis*, were prescribed CDC-recommended treatment at their initial visit. The remainder were treated up to 5 days later [57,68]. Reviews of medical records from private sector settings have shown that patients who had symptoms of *N gonorrhoea* were more likely to be presumptively treated at the initial visit using CDC-recommended regimens, and that asymptomatic patients were more likely to be treated at the follow-up visit after test results were available [57,69]. Regarding treatment of PID, a condition that is usually diagnosed presumptively, 52% of California physicians (78% practicing in private sector settings) reported that they did not use CDC treatment guidelines [70].

Barriers to appropriate treatment include lack of recommended drugs on MCO formularies, the higher cost of some single-dose regimens [29], and keeping up with revised recommendations (eg, emerging fluoroquinolone resistance of *N gonorrhoea*) [71]. In addition to these barriers, recalling patients who had positive STD tests for treatment can be difficult, especially in settings where resources for telephone or in-person outreach are limited, but this is uncommon in most MCOs. Several interventions have been used to increase appropriate treatment in MCOs, including (1) formal adoption of CDC STD treatment guidelines, followed by active dissemination through booklets, wall charts, pocket guides, hand-held computers, and print- and Web-based clinical guidelines [32,57]; (2) issuing new treatment alerts in response to emerging drug resistance patterns [71]; (3) including CDC-recommended drugs on MCO formularies; (4) including STD treatments in prescription order-entry systems [72]; (5) automatically printing recommended treatment on positive test result reports or on health department case report cards [57,58]; and (6) didactic, online, or in-service clinician training [61,73]. Several policy interventions have also been implemented, including (1) requiring that CDC guidelines be used in Missouri's Medicaid MCOs; (2) establishing memoranda of understanding between Medicaid MCOs and public health agencies that specify treatment standards; and (3) reimbursing treatment of MCO enrollees who seek anonymous STD care in public clinics [9,16].

Risk-reduction counseling and patient education

Patients at risk for or infected with STD should be offered counseling or education to reduce risky sexual behaviors [30]. Several studies have assessed risk-reduction counseling provided by private providers. One study revealed that during STD-related treatment visits, 78% of physicians surveyed always tell their patients to avoid sex and 76% tell their patients to use condoms [74]. Studies of ambulatory care visits in private sector settings showed that HIV/STD counseling was documented in the medical records of only 30% to 35% of all visits in which HIV or STD tests were performed [26,75]. Of physicians practicing at Medicaid MCOs, 98% reported that they provide prevention counseling while taking a sexual history despite the fact that only 81% of their affiliated medical groups and 57% of their MCOs explicitly recommended this practice [29].

In a 1999 survey of primary care providers in staff and network MCOs, more than 30% cited a limited number of staff members to counsel patients or difficulties keeping up-to-date on how to manage patients at risk for STD as challenges to STD management [41]. Other challenges include patient or provider discomfort with or lack of training on counseling [8,37], competing clinical priorities during brief visits, lack of staff dedicated to counseling and education, lack of decision-support tools such as counseling checklists and reminder systems, and the absence of guidelines, policies, protocols, and reimbursement (see Box 1) [26,46]. For example, a 1998 Washington State survey found that the indemnity health plans that dominated in the state were less likely to cover STD counseling (29%) than the less common HMOs (100%) [42]. Other studies have observed that clinicians may forego counseling for enrollees of capitated MCOs that do not provide added reimbursement for this service [9,14].

Various interventions have attempted to increase patient education and counseling in MCOs. Simple approaches include providing clinician training in risk-reduction counseling and communication about sexual issues [76]. One group-model MCO observed improved STD prevention in adolescents after a standard risk assessment and education tools were implemented [43]. Another group-model MCO saw sustained improvements in sexual health knowledge and counseling among providers after training was offered, staff roles were clarified, tools and materials were provided, and reminder and feedback systems were implemented [77]. Patient supports include pamphlets, videos, hot lines, Web sites, or referrals to group counseling or community support groups [78]. One potentially time-saving tool is a patient-administered, computer-assisted program that tailors counseling messages to individual patient risk factors [44]. To foster adolescent risk assessment, counseling, and education, North Carolina requires Medicaid MCOs to have adequate numbers of adolescent specialists [45]. Some Medicaid agencies include counseling and patient education in MCO service contracts [45].

Case reporting

Laboratory and provider reporting of *N gonorrhoea*, *C trachomatis*, and syphilis is mandatory in every state [10]. STD reporting appears to be more complete and timely from public STD clinics than from private sector and MCO providers [15,79]. Most physicians surveyed in various private sector settings and Medicaid MCOs are aware that laboratories report STD cases to health authorities [28,48,80]. Nevertheless, about 9% to 28% of laboratory-confirmed cases of *C trachomatis* and *N gonorrhoea* are not reported [58,81,82]. In an evaluation of MCO reporting practices in three states, most cases were reported 1 to 3 weeks after specimen collection, and reporting was faster when laboratories electronically reported cases to health departments [58].

Several factors may preclude reporting, including (1) lack of provider awareness about reporting obligations; (2) confidentiality concerns with billing, medical records, and health department staff; (3) lack of reimbursement; (4) lack of centralized systems to facilitate reporting; and (5) limited public health perspective of private sector providers [58,82,83]. MCOs have used various approaches to promote complete and timely reporting, including (1) having MCO staff members dedicated to reporting functions, (2) use of secure methods to electronically transfer positive laboratory test reports to health departments, (3) attachment of case report cards to positive laboratory results received by clinicians, and (4) initiation of regular communication with health departments about types of cases that activate sex partner notification [58]. Some California MCOs have developed systems to automatically track and report STD cases to expedite reporting and measure enrollee STD burden [9]. Policy-level interventions that may improve reporting include reimbursing clinicians for time spent on reporting and establishing memoranda of understanding that detail reporting roles of providers, laboratories, and health department staff. Some states have formal contracts that require out-of-state laboratories to report cases to the state where the patient resides, which is an important issue as large regional laboratories now serve MCOs in several states [9,84].

Management of exposed sex partners

Prompt evaluation and treatment of the sex partners of patients who are infected with STD is recommended [30]. In the 1998 national primary care provider survey, 80% reported always asking patients who are infected with STD to notify their partners, but less than half of the physicians always reported patients' names to health departments to initiate partner services, and less than 5% reported always contacting partners themselves [74,85]. A minority of private providers in Seattle addressed sex partner management [86]. Among physicians at Medicaid MCOs, 62% reported testing and treating a partner regardless of MCO membership, despite the fact that only 61% of their medical groups and 10% of their MCOs explicitly recommended this practice [29]. Few MCO patients who have STD are provided partner management services by health department staff, even in high-morbidity areas of the United States [5,29,87].

MCO clinicians cite several challenges to managing sex partners, including (1) the lack of clear policies about out-of-plan partners, (2) medicolegal liability concerns, (3) cost-containment pressures, (4) lack of reimbursement, and (5) time or staffing constraints [5,16]. Other barriers include patients' and providers' lack of comfort in discussing partners and concern about maintaining confidentiality or adverse consequences to relationships when partners are notified. Chronic shortages of health department disease-investigation staff force most health departments to focus on partners of patients who are infected with HIV, syphilis, or *N gonorrhoea* [87].

To support partner management, some MCOs have developed more explicit policies and procedures, such as providing physicians with prescription-writing authority to treat sex partners not enrolled in the MCO and methods to seek third-party reimbursement for managing uninsured partners [5,9,26,88]. A recent trial showed that it was acceptable to allow partners to get treatment at commercial pharmacies without visiting a physician and that it increased treatment [89]. In a few states, laws or regulations allow clinicians to prescribe treatment for the sex partners of their patients even if the partners are not their patients, or to permit their patients to deliver treatment to partners [90]. Other MCOs have provided one-page "after visit summaries" to patients infected with STD that list actions to take with sex partners, and have explored using telephone advice nurses to explain sex partner management services to patients who have positive STD tests (Mullolly, submitted for publication).

Discussion

Bacterial STD care remains a low priority in most MCOs, except in some Medicaid MCOs and innovative staff-model MCOs that enroll large numbers of adolescents and young women or emphasize preventive care. Few of the potential advantages that MCOs have in addressing a population health issue like STD control have been achieved on a large scale [14,16,17]. This low-priority status derives partly from the perception that MCO populations have a low prevalence of and are at low risk for bacterial STD, despite data demonstrating fairly high prevalence of *C trachomatis*. It is therefore not surprising that most interventions have addressed *C trachomatis*. However, in some MCOs that serve many persons at high risk for *N gonorrhoea* and syphilis, such as those of low-income who seek care in MCO emergency departments or MSMs who have multiple sex partners, *N gonorrhoea* and syphilis control may merit more attention.

MCOs may show little organizational commitment to STD because most management involves low-cost care for acute conditions, which yields less financial burden or patient volume than the more prevalent chronic conditions. Other factors that contribute to low-priority status include limited commitment, investment, and experience in the public health aspects of communicable disease control (such as sex partner services), and concerns that STD services (such as routine sexual risk assessment, risk-reduction counseling, and screening of asymptomatic patients) are inadequately reimbursed, not cost-effective, or challenging to deliver [9]. Finally, the stigma surrounding STD may make MCOs or large health care purchasers that contract with MCOs reluctant to openly champion quality improvement efforts, and patients reluctant to request services.

Treatment regimens used in MCOs for laboratory-confirmed STD cases are largely consistent with national guidelines. Reporting of notifiable laboratory-confirmed *C trachomatis* and *N gonorrhoea* cases is fairly complete in the few MCOs evaluated, especially when laboratories or centralized MCO staff members take primary responsibility for reporting. Delivery of routine sexual risk assessment, risk-reduction counseling, screening, and sex partner management show room for improvement in many MCOs, probably because most clinicians prioritize diagnosis and treatment of symptomatic patients over prevention.

The challenges in delivering STD services are similar to those delivering other primary care and preventive services, including (1) time constraints during short encounters, (2) cost pressures, (3) clinical system design and information systems that do not support clinical reminders, and (4) staffing that underuses nonphysician staff members for routine risk assessment, counseling and patient education, and case reporting. Although several MCOs have introduced interventions to improve delivery of these services, most have addressed just one or two STDs, and few have been rigorously evaluated. Providers and health systems should consider evaluating and tailoring the current interventions used with their own patients, practices, and STD priorities. Operations research on intervention effectiveness, cost-effectiveness, feasibility, scale-up, and sustainability is also needed.

Several promising developments may address the challenges to delivering quality STD care in MCOs. First, MCOs are poised to adopt several new STD technologies, including new highly sensitive nucleic acid amplification and urine-based tests for bacterial STD; computer-based risk assessment and counseling tools; electronic clinical information systems that ease tracking of patient services and outcomes; and an explosion of Web-based information for clinicians and patients and their partners. Second, the growing focus on accountability and quality improvement may urge health care purchasers and consumers to demand standards of care in MCO contracts and adequate financial incentives for under-resourced services, such as risk assessment, screening, counseling, and sex partner management. The MCO performance measure for *C trachomatis* and its ranking of *C trachomatis* screening as a high-priority preventive service will continue to spotlight *C trachomatis* screening as a quality improvement focus [55]. Third, new models that have improved delivery of primary care and preventive services through changes in clinical decision support, delivery system design, clinical information systems, and self-management supports could be readily applied to STD care [91]. For example, clinical delivery systems could be modified to ensure that all patients routinely receive sexual risk assessment before they are seen by their clinician. Clinical information systems could generate reminders for patients due for screening or infected patients due for risk-reduction counseling. Clinicians could urge patients who are infected with STD to notify sex partners as a self-management goal.

Summary

Most STD cases in the United States are managed in health sectors dominated by commercial and Medicaid MCOs. To sustain the recent declines in bacterial STD incidence in the United States and to control expansion of the prevalent viral STD, MCOs will need to contribute substantially to control efforts. Applied researchers and quality improvement specialists must work with clinicians, patients, and health systems to develop and scale-up interventions to improve STD prevention and control.

References

[1] Cates W Jr. Estimates of the incidence and prevalence of sexually transmitted diseases in the United States. American Social Health Association Panel. Sex Transm Dis 1999;26(4 Suppl): S2–7.
[2] Weinstock H, Berman S, Cates W Jr. Sexually transmitted diseases among American youth: incidence and prevalence estimates, 2000. Perspect Sex Reprod Health 2004;36(1):6–10.
[3] Donovan B. Sexually transmissible infections other than HIV. Lancet 2004;363(9408): 545–56.
[4] Centers for Disease Control and Prevention. Sexually transmitted diseases treatment guidelines 2002. MMWR 2002;51(RR-6):1–78.
[5] Gunn RA, Rolfs RT, Greenspan JR, et al. The changing paradigm of sexually transmitted disease control in the era of managed health care. JAMA 1998;279(9):680–4.
[6] Eng TR, Butler WT. Current STD-related services. In: Eng TR, Butler WT, editors. The hidden epidemic: confronting sexually transmitted diseases. Washington (DC): National Academy Press; 1997. p. 175–219.
[7] Brackbill RM, Sternberg MR, Fishbein M. Where do people go for treatment of sexually transmitted diseases? Fam Plann Perspect 1999;31(1):10–5.
[8] Chaulk CP, Zenilman J. Sexually transmitted disease control in the era of managed care: "magic bullet" or "shadow on the land"? J Public Health Manag Pract 1997;3(2):61–70.
[9] Gonen JS. Confronting STDs: a challenge for managed care. Womens Health Issues 1999; 9(2 Suppl):S36–46.
[10] Centers for Disease Control and Prevention. Sexually transmitted disease surveillance 2003. Available at: http://www.cdc.gov/std/stats/. Accessed April 18, 2005.
[11] The Henry J. Kaiser Family Foundation. Trends and indicators in the changing health care marketplace, 2004 update. Available at: http://www.kff.org/insurance/7031/index.cfm. Accessed April 18, 2005.
[12] Hurley RE, Somers SA. Medicaid and managed care: a lasting relationship? Health Aff 2003; 22:77–88.
[13] Cates JR, Alexander L, Cates W Jr. Prevention of sexually transmitted diseases in an era of managed care: the relevance for women. Womens Health Issues 1998;8(3):169–86.
[14] Eng TR. Summary of workshop on the role of managed care organizations in STD prevention. In: Eng TR, Butler WT, editors. The hidden epidemic: confronting sexually transmitted diseases. Washington (DC): National Academy Press; 1997. p. 370–82.
[15] Eng TR. Prevention of sexually transmitted diseases. A model for overcoming barriers between managed care and public health. The IOM Workshop on the Role of Health Plans in STD Prevention. Am J Prev Med 1999;16(1):60–9.
[16] Lafferty WE, Kimball AM, Bolan G, et al. Medicaid managed care and STD prevention: opportunities and risks. J Public Health Manag Pract 1998;4:52–8.
[17] Chorba TL, Scholes D, BlueSpruce J, et al. Sexually transmitted diseases and managed care: an inquiry and review of issues affecting service delivery. Am J Med Qual 2004;19(4):145–56.
[18] Datta SD, Sternberg M, Johnson RE, et al. Prevalence of chlamydia and gonorrhea in the United States among persons aged 14–39, 1999–2000 [abstract 0349]. The 2003 International Society for Sexually Transmitted Disease Research (ISSTDR) Congress: Ottawa (Canada): 2003. p. 122–3.
[19] Miller WC, Ford CA, Morris M, et al. Prevalence of chlamydial and gonococcal infections among young adults in the United States. JAMA 2004;291(18):2229–36.
[20] Walsh C, Irwin KL. Combating the silent chlamydia epidemic. Contemp Ob Gyn 2002; Apr:90–8.

[21] Shafer MA, Tebb KP, Pantell RH, et al. Effect of a clinical practice improvement intervention on Chlamydial screening among adolescent girls. JAMA 2002;288(22):2846–52.
[22] Shafer MA, Tebb KP, Ko TH. Extending preventive care to pediatric urgent care: a new venue for CT screening [abstract A06f]. In: Program and abstract of the 2004 National STD Prevention Conference. Philadelphia; 2004. p. A.24–5.
[23] Burstein GR, Snyder MH, Conley D, et al. Adolescent chlamydia testing practices and diagnosed infections in a large managed care organization. Sex Transm Dis 2001;28(8): 477–83.
[24] Armstrong J, Leeds-Richter S, Sangi-Haghpeykar H. Prevalence of chlamydia trachomatis (CT) in a commercially insured population. Presented at the 2002 National STD prevention conference. San Diego, CA, March 4–7, 2002.
[25] Burstein GR, Snyder MA, Conley D, et al. Screening rates before and after the introduction of the chlamydia HEDIS (Health Plan Employer Data and Information Set) Measure in a managed care organization [abstract A06B]. In: Program and abstracts of the 2004 National STD Conference. Philadelphia; 2004. p. A.22.
[26] Michigan Peer Review Organization. Prevention, screening, and treatment of STD in Minnesota publicly funded managed care programs. Available at: www.dhs.state.mn.us/healthcare/studies. Accessed April 18, 2005.
[27] Blocker ME, Levine WC, St Louis ME. HIV prevalence in patients with syphilis, United States. Sex Transm Dis 2000;27(1):53–9.
[28] Pourat N, Razack N, Brown ER, et al. Sexually transmitted disease services in California's Medi-Cal managed care. Los Angeles (CA): UCLA Center for Health Policy Research; 2004.
[29] Pourat N, Brown ER, Razack N, et al. Medicaid managed care and STDs: missed opportunities to control the epidemic. Health Aff 2002;21(3):228–39.
[30] Scholes D, Anderson LA, Operskalski BH, et al. STD prevention and treatment guidelines: a review from a managed care perspective. Am J Manag Care 2003;9(2):181–9.
[31] Workowski KA, Levine WC, Wasserheit JN. US Centers for Disease Control and Prevention guidelines for the treatment of sexually transmitted diseases: an opportunity to unify clinical and public health practice. Ann Intern Med 2002;137(4):255–62.
[32] Stiffman M, Magid D, Irwin K, et al. Use of and adherence to CDC-recommended treatment guidelines for chlamydia and genital warts: A survey of managed care providers. Building Bridges V: Managed Care Research Forum. Seattle (WA), April 26–27, 2001.
[33] Tao G, Irwin KL, Kassler WJ. Missed opportunities to assess sexually transmitted diseases in US adults during routine medical checkups. Am J Prev Med 2000;18(2):109–14.
[34] The Henry J.Kaiser Family Foundation. Talking about STDs with health professionals: women's experiences. 1997. Available at: http://www.kff.org/womenhealth/1313-index.cfm. Accessed April 18, 2005.
[35] Landry DJ, Forrest JD. Public health department providing sexually transmitted disease services. Fam Plan Perspect 1996;28(6):261–6.
[36] Greene KH, Eng TR, Mattingly PH, et al. STD-related services among managed care organizations serving high-risk population. In: Eng TR, Butler WT, editors. The hidden epidemic: confronting sexually transmitted diseases. Washington (DC): National Academy Press; 1997. p. 383–93.
[37] Bull SS, Rietmeijer C, Fortenberry JD, et al. Practice patterns for the elicitation of sexual history, education, and counseling among providers of STD services: results from the gonorrhea community action project (GCAP). Sex Transm Dis 1999;26:584–9.
[38] Torkko KC, Gershman K, Crane LA, et al. Testing for Chlamydia and sexual history taking in adolescent females: results from a statewide survey of Colorado primary care providers. Pediatrics 2000;106:E32.
[39] Lafferty WE, Downey L, Holan CM, et al. Provision of sexual health services to adolescent enrollees in Medicaid managed care. Am J Public Health 2002;92(11):1779–83.
[40] Eubanks C, Lafferty WE, Kimball AM, et al. Privatization of STD services in Tacoma, Washington: a quality review. Sex Transm Dis 1999;26(9):537–42.

[41] Irwin KL, Anderson LA, Stiffman M, et al. Leading barriers to STD care in two managed care organizations [abstract]. In: Proceedings of 2002 National STD Prevention Meeting. San Diego, March 4–7, 2002. p. 96.

[42] Kurth A, Bielinski L, Graap K, et al. Reproductive and sexual health benefits in private health insurance plans in Washington State. Fam Plann Perspect 2001;33(4):153–60, 179.

[43] Boekeloo BO, Schamus LA, Simmens SJ, et al. A STD/HIV prevention trial among adolescents in managed care. Pediatrics 1999;103:107–15.

[44] Kurth A, Spielberg F, Fortenberry JD, et al. Computer-assisted risk assessment & education: "CARE" CD-ROM [abstract 0494]. Presented at the International Society of STD Research Conference. Ottawa, Canada, July 27–30, 2003.

[45] Blake S, Kenney K. Contract specifications for sexually transmitted disease (STD) services in Medicaid managed care plans: a focused study for the centers for disease control and prevention. Washington, DC: George Washington University Center for Health Services Research and Policy; 1998.

[46] Schauffler HH. Policy tools for building health education and preventive counseling into managed care. Am J Prev Med 1999;17(4):309–14.

[47] Tao G, Patterson E, Lee LM, et al. Estimating prenatal syphilis and HIV screening rates for commercially insured women. Am J Prev Med 2005;28(2):175–81.

[48] St Lawrence JS, Montano DE, Kasprzyk D, et al. STD screening, testing, case reporting, and clinical and partner notification practices: a national survey of US physicians. Am J Public Health 2002;92(11):1784–8.

[49] Cook RL, Wiesenfeld HC, Ashton MR, et al. Barriers to screening sexually active adolescent women for chlamydia: a survey of primary care physicians. J Adolesc Health 2001;28(3): 204–10.

[50] Boekeloo BO, Snyder MH, Bobbin M, et al. Provider willingness to screen all sexually active adolescents for chlamydia. Sex Transm Infect 2002;78(5):369–73.

[51] Thrall JS, McCloskey L, Spivak H, et al. Performance of Massachusetts HMOs in providing Pap smear and sexually transmitted disease screening to adolescent females. J Adolesc Health 1998;22:184–9.

[52] Shih S, Scholle S, Irwin KL, et al. Chlamydia screening among sexually active young female enrollees of health plans—United States, 1999–2001. MMWR 2004;53(42):983–5.

[53] Johnson RE, Newhall WJ, Papp JR, et al. Screening tests to detect Chlamydia trachomatis and Neisseria gonorrhoeae infections–2002. MMWR 2002;51(RR-15):1–27.

[54] Michigan Peer Review Organization. Sexual health care: motivators and barriers. Available at: www.dhs.state.mn.us/healthcare/studies. Accessed April 18, 2005.

[55] Coffield AB, Maciosek MV, McGinnis JM, et al. Priorities among recommended clinical preventive services. Am J Prev Med 2001;21:66–7.

[56] Civic D, Scholes D, Grothaus L, et al. Adolescent HMO enrollees' utilization of out-of-plan services. J Adolesc Health 2001;28(6):491–6.

[57] Centers for Disease Control and Prevention. Evaluation of sexually transmitted disease control practices for male patients with urethritis at a large group practice affiliated with a managed care organization–Massachusetts, 1995–1997. MMWR 2001;50(22):460–2.

[58] Centers for Disease Control and Prevention. Reporting of laboratory-confirmed chlamydia infection and gonorrhea by providers affiliated with three large managed care organizations–United States, 1995–1999. MMWR 2002;51(12):256–9.

[59] Bull SS, Jones CA, Granberry-Owens D, et al. Acceptability and feasibility of urine screening for chlamydia and gonorrhea in community organizations: perspectives from Denver and St Louis. Am J Public Health 2000;90:285–6.

[60] Szebenyi SE, Upstill CE, Saleh SS, et al. Stop STDs! Improving prevention and screening of sexually transmitted infections and HIV: final report to the New York State Department of Health Office of Managed Care. September 15, 2004.

[61] Casebeer L, Allison J, Spettell CM. Designing tailored Web-based instruction to improve practicing physicians' chlamydial screening rates. Acad Med 2002;77(9):929.

[62] Scholes D, Stergachis A, Heidrich FE, et al. Prevention of pelvic inflammatory disease by screening for cervical chlamydial infection. N Engl J Med 1996;334(21):1362–6.
[63] Asbel L, Jeanette R, Goldberg M, et al. Randomized trial comparing different outreach strategies for Chlamydia screening. Presented at the 2002 National STD prevention conference. San Diego, CA, March 4–7, 2002.
[64] Magid DJ, Stiffman M, Anderson LA, et al. Adherence to CDC STD guideline recommendations for the treatment of Chlamydia trachomatis infection in two managed care organizations. Sex Transm Dis 2003;30(1):30–2.
[65] Tun W, Stiffman M, Magid D, et al. Evaluation of clinician adherence to CDC's guidelines for the treatment of Chlamydia trachomatis in two large health plans–Colorado and Minnesota, 2000. In: Proceedings of the 52nd Annual EIS Conference. Atlanta, GA, March 31–April 4, 2003.
[66] Kelly JJ, Dalsey WC, McComb J, et al. Follow-up program for emergency department patients with gonorrhea or chlamydia. Acad Emerg Med 2000;7:1437–9.
[67] Mehta SD, Rothman RE, Kelen GC, et al. Unsuspected gonorrhea and chlamydia in patients of an urban adult emergency department: a critical population for STD control intervention. Sex Transm Dis 2001;28:33–9.
[68] Ratelle S, Yokoe D, Whelan M, et al. Management of urethritis in health maintenance organization members receiving care at a multispecialty group practice in Massachusetts. Sex Transm Dis 2001;28(4):232–5.
[69] Wiest DR, Spear SJ, Bartfield JM. Empiric treatment of gonorrhea and chlamydia in the ED. Am J Emerg Med 2001;19(4):274–5.
[70] Hessol NA, Priddy FH, Bolan G, et al. Management of pelvic inflammatory disease by primary care physicians. A comparison with Centers for Disease Control and Prevention guidelines. Sex Transm Dis 1996;23(2):157–63.
[71] Centers for Disease Control and Prevention. Increases in fluoroquinolone-resistant Neisseria gonorrhoeae among men who have sex with men—United States, 2003, and revised recommendations for gonorrhea treatment, 2004. MMWR 2004;53(16):335–8.
[72] Papshev D, Peterson AM. Electronic prescribing in ambulatory practice: promises, pitfalls, and potential solutions. Am J Manag Care 2001;7(7):725–36.
[73] Ellen J, Douglas J, Allen G, et al. Effect of the STD/HIV prevention training center network's core clinical course on clinicians' STD care-related practices. Presented at STIs at the Millennium. Baltimore, MD, May 3–7, 2000.
[74] McCree DH, Liddon NC, Hogben M, et al. National survey of doctors' actions following the diagnosis of a bacterial STD. Sex Transm Infect 2003;79(3):254–6.
[75] Tao G, Branson BM, Anderson LA, et al. Do physicians provide counseling with HIV and STD testing at physician offices or hospital outpatient departments? AIDS 2003;17(8):1243–7.
[76] Ratelle S, Dyer J, Cherneskie T, et al. Assessing the training needs of managed care providers: implications for STD clinical training targeting this hard-to-reach group [abstract A05A]. In: Proceedings of the 2004 National STD Prevention Conference. Philadelphia, March 8–11, 2004. p. A17.
[77] Bluespruce J, Dodge WT, Grothaus L, et al. HIV prevention in primary care: impact of a clinical intervention. AIDS Patient Care STDS 2001;15:243–53.
[78] Robin L, Dittus P, Whitaker D, et al. Behavioral interventions to reduce incidence of HIV, STD, and pregnancy among adolescents: a decade in review. J Adolesc Health 2004;34(1):3–26.
[79] Anderson JE, McCormick L, Fichtner R. Factors associated with self-reported STDs: data from a national survey. Sex Transm Dis 1994;21:303–8.
[80] Roush S, Birkhead G, Koo D, et al. Mandatory reporting of diseases and conditions by health care professionals and laboratories. JAMA 1999;282:164–70.

[81] Backer HD, Bissell SR, Vugia DJ. Disease reporting from an automated laboratory-based reporting system to a state health department via local county health departments. Public Health Rep 2001;116:257–65.
[82] Tao G, Carr P, Stiffman M, et al. Incompleteness of reporting of laboratory-confirmed chlamydial infection by providers affiliated with a managed care organization, 1997–1999. Sex Transm Dis 2004;31(3):139–42.
[83] Smucker DR, Thomas JC. Evidence of thorough reporting of sexually transmitted diseases in a southern rural county. Sex Transm Dis 1995;22:149–54.
[84] Mauery RD, Kamoie B, Blake SC, et al. Communicable disease reporting laws: managed care organizations' laboratory contracting practices and their implications for state surveillance and reporting statutes. Center for Health Services Research & Policy. Washington, DC: The George Washington University School of Public Health & Health Services; 2003.
[85] Hogben M, St Lawrence JS, Montano DE, et al. Physicians' opinions about partner notification methods: case reporting, patient referral, and provider referral. Sex Transm Infect 2004;80(1):30–4.
[86] Golden MR, Whittington WL, Gorbach PM, et al. Partner notification for chlamydial infections among private sector clinicians in Seattle-King County: a clinician and patient survey. Sex Transm Dis 1999;26(9):543–7.
[87] Golden MR, Hogben M, Handsfield HH, et al. Partner notification for HIV and STD in the United States: low coverage for gonorrhea, chlamydial infection, and HIV. Sex Transm Dis 2003;30:490–6.
[88] St. Lawrence JS, Hogben M, Golden M, et al. Partner-delivered partner therapy for STD: evidence and prospects for implementation [abstract D01F]. In: Proceedings of the 2004 National STD Prevention Conference. Philadelphia, March 8–11, 2004.
[89] Golden MR, Whittington WL, Handsfield HH, et al. Partner management for gonococcal and chlamydial infection: expansion of public health services to the private sector and expedited sex partner treatment through a partnership with commercial pharmacies. Sex Transm Dis 2001;28:658–65.
[90] Golden MR, Anukam U, Williams DH, et al. The Legal status of patient-delivered partner therapy for sexually transmitted infections in the United States: a national survey of state medical and pharmacy boards. Sex Transm Dis 2005;32(2):112–4.
[91] Bodenheimer T, Wagner EH, Grumbach K. Improving primary care for patients with chronic illness. JAMA 2002;288(14):1775–9.

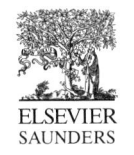

Innovative Approaches to the Prevention and Control of Bacterial Sexually Transmitted Infections

Matthew R. Golden, MD, MPH[a,b,*], Lisa E. Manhart, PhD[c]

[a]*Center for AIDS and STD, University of Washington, Harborview Medical Center, 325 9th Avenue, Box 359777, Seattle, WA 98104, USA*
[b]*Public Health—Seattle & King County, 999 3rd Avenue, Ste. 1200, Seattle, Washington 98104, USA*
[c]*Center for AIDS and STD, University of Washington, Harborview Medical Center, 325 9th Avenue, Box 359931, Seattle, WA 98104, USA*

Rates of gonorrhea and syphilis in the United States and Western Europe have declined dramatically over the last 30 years and are now at or near their lowest levels since World War II [1]. Existing data suggest that the prevalence of genital chlamydial infections has also declined in parts of the United States and in Sweden [1,2], the areas with the longest-standing chlamydial screening programs. Despite this progress, sexually transmitted infections (STIs) continue to present new challenges. After years of decline, overall rates of gonorrhea and chlamydial infection have recently plateaued in the United States, and appear to be increasing in some areas [1]. An epidemic of syphilis in the former Soviet Union threatens Europe [3], even as newly initiated chlamydial screening programs in some European nations tax the limited resources available to control STIs [4]. Meanwhile, a global epidemic of STIs is underway among men who have sex with men (MSMs) and shows no signs of abating [1,5]. Meeting these new challenges will require that clinicians and public health officials adopt new STI prevention measures.

This article reviews recent, innovative approaches to the control of STIs as they pertain to the United States and other developed nations, focusing

---

This work was supported by NIH K23 AI01846 (Golden) and NIH AI 27757.
* Corresponding author. Center for AIDS and STD, University of Washington, Harborview Medical Center, 325 9th Avenue, Box 359777, Seattle, WA 98104, USA.
  E-mail address: golden@u.washington.edu (M.R. Golden).

on bacterial STIs and presenting a public health perspective on what role these approaches might play in disease control. STI vaccines and suppressive therapy for genital herpes are discussed elsewhere in this issue and therefore are not reviewed here. This article attempts to refer to controlled trials whenever possible. However, the discussion is not restricted to evidence from such studies, nor does this article attempt to catalog results from all such trials. A systematic review of randomized trials to prevent STI has recently been published [6].

Behavioral interventions

Behaviors such as number of sex partners, partner selection, types of sex practiced (ie, sexual repertoire), condom use, obtaining health care, adherence to therapy, and partner notification all affect a person's vulnerability to STIs or likelihood of transmitting an STI to others. Thus, it stands to reason that clinicians and public health officials who seek to prevent STI would attempt to alter these risk behaviors.

Toward that end, STI prevention research has increasingly focused on efforts to change behavior over the last 2 decades. Most intervention studies in this area have involved individual or group counseling. A meta-analysis of behavioral intervention studies found that these interventions can induce changes in self-reported risk behaviors. Among MSM and sexually experienced adolescents, these interventions reduced the likelihood that participants would engage in unprotected sexual intercourse by approximately 30% (MSM summary odds ratio 0.69, 95% CI 0.56–0.86; adolescent summary odds ratio 0.66; 95% CI 0.55–0.79) [7,8]. A somewhat smaller reduction in a sexual risk behavior index was observed among heterosexual adults (summary odds ratio 0.81, 95% CI 0.69–0.95) [9].

Fewer data are available on the impact of behavioral interventions on STI incidence. These types of studies are particularly important because reduced risk behaviors have not always translated into a corresponding reduction in STI incidence [10–12]. Several intervention trials conducted among heterosexual STD clinic patients have demonstrated reductions in STI incidence (Table 1) [10,12–24]. These interventions have varied substantially in their intensity and somewhat in their methodological rigor. Less rigorous, low-intensity, single-session group interventions conducted in the early 1990s appeared to decrease STI incidence [13,15–17]. A subsequent large, multicenter trial comparing client-centered counseling to a didactic educational message (Project RESPECT) demonstrated that a brief, individual counseling intervention was effective in preventing STIs [14]. The effect of this intervention persisted at 1 year, but appeared to wane with time. More intensive group counseling interventions have also been shown to be effective in preventing STIs among heterosexuals [18,20,23–25]. Limited data are available on the effect of behavioral interventions on STI

Table 1
Selected trials of behavioral interventions to prevent sexually transmitted infection

Author	Population	Intervention	Outcome (intervention versus control)	Comment
Individual counseling interventions				
Cohen et al [13]	903 STD clinic patients in Los Angeles	Single session to promote condom use through one of three interventions: (1) condom skills, (2) social influences; (3) free access to condoms	No impact on STI rates overall; condom skills associated with lower rate of infection compared with control group in men 12.5% versus 25%. (RR 0.5, 95% CI 0.29–0.85)	Group randomization by clinic session; outcomes defined from medical record review (ie, passive ascertainment)
Boyer et al [10]	393 patients at San Francisco STD clinic	Four 60-min counseling sessions over 4 wk	STI at follow-up occurred in 13% versus 11% ($P = 0.57$); decreased unprotected sex at 3 mo in men only; no difference in unprotected sex at 5 mo	38% of potentially eligible participated
Kamb et al [14]	5758 heterosexuals evaluated at five inner-city United States STD clinics patients	Four session-enhanced counseling versus two session-enhanced counseling versus two session-didactic counseling	STI at 6 mo occurred in 7.2% four session enhanced counseling, 7.3% two session enhanced counseling, and 10.4% of didactic counseling ($P < .01$ enhanced versus didactic)	Enhanced counseling intervention involved "client centered" counseling, emphasizing the need to define a risk reduction plan; magnitude of benefit declined over time
Koblin et al [12]	4295 men who have sex with men	Ten counseling sessions over 4–6 mo followed by maintenance session every 3 mo; control condition involved twice yearly counseling	HIV acquisition 1.9 per 100 person years versus 2.3 per 100 person years (OR 0.82, 95% CI 0.64–1.05)	Difference in HIV acquisition appeared greatest in first 12–18 mo of follow-up: unprotected anal intercourse with HIV positive or HIV status-unknown partner lower in intervention arm (OR 0.85, 95% CI 0.78–0.94)

(continued on next page)

Table 1 (continued)

Author	Population	Intervention	Outcome (intervention versus control)	Comment
Group counseling interventions				
Cohen [15]	Sample of 192 STD clinic patients in Los Angeles	Group discussion of condom skills	STI at 1 year follow-up 11.3% versus 20% ($P = .10$)	Groups assigned based on health educator schedule (ie, not randomized); all clinic patients seen during study period included; sampling procedures for chart review and what STIs included as reinfections not clearly identified; outcome reported with $P = .05$ based on one-tailed test
Cohen et al [16]	551 Los Angeles STD clinic patients	Group discussion, videotape and role playing in STD clinic waiting room	Gonorrhea, chlamydial infection; reinfection defined as any of the following: (1) syphilis, nongonococcal urethritis, primary herpes, PID; (2) newly diagnosed genital warts or bacterial vaginosis; (3) contact to gonorrhea, chlamydial infection, or syphilis in the absence of condom use; reinfection 6% versus 13% (RR 0.49, 95% CI 0.26–0.90)	Intervention versus control assigned to vary morning and evening on different days of the wk (ie, not random); all clinic patients seen during study period included; STI outcome based on chart review (ie, passive ascertainment); condom use protective for STI
O'Donnell et al [17]	2004 men attending STD clinics in New York City	Video-based patient education	STI reported in 22.5% versus 26.8% ($P < .05$)	STI outcome identified through disease reporting and matching to participant identifiers; group randomization by day

NIMH Prevention Trial Group [18]	3706 primarily heterosexual persons recruited at community-based clinics in five United States cities	Seven session small group counseling	No difference in prevalence of gonorrhea or chlamydial infection at 12 mo; among men recruited from STD clinics, those in the intervention arm had fewer episodes of gonorrhea during follow-up (see comment) than those in the control arm (6.4% versus 6.3%, $P < .03$); intervention associated with fewer acts of unprotected vaginal or anal intercourse ($P < .001$)	Difference in gonorrhea based on chart review
Branson et al [19]	964 STD clinic patients	Four 1-h group counseling sessions compared to two 20-min individual counseling sessions	No difference in occurrence of STI (gonorrhea, chlamydial infection, syphilis, or HIV) or in number of sex partners or condom use between study arms	Lower attendance at group counseling sessions among younger persons and those who had STI at baseline visit
Shain et al [20]	617 Latino and African Americans with nonviral STIs diagnosed at an STD clinic in Texas	Three 3–4 h small group sessions	Gonorrhea or chlamydial infection 16.8% versus 26.9%, $P = .008$	Intervention associated with fewer sex partners and more condom use
Hobfoll et al [21]	935 single or short-term cohabitating women on welfare or without medical insurance seen in two Midwestern United States clinics	Two intervention arms consisting of six small group sessions emphasizing HIV prevention or general health promotion versus standard care	No difference in STI at follow-up	Intervention associated with decreased unprotected sex

(continued on next page)

Table 1 (continued)

Author	Population	Intervention	Outcome (intervention versus control)	Comment
DiClemente et al [22]	522 African American adolescent girls recruited from community health agencies in Alabama	Four 4-h group sessions	No difference in STI at follow-up observed; analysis adjusting for baseline variables and covariates associated the intervention with a significantly lower risk of chlamydial infection, with a trend toward a lower risk of gonorrhea and trichomonas	Intervention significantly associated with increased condom use relative to control condition
Shain et al [23]	775 female STD clinic patients with nonviral STI	Three 3-4 h group sessions over 3 wk (standard intervention as in reference 16), standard intervention + five optional 90-min group follow-up counseling sessions at monthly intervals versus control	By 2 years, gonorrhea or chlamydial infection occurred in 26% of standard intervention women, 24% of enhanced intervention women, and 40% of controls ($P < .001$)	Women who had STI at 1-y follow-up were more likely to have STI at 2-y; attending optional follow-up counseling associated with a lower risk of STI
Boyer et al [24]	2157 female United States military recruits	Four 2-h group sessions over 12 wk	Gonorrhea, chlamydial infection, trichomonas or unintended pregnancy 24% versus 18% (OR 1.41, 95% CI 1.01–1.98)	Participants randomized by platoon
Wingood et al [25]	366 HIV positive women in Georgia and Alabama	Four 4-h group sessions over 4 wk	Gonorrhea or chlamydial infection 10.2% versus 4.0% ($P = .02$); intervention associated with lower mean number of episodes of unprotected vaginal intercourse ($P = .04$)	

Studies are randomized controlled trials unless otherwise noted in the comments section.
Abbreviations: NIMH, National Institute of Mental Health; OR, odds ratio; PID, pelvic inflammatory disease; RR, relative risk.

or HIV incidence in MSM. Unfortunately, these data are discouraging, with a large, intense ten-session intervention trial demonstrating no significant impact on HIV incidence [12].

Despite some convincing demonstrations that behavioral interventions can prevent STI in heterosexuals, such interventions have not been widely instituted. Project RESPECT influenced HIV counseling standards in the United States, but few STD clinics in the United States appear to have adopted the study's model [26], which involved having patients define a risk reduction plan and a subsequent review of plan adherence during a face-to-face posttest counseling session. We are unaware of any counseling intervention being widely applied as part of routine public health activities, and it seems likely that behavioral interventions have had little meaningful public health impact to date, even if some have probably affected the health of individual participants.

The failure to translate behavioral interventions into practice is certainly multifactorial. However, two problems may be dominant: the absence of infrastructure to widely institute targeted interventions (ie, move interventions beyond research settings and STD clinics) and cost. In the absence of substantial new public health funding, behavioral interventions will either need to be inexpensive, or will need to narrowly focus on the groups at greatest risk for STI.

Project RESPECT was designed to be an effective, low-cost, low-intensity intervention. It was effective, but probably was not low enough in cost, at least not for universal application among STD clinic patients. The brief, untargeted group interventions undertaken in STD clinic waiting rooms that demonstrated promise in the early 1990s [13,15–17] fell out of favor as a research topic without ever becoming part of public health practice. It may be time to reassess the utility of these types of interventions and more rigorously assess their efficacy and cost-effectiveness. Other alternative, potentially low-cost approaches to promulgating behavioral interventions might include efforts to use computer counseling tools [27], or to focus publicly financed intervention efforts on training private sector clinical providers to deliver interventions to their patients (which will shift costs from health departments to insurers).

More intensive interventions appear promising among selected, high-risk populations. Existing evidence suggests two target groups: persons who have a recent history of STI and heterosexual women who have HIV. Shain et al [20,23] instituted a multisession group intervention focusing on the prevention of recurrent STI in minority women, and demonstrated that such an intervention is feasible and effective. Persons who have a recent history of STI or those who have repeated episodes of STI are a logical target group for more intensive interventions. Formal cost-effectiveness analyses assessing these efforts relative to other public health activities are warranted. The other group for which studies with biological outcomes support intensive behavioral interventions is heterosexual women who have HIV [25]. With this group, the need to change behavior is compelling as a means to diminish transmission of HIV to uninfected partners [28].

Beyond cost, the institution of intensive interventions is hindered by the logistical barriers to accessing and intervening with a meaningful proportion of persons at highest risk for acquiring or transmitting STI. To the extent that behavioral interventions appear to be cost-effective, health departments need to devise means to apply them to a wide population of high-risk persons. Restricting the implementation of successful interventions to public STD clinics will not be sufficient. Only a small number of persons diagnosed with gonorrhea or chlamydial infection in the United States are treated in STD clinics [29]. Thus, interventions will need to extend beyond these clinics if they are to impact the public health.

Microbicides

Microbicides may be a promising STI prevention intervention. They may be more appealing and easier to use than condoms, and, unlike condoms, are likely to be female-controlled. To date, studies of microbicides have focused solely on intravaginal use of nonoxynol-9 (N-9). Although early trials of N-9 for preventing gonococcal or chlamydial infection were encouraging [30–34], subsequent trials using more rigorous designs produced conflicting results. In these later trials, N-9 was associated with a significant increase in risk of genital ulcers and irritation of the genital tract epithelium [35,36]. Eager to reduce these adverse effects, investigators tested reduced concentrations and different formulations of N-9 [37,38]. Unfortunately, by reducing the concentration of active N-9, they also eliminated the benefit, and studies of reduced N-9 concentrations reported an elevated risk of gonorrhea acquisition in women using N-9. The most recent trial actually reported a significant increase in the risk of HIV-1 seroconversion among women using a 3.5% N-9 gel and no effect on either gonococcal or chlamydial infection [39], leading to the conclusion that N-9 products produced no significant reduction in risk of STI/HIV, but showed some evidence of harm through inducing genital lesions [40]. N-9 is clearly not a safe and effective microbicide.

Other microbicides are under development, and several are currently in phase 2 and phase 3 trials. Most are being evaluated primarily for effectiveness against HIV rather than STI. As a result, most candidate microbicides are based on antiviral compounds used as clinical antiretroviral therapies for HIV, particularly reverse transcriptase inhibitors. Compounds designed to inhibit attachment and fusion of HIV to host cells are promising [41], but will likely not be effective against bacterial STI. Other formulations currently under evaluation include an alcohol-based emollient gel, cyanovirin-N, beta-cyclodextrin, cellulose acetate phthalate, naphthalene sulfonic acid, C31G, and RNA interference (RNAi). Acceptability studies for many of these agents are also underway and will guide implementation of effective agents. In addition to intravaginal formulations, rectal microbicides and external male microbicides (applied to the penile shaft) are being tested.

Innovations to improve case-finding and treatment

Case-finding and treatment is a traditional mainstay in the control of curable communicable diseases, including STI, and is increasingly regarded as the cornerstone of public health efforts to control noncurable STIs, such as HIV and genital herpes [28,42,43]. A first step in developing an STI control program is typically to provide basic curative medical care to persons who have symptomatic infections. Under at least some circumstances, improving syndromic care has been shown to affect the prevalence of syphilis, trichomonas, and gonorrhea in community-level randomized trials [44]. Beyond the provision of basic medical care, selective screening and partner notification and treatment have been fundamental components of public health efforts to control STI. The development of nucleic acid amplification tests (NAATs), with the associated ability to test urine and self-obtained vaginal swab or flush specimens, and the advent of safe, single-dose oral therapies for gonorrhea and chlamydial infections have led to several innovations in screening and partner treatment.

Efforts to promote female screening in medical care settings

The Centers for Disease Control and Prevention (CDC) and the US Preventive Services Task Force recommend that all women aged 25 years or younger be tested annually for *Chlamydia trachomatis* [45]. However, analysis of the Health Plan Employer Data and Information Set, which contains information on over 400 HMOs and point-of-service plans, found that only 26% of women aged 16 to 26 years were tested in 2001 [42]. One means to improve the control of chlamydial infection would be to promote increased adherence with screening guidelines among insured women. A clinic-level randomized trial undertaken in ten Northern California clinics demonstrated that a practice improvement intervention could increase rates of chlamydial screening [46]. However, a subsequent, larger trial undertaken in Washington State failed to demonstrate such an increase [47]. Practice-level interventions have been successfully employed to promote childhood immunizations [48] and asthma care [49], but have not typically been promoted by public health officials. Interventions that seek to promote provider adherence with screening guidelines might be cost-effective areas for public–private sector collaboration, particularly if the alternative is more publicly financed testing.

Male chlamydial screening

Although CDC and the US Preventive Services Task Force have issued guidelines promoting chlamydial screening of women [45], no similar guidelines exist in the United States for men. (The United Kingdom chlamydial screening program promotes screening for men and women equally [4]). Arguments in favor of screening men include their obvious importance in maintaining heterosexual transmission, the high prevalence of largely asymptomatic infection observed in some populations [50–53], and the failure of ongoing chlamydial control activities to drive chlamydial prevalence below current levels [1]. Arguments against chlamydial screening of men include the fact that chlamydial infection is less prevalent among young men than among young women in the United States [53] and in most screened populations [1,53–57]; that men experience little significant morbidity as a consequence of asymptomatic infection; and that inadequate resources are currently devoted to chlamydial testing in women, where the benefit is more direct. Cost-effectiveness analyses have suggested that screening of men may be worthwhile in selected, higher-prevalence populations [58] or when diagnostic testing is limited to men who have a positive leukocyte esterase test [59,60]. Dynamic mathematical modeling of chlamydial control activities suggests that universal, age-based screening of men would somewhat decrease the prevalence of infection below the level achieved through screening women alone, but might be less effective than a comparable effort focusing on enhanced partner treatment, and would be costly compared with screening of women [61,62].

At present, no consensus exists in support of male screening, and operationalizing universal screening of men would likely prove costly and difficult. However, selective, opportunistic screening of young men in high prevalence venues, such as STD clinics and juvenile detention centers, seems reasonable. In addition, annual screening of MSM for rectal chlamydial infection, syphilis, HIV, and rectal and pharyngeal gonorrhea seems warranted [63,64].

Sexually transmitted infection testing in unconventional locations

Largely because of the advent of NAATs, health departments have established programs to test for STIs in a wide spectrum of nonclinical settings, including correctional facilities [1], schools [65,66], substance abuse treatment centers [67], emergency rooms [68–72], job training programs [73], bathhouses [74,75], and street outreach programs [76,77]. Screening programs for *C trachomatis* in correctional facilities and in schools merit particular comment.

STI screening among "law breakers" was proposed by Thomas Parran [78] in 1937. Syphilis screening continues to be productive in some correctional settings, but is highly variable [79]. In contrast, the prevalence of *C trachomatis* in juvenile detention facilities is consistently high [55,80]. In 2003, 15.9% of 53,000 adolescent women tested in selected correctional sites were positive for *C trachomatis* [1]. The prevalence of asymptomatic chlamydial infection among men tested in juvenile detention facilities also appears to be high, though perhaps more variable from place to place [81]. However, as of 1997, fewer than 20% of jails in the United States routinely offered gonorrhea or chlamydial testing to inmates in the absence of symptoms, and fewer than 50% routinely performed syphilis screening tests. Screening inmates at booking is challenging, but would ensure the widest program coverage. Establishing screening programs in juvenile detention settings should be regarded as a high priority for publicly supported STI testing programs.

Some school-based programs have been highly successful in identifying large numbers of adolescent girls who have chlamydial infection or gonorrhea [65,66], whereas others have been characterized by low rates of participation and a low prevalence of infection [82]. The prevalence of bacterial STI varies between geographic areas and between schools within a school district, suggesting that selective institution of screening programs may be the most cost-effective strategy for developing school-based testing programs. Although implementing such programs can be fraught with political challenges, some programs have been highly successful [57,65,83], and school-based testing may be the best means to access large at-risk adolescent populations.

Rescreening

People who have STIs get STIs. Across a wide range of studies, few factors have been as strongly associated with the risk of STI as a recent history of STI [15,16,84–87]. Clinical and public health efforts to focus on persons who experience repeated infections reflect the elevated risk of adverse sequelae associated with recurrent episodes of pelvic inflammatory disease in women, and the presumed importance of persons who experience repeated infection in sustaining transmission of STI in the population.

Prospective studies with active follow-up have observed chlamydial infection in 7% to 25% of women and 13% of men tested 3 to 6 months after treatment for genital *C trachomatis* infection [88–92], and rescreening of young women who have chlamydial infection has been shown to be cost-effective [93]. Although fewer data are available on gonorrhea, recurrent infections have been reported in 12% to 24% of women and 9% of men tested 1 to 6 months after treatment [92,94,95].

The argument in favor of rescreening is strong, but is not new [96]. In the 1970s, CDC promoted rescreening of persons who had gonorrhea [97]. The effort was largely abandoned, probably because of poor success and associated high costs [98]. Recent epidemiologic trends and technical innovations should prompt a reconsideration of rescreening. First, in much of the United States and Europe, gonorrhea is now rare in heterosexuals; *Neisseria gonorrhoeae* was detected in less than 1% of women tested in family planning clinics in the United States in 2000 [99]. This means that the incremental cost of rescreening relative to initial screening has probably decreased. Moreover, if further progress in the control of the infection is to occur, public health efforts will need to be more focused on those at greatest risk. Persons who have a recent history of gonorrhea are a readily definable high-risk group. Second, the advent of NAATs makes screening simpler. It is possible to screen people without an examination or even through the mail.

Studies of rescreening for gonorrhea and chlamydial infection suggest that major operational barriers persist (Table 2). At least among STD clinic patients, simply advising patients to return and giving them an appointment seems to prompt fewer than 15% to be retested [102]. Mailing specimen collection kits to patients without any sort of verbal reminder may be marginally more effective in prompting people to retest [100]. Telephone calls to remind people to be retested is effective at prompting people to rescreen [102], and giving them the additional option of mailing in a specimen for retesting may somewhat increase the proportion retested [101]. Whether reminder calls are cost-effective is uncertain. Moreover, no study to date has successfully retested more than one third of persons targeted for retesting, and most have tested substantially fewer. Thus, although rescreening is merited on the basis of substantial evidence that persons who have STIs are at high risk for infection in the months following their treatment, mechanisms to ensure retesting have not been established. Furthermore, how to promote retesting outside of STD clinics has not been studied.

Cluster tracing and peer referral

Partner notification (PN) programs for syphilis have long included efforts to test cases' nonsexual contacts (ie, "suspects") and the social and sexual contacts named by uninfected persons initially identified through PN activities (ie, "associates"), a process called cluster tracing or cluster case finding [103]. More recently, increasing research on sexual networks has prompted renewed interest in focusing on social networks as a means to identify persons who have undiagnosed syphilis or HIV [104]. Such efforts have met with mixed success. Studies conducted in the 1990s reported interviewing between 9.1 and 500 syphilis cases to identify one new case of syphilis among suspects or associates [105–109].

A variant on traditional cluster tracing is peer referral. Peer referral involves recruiting persons from an at-risk social network to refer other members of the network for HIV or STI testing. Peer recruiters are typically given some incentive for referring others. A small study of HIV positive patients treated in an inner-city Los Angeles HIV clinic suggests that this

Table 2
Studies of rescreening

Author	Population	Intervention(s)	Percent retested	Comment
Judson Wolf [98]	438 STD clinic patients treated for gonorrhea (347 men)	Patients received appointment cards, telephone reminders, letter reminders, and field visits	27% tested at 6 wk; five (4.3%) tested positive	All patients also advised to have test-of-cure at 3–5 d; 70% did so
Bloomfield et al [100]	399 persons diagnosed with chlamydial infections (200 STD clinic patients)	Specimen collection kits mailed to patients 1–6 mo following treatment without prior notification or telephone calls	16% kits returned; two specimens (3.2%) tested positive	66 kits returned; return rate 22.4% for kits successfully delivered
Sparks et al [101]	122 persons treated for gonorrhea or chlamydial infection in an STD clinic or emergency room	RCT comparing reminder call to return for retesting >10 wk after treatment to reminder call plus the offer of mailing a specimen for retesting	45% of persons offered the option of mailing a specimen and 32% of those only reminded to come to the clinic retested (OR 1.7, 95% CI 0.8–3.8); Six (10%) of 58 persons retested positive	42% of potentially eligible persons could not be contacted for the study; all enrolled patients spoke with study personnel by telephone
Malotte et al [102]	Study 1: 421 STD clinic patients treated for gonorrhea or chlamydial infection	RCT 3 arms: 1) Appointment card & 5-min counseling 2) Arm 1 + $20 3) Motivational interviewing (MI) 13–25-min counseling, letter or phone call	Proportion retested: 11.4% 13.2% 23.9%	Significantly more people retested in arm 3 compared to arm 1 (OR 2.5, 95% CI 1.3–4.8)

(continued on next page)

Table 2 (*continued*)

Author	Population	Intervention(s)	Percent retested	Comment
	Study 2: 81 STD clinic patients treated for gonorrhea or chlamydial infection	1) Appointment card and 5-min counseling 2) Arm 1 + telephone reminder 3) MI without reminder	3.4% 33.3% 12% 8.9% of people infected at follow-up testing	Significantly more people tested in arm 2 compared to arm 1 (OR 12.3, 95% CI 1.4–112) Proportion of potentially eligible persons enrolled not reported

Abbreviations: MI, motivational interview; OR, odds ratio; RCT, randomized controlled trial.

approach may be effective. In that study, 31 HIV-positive patients referred 79 peers for testing and counseling, of whom 37 (47%) tested HIV positive [110,111]. This success does not appear to have been replicated, and further research on this intervention is merited.

Expedited partner therapy

Public health departments in high morbidity areas of the United States currently provide traditional partner notification services to fewer than 20% of persons treated for gonorrhea or chlamydial infection [112]. Diagnosing clinicians almost always tell patients to notify their partners, but they seldom know whether partners actually get treated. For example, a study of 140 clinicians interviewed after reporting a case of chlamydial infection to the health department in King County, Washington, found that only 17% knew whether their patient's partners had been treated [113]. Thus, in essence, the current standard of care in the United States is that patients are left to ensure their partners' treatment with no assistance and little guidance. Existing data suggest that roughly half of sex partners are treated [113–119]. The inadequacies of this system are self-evident, and the Institute of Medicine concluded that the United States' partner notification system was in need of redesign [120].

Expedited partner therapy (EPT) is a promising alternative to this existing PN system. EPT is a global term for approaches to treating the sex partners of persons who have STI that bypass the traditional requirement that all partners receive a complete medical evaluation before therapy. Such approaches include having public health personnel deliver medications to sex partners [121], contracts with pharmacies to provide medication to sex partners without the partners' prior examination [92,122], or having patients deliver prescriptions to their partners. In most instances EPT has involved patient-delivered partner therapy (PDPT), the practice of dispensing medications to patients for them to give to their sex partners.

Surveys of clinicians treating persons for gonorrhea or chlamydial infection suggest that approximately half of all providers in the United States have employed PDPT, but that most do so infrequently [113,123]. Observational studies conducted in the 1980s and early 1990s found that women provided with PDPT experienced lower rates of recurrent chlamydial infection [124,125]. Three randomized controlled trials subsequently tested the hypothesis that EPT, usually PDPT, could decrease the prevalence of infection in index patients (those originally diagnosed with the STI) at follow-up testing [92,126,127]. Two of these trials showed a statistically significant decrease in infection at follow-up in persons given EPT compared with controls [92,127], whereas the third reported a nonsignificant trend toward lower rates of chlamydial infection in women receiving PDPT (Table 3) [126]. Recipients of EPT were also significantly more likely to report that their partners were treated. These trials

Table 3
Summary of randomized controlled trials of expedited partner therapy to prevent recurrent gonorrhea or chlamydial infection

Author	Population	Intervention(s)	Outcome	Comment
Schillinger et al [126]	1787 women treated for chlamydial infection in diverse clinical settings in five United States cities	Azithromycin PDPT versus patient referral[a]	Chlamydia diagnosed in 12% PDPT versus 15% self-referral at 1-or 4-mo follow-up (OR 0.80, 95% CI 0.62–1.05)	Study did not achieve goal enrollment; behavioral outcomes not reported
Golden et al [92]	2751 persons (24% men) reported with gonorrhea or chlamydial infection in King County, Washington	Expedited partner treatment versus standard partner referral; expedited therapy included PDPT with azithromycin for chlamydial infection or azithromycin & cefixime for gonorrhea; 9% expedited care partners treated without prior exam through direct study staff contact; standard partner referral involved patient referral[a] with an offer of assistance notifying sex partners	Infection at 10–18 wk follow-up detected in 9.9% of subjects who received expedited partner treatment subjects and 13% who received standard partner referral (RR 0.76, 95% CI 0.59–0.98); persons receiving expedited partner care significantly more likely to report all partners were treated	Subgroup analysis showed expedited partner therapy significantly more effective for gonorrhea (RR 0.32, 95% CI 0.13–0.77) than for chlamydial infection (RR 0.82, 95% CI 0.62–1.07)
Kissinger et al [127]	977 men treated for urethritis in New Orleans STD clinic; 60% infected with gonorrhea and 20% chlamydial infection	3 arms: PDPT with azithromycin + ciprofloxacin or cefixime, BR, or PR[a]	Partner treatment reported by 56% PDPT, 44% BR, and 34% PR ($P < .001$); infection at follow-up detected in 23% PDPT, 14% BR, and 43% PR ($P < 0.001$)	Follow-up interviews performed on 80% of men; STI testing performed on in 30% of men

Abbreviations: BR, information booklet; OR, odds ratio; PDPT, partner-directed patient therapy; PR, patient referral; RR, relative risk.
[a] Patient referral means patients were advised to notify their sex partners and to advise the partners to seek medical care.

demonstrate that PDPT decreases the occurrence of persistent or recurrent gonorrhea or chlamydial infection in men and women but that the benefit is greater for gonorrhea, likely reflecting lower cure rates for chlamydial infection than for gonorrhea among women receiving conventional therapies.

The risk for significant treatable comorbidities, including PID, in heterosexual partners treated through PDPT appears to be low, suggesting that fear of missed opportunities to treat co-occurring STIs should not be a major impediment to the widespread use of PDPT [128]. Comorbidities in men treated as partners to women who have trichomonas are more common. State health departments in California and Washington State have already issued PDPT guidelines. However, the legal status of PDPT is uncertain in many states [129], and more widespread use of this intervention will likely require efforts to clearly define where and under what circumstances the practice is lawful.

Mass treatment and selective mass treatment

STI is sometimes concentrated in specific populations or geographic areas that are the focus of intensive prevention and disease control efforts. Unfortunately, these populations are often difficult to reach with traditional diagnostic testing and follow-up treatment, and syndromic therapy neglects many persons who have asymptomatic or subclinical infection. One means to control infections in such high-risk populations may be to treat all persons at risk.

Over the last 35 years, at least four studies have investigated mass treatment (MT) or selective mass treatment (SMT) (Table 4). Two studies described SMT interventions undertaken among female sex workers (FSWs) [130,132], and two were population-level mass treatment interventions [131,133]. Together, these reports strongly suggest that SMT can decrease STI prevalence in those treated, but that the effect is transient. MT of whole populations likewise seems to result in a transient decrease in prevalence. An increase in syphilis morbidity occurred following a single round of syphilis MT in Vancouver [133], and a similar increase in gonorrhea morbidity was observed among Naval servicemen following a single round of SMT of FSWs for gonorrhea [130]. These increases likely reflect a rebound phenomenon as STI equilibrium prevalence is reestablished following an unsustained intervention [134].

SMT and MT can be effective, although in most instances they probably need to be ongoing, rather than a one-time intervention. The potential development of antimicrobial resistance after MT and SMT is an additional concern requiring ongoing assessment when these interventions are employed. SMT of high-risk persons may be a reasonable intervention in some resource-poor, high-morbidity areas, though targeted periodic screening interventions may have a similar impact with less treatment-associated

Table 4
Studies of mass treatment or selective mass treatment of sexually transmitted infection

Author	Population	Intervention(s)	Outcome	Comment
Holmes et al [130]	Mass treatment of registered FSWs in Olongapo, Philippines	SMT of FSWs with ampicillin-probenecid for gonorrhea; mass treatment performed only once	Transient drop in gonorrhea prevalence in screened CSWs from 4% to 1.6% ($P < .001$); prevalence climbed to above premass treatment after intervention; SMT had no impact on number of gonorrhea cases passively detected in U.S. Navy servicemen during period of observation	Program of PN of CSW named by servicemen and scheduled CSW screening and treatment associated with a decline in gonorrhea prevalence among CSW, and in cases detected among Navy servicemen; SMT undertaken in context of existing PN and CSW screening program
Wawer et al [131]	10 community clusters in Uganda	Five community clusters randomly assigned to receive azithromycin, ciprofloxacin, metronidazole MS; control communities received vitamins and antihelmintics	Lower prevalence of syphilis (RR 0.80, 955 CI 0.71–0.89) and trichomonas (RR 0.59, 95% CI 0.38–0.91); magnitude of decline in chlamydial infection and gonorrhea significantly greater in intervention communities: prevalence of gonorrhea, chlamydial infection, and trichomonas in intervention communities significantly lower in postpartum women; no difference in HIV incidence	

Kaul et al [132]	466 Kenyan FSWs	230 randomly assigned to receive monthly azithromycin 1 g or placebo	Women who received azithromycin experienced a lower incidence of *N gonorrhoeae* (0.46, 95% CI 0.31–0.68), *C trachomatis* (0.38, 95% CI 0.26–0.57), and *T vaginalis* (0.56, 95% CI 0.40–0.78); no difference in syphilis or HIV incidence	No difference in syphilis or HIV incidence
Rekart et al [133]	4384 persons at risk for syphilis in Vancouver, BC	Azithromycin 1 g delivered by FSW, their clients, and others residing in a high prevalence area	Transient decline in monthly number of syphilis cases reported from 6.7 versus 10.2 ($P = .016$), with increase in number of monthly syphilis cases then rising to above that observed in the preintervention period	Model suggests rise in postintervention syphilis morbidity reflects rebound effect [134]

Abbreviations: CSW, commercial sex worker; FSW, female sex worker; MS, mass treatment; PN, partner notification; SMT, selective mass treatment.

morbidity [130]. SMT and MT do not currently appear to be promising interventions for use in developed nations.

Internet-based interventions

Since the late 1990s, the Internet has emerged as an important mechanism through which people form sexual partnerships. Early reports documented the role of Internet-based partnerships in a newly emerging syphilis epidemic among MSM, and a potential role for online-contact tracing in the control of that epidemic [135]. Internet use to recruit sex partners is extremely common among MSM and is likely increasing [136]. In 2000, 35% of MSM STD clinic patients in San Francisco reported meeting a partner on the Internet in the preceding year [137], whereas a random digit-dial study of 400 Seattle MSM conducted in 2003 found that 13.5% had met an anal sex partner on the Internet in the preceding 12 months (unpublished data). The importance of the Internet among heterosexuals is less certain. Although some heterosexuals meet partners over the Internet [138], it seems to be much less common than among MSM [139].

Public health authorities have used the Internet to disseminate information, promote safer sex, facilitate STI testing, and trace contacts to STI [137]. Syphilis contact tracing has met with some success [135,136,141], and patient interest in using the Internet to provide sex partners with information about STI is high [142]. Banners placed on Internet sex sites are frequently accessed, and Internet chats and question-and-answer sites have successfully engaged MSM. Additionally, an online syphilis testing program that allows patients to receive requisitions for testing through the Internet have allowed public health authorities in San Francisco to test small numbers of high-risk MSM [140]. However, Internet-based counseling interventions involving multiple sessions have been hampered by low rates of follow-up [143].

The Internet has clearly emerged as an important means through which people, particularly MSM, meet sex partners. Existing evidence suggests that the Internet can be used by public health authorities for purposes of partner notification and to disseminate educational and counseling messages. However, evaluations of Internet-based counseling or educational interventions do not yet exist.

Summary

Bacterial STI continues to be a major problem in developed nations. Research and evolving standards of public health practice are cause for optimism and concern. Innovations in case-finding and treatment, particularly the application of NAATs to test for chlamydial infection in nonclinical settings, are successes that merit more widespread application. EPT, selective STI screening in men, and rescreening are all promising, but are not yet in widespread use and may face significant operational barriers.

To date, public health efforts to alter sexual behavior, at least through specific interventions, are more discouraging. Although some behavioral interventions have been effective, none has been widely instituted. Moreover, the likelihood that existing behavioral interventions will be widely applied seems remote. Future research efforts in this area will need to focus less on proof-of-concept efficacy trials and more on developing and testing sustainable, cost-effective interventions that focus on those at greatest risk and that can be scaled-up within the existing public health infrastructure.

References

[1] Centers for Disease Control and Prevention. Sexually Transmitted Disease Surveillance. Atlanta (GA): Centers for Disease Control and Prevention; 2003. Available at: http://www.cdc.gov/std/stats/toc2003.htm.

[2] Herrmann B, Egger M. Genital Chlamydia trachomatis infections in Uppsala County, Sweden, 1985–1993: declining rates for how much longer? Sex Transm Dis 1995;22:253–60.

[3] Tichonova L, Borisenko K, Ward H, et al. Epidemics of syphilis in the Russian Federation: trends, origins, and priorities for control. Lancet 1997;350:210–3.

[4] LaMontagne DS, Fenton KA, Randall S, et al. Establishing the National Chlamydia Screening Programme in England: results from the first full year of screening. Sex Transm Infect 2004;80:335–41.

[5] Hughes G, Fenton KA. Recent trends in gonorrhoea - an emerging public health issue? Euro Surveill 2000;5:1–2.

[6] Manhart L, Holmes KK. Randomized controlled trials of individual-level, population-level, and multilevel interventions for preventing sexually transmitted infections: what has worked? J Infect Dis 2004;190(Suppl 1):S1–17.

[7] Johnson WD, Hedges LV, Ramirez G, et al. HIV prevention research for men who have sex with men: a systematic review and meta-analysis. J Acquir Immune Defic Syndr 2002; 30(Suppl 1):S118–29.

[8] Mullen PD, Ramirez G, Strouse D, et al. Meta-analysis of the effects of behavioral HIV prevention interventions on the sexual risk behavior of sexually experienced adolescents in controlled studies in the United States. J Acquir Immune Defic Syndr 2002;30(Suppl 1):S94–105.

[9] Neumann MS, Johnson WD, Semaan S, et al. Review and meta-analysis of HIV prevention intervention research for heterosexual adult populations in the United States. J Acquir Immune Defic Syndr 2002;30(Suppl 1):S106–17.

[10] Boyer CB, Barrett DC, Peterman TA, et al. Sexually transmitted disease (STD) and HIV risk in heterosexual adults attending a public STD clinic: evaluation of a randomized controlled behavioral risk-reduction intervention trial. AIDS 1997;11:359–67.

[11] Imrie J, Stephenson JM, Cowan FM, et al. A cognitive behavioural intervention to reduce sexually transmitted infections among gay men: randomised trial. BMJ 2001;322:1451–6.

[12] Koblin B, Chesney M, Coates T. Effects of a behavioural intervention to reduce acquisition of HIV infection among men who have sex with men: the EXPLORE randomised controlled study. Lancet 2004;364:41–50.

[13] Cohen DA, Dent C, MacKinnon D, et al. Condoms for men, not women. Results of brief promotion programs. Sex Transm Dis 1992;19:245–51.

[14] Kamb ML, Fishbein M, Douglas JM Jr, et al. Efficacy of risk-reduction counseling to prevent human immunodeficiency virus and sexually transmitted diseases: a randomized controlled trial. Project RESPECT Study Group. JAMA 1998;280:1161–7.

[15] Cohen DA. Condom skills education and sexually transmitted disease reinfection. J Sex Res 1991;28:139–44.

[16] Cohen DA, MacKinnon DP, Dent C, et al. Group counseling at STD clinics to promote use of condoms. Public Health Rep 1992;107:727–31.
[17] O'Donnell CR, O'Donnell L, San Doval A, et al. Reductions in STD infections subsequent to an STD clinic visit. Using video-based patient education to supplement provider interactions. Sex Transm Dis 1998;25:161–8.
[18] The National Institute of Mental Health (NIMH) Multisite HIV Prevention Trial Group. The NIMH Multisite HIV Prevention Trial: reducing HIV sexual risk behavior. Science 1998;280:1889–94.
[19] Branson BM, Peterman TA, Cannon RO, et al. Group counseling to prevent sexually transmitted disease and HIV: a randomized controlled trial. Sex Transm Dis 1998;25: 553–60.
[20] Shain RN, Piper JM, Newton ER, et al. A randomized, controlled trial of a behavioral intervention to prevent sexually transmitted disease among minority women. N Engl J Med 1999;340:93–100.
[21] Hobfoll SE, Jackson AP, Lavin J, et al. Effects and generalizability of communally oriented HIV-AIDS prevention versus general health promotion groups for single, inner-city women in urban clinics. J Consult Clin Psychol 2002;70:950–60.
[22] DiClemente RJ, Wingood GM, Harrington KF, et al. Efficacy of an HIV prevention intervention for African American adolescent girls: a randomized controlled trial. JAMA 2004;292:171–9.
[23] Shain RN, Piper JM, Holden AE, et al. Prevention of gonorrhea and Chlamydia through behavioral intervention: results of a two-year controlled randomized trial in minority women. Sex Transm Dis 2004;31:401–8.
[24] Boyer CB, Shafer MA, Shaffer RA, et al. Evaluation of a cognitive-behavioral, group, randomized controlled intervention trial to prevent sexually transmitted infections and unintended pregnancies in young women. Prev Med 2005;40:420–31.
[25] Wingood GM, DiClemente RJ, Mikhail I, et al. A randomized controlled trial to reduce HIV transmission risk behaviors and sexually transmitted diseases among women living with HIV: The WiLLOW Program. J Acquir Immune Defic Syndr 2004;37:S58–67.
[26] Castrucci BC, Kamb ML, Hunt K. Assessing the Center for Disease Control and Prevention's 1994 HIV counseling, testing, and referral: standards and guidelines: how closely does practice conform to existing recommendations? Sex Transm Dis 2002;29: 417–21.
[27] Kurth A, Spielberg F, Fortenberry JD, et al. Computer-assisted risk assessment and education. Presented at the International Society for Sexually Transmitted Diseases Research Congress. Ottawa, Canada, July 27–30, 2003.
[28] Centers for Disease Control and Prevention. Advancing HIV prevention: new strategies for a changing epidemic—United States, 2003. MMWR Morb Mortal Wkly Rep 2003;52: 329–32.
[29] Brackbill RM, Sternberg MR, Fishbein M. Where do people go for treatment of sexually transmitted diseases? Fam Plann Perspect 1999;31:10–5.
[30] Cutler JC, Singh B, Carpenter U, et al. Vaginal contraceptives as prophylaxis against gonorrhea and other sexually transmissible diseases. Adv Plan Parent 1977;12:45–56.
[31] Rendon AL, Covarrubias J, McCarney KE, et al. A controlled comparative study of phenylmercuric acetate, nonoxynol-9 and placebo vaginal suppositories as prophylactic agents against gonorrhea. Current Therapeutic Research 1980;27:780–3.
[32] Rosenberg MJ, Rojanapithayakorn W, Feldblum PJ, et al. Effect of the contraceptive sponge on chlamydial infection, gonorrhea, and candidiasis. A comparative clinical trial. JAMA 1987;257:2308–12.
[33] Louv WC, Austin H, Alexander WJ, et al. A clinical trial of nonoxynol-9 for preventing gonococcal and chlamydial infections. J Infect Dis 1988;158:518–23.
[34] Niruthisard S, Roddy RE, Chutivongse S. Use of nonoxynol-9 and reduction in rate of gonococcal and chlamydial cervical infections. Lancet 1992;339:1371–5.

[35] Kreiss J, Ngugi E, Holmes K, et al. Efficacy of nonoxynol 9 contraceptive sponge use in preventing heterosexual acquisition of HIV in Nairobi prostitutes. JAMA 1992;268: 477–82.
[36] Roddy RE, Zekeng L, Ryan KA, et al. A controlled trial of nonoxynol 9 film to reduce male-to-female transmission of sexually transmitted diseases. N Engl J Med 1998;339: 504–10.
[37] Roddy RE, Zekeng L, Ryan KA, et al. Effect of nonoxynol-9 gel on urogenital gonorrhea and chlamydial infection: a randomized controlled trial. JAMA 2002;287:1117–22.
[38] Richardson BA, Lavreys L, Martin HL Jr, et al. Evaluation of a low-dose nonoxynol-9 gel for the prevention of sexually transmitted diseases: a randomized clinical trial. Sex Transm Dis 2001;28:394–400.
[39] Van Damme L, Ramjee G, Alary M, et al. Effectiveness of COL-1492, a nonoxynol-9 vaginal gel, on HIV-1 transmission in female sex workers: a randomised controlled trial. Lancet 2002;360:971–7.
[40] Wilkinson D, Tholandi M, Ramjee G, et al. Nonoxynol-9 spermicide for prevention of vaginally acquired HIV and other sexually transmitted infections: systematic review and meta-analysis of randomised controlled trials including more than 5000 women. Lancet Infect Dis 2002;2:613–7.
[41] Moore JP. Topical microbicides become topical. N Engl J Med 2005;352:298–300.
[42] Centers for Disease Control and Prevention. Chlamydia screening among sexually active young female enrollees of health plans—United States, 1999–2001. MMWR Morb Mortal Wkly Rep 2004;53:983–5.
[43] Corey L, Handsfield HH. Genital herpes and public health: addressing a global problem. JAMA 2000;283:791–4.
[44] Sangani P, Rutherford G, Wilkinson D. Population-based interventions for reducing sexually transmitted infections, including HIV infection. Cochrane Database Syst Rev 2004;(2):CD001220.
[45] Centers for Disease Control and Prevention. Sexually transmitted diseases treatment guidelines 2002. MMWR Recomm Rep 2002;51(RR-6):1–78.
[46] Shafer MA, Tebb KP, Pantell RH, et al. Effect of a clinical practice improvement intervention on Chlamydial screening among adolescent girls. JAMA 2002;288:2846–52.
[47] Scholes D, Grothaus L, McClure J, et al. A randomized trial of strategies to increase chlamydia screening in young women. Am J Prev Med, in press.
[48] Bordley WC, Margolis PA, Stuart J, et al. Improving preventive service delivery through office systems. Pediatrics 2001;108:E41.
[49] Heinrich P, Homer CJ. Improving the care of children with asthma in pediatric practice: the HIPPO project. Helping Improve Pediatric Practice Outcomes. Pediatr Ann 1999;28:64–72.
[50] Oh MK, Smith KR, O'Cain M, et al. Urine-based screening of adolescents in detention to guide treatment for gonococcal and chlamydial infections. Translating research into intervention. Arch Pediatr Adolesc Med 1998;152:52–6.
[51] Mrus JM, Biro FM, Huang B, et al. Evaluating adolescents in juvenile detention facilities for urogenital chlamydial infection: costs and effectiveness of alternative interventions. Arch Pediatr Adolesc Med 2003;157:696–702.
[52] Pack RP, Diclemente RJ, Hook EW III, et al. High prevalence of asymptomatic STDs in incarcerated minority male youth: a case for screening. Sex Transm Dis 2000;27: 175–7.
[53] LaMontagne DS, Fine DN, Marrazzo JM. Chlamydia trachomatis infection in asymptomatic men. Am J Prev Med 2003;24:36–42.
[54] Fenton KA, Korovessis C, Johnson AM, et al. Sexual behaviour in Britain: reported sexually transmitted infections and prevalent genital Chlamydia trachomatis infection. Lancet 2001;358:1851–4.
[55] Bauer HM, Chartier M, Kessell E, et al. Chlamydia screening of youth and young adults in non-clinical settings throughout California. Sex Transm Dis 2004;31:409–14.

[56] Nsuami M, Cammarata CL, Brooks BN, et al. Chlamydia and gonorrhea co-occurrence in a high school population. Sex Transm Dis 2004;31:424–7.
[57] Salmon M. Implementing gonorrhea and chlamydia screening in Philadelphia public high schools. Presented at the 2004 National STD Prevention Conference. Philadelphia, PA, March 8–11, 2004.
[58] Blake DR, Gaydos CA, Quinn TC. Cost-effectiveness analysis of screening adolescent males for Chlamydia on admission to detention. Sex Transm Dis 2004;31:85–95.
[59] Genc M, Ruusuvaara L, Mardh PA. An economic evaluation of screening for Chlamydia trachomatis in adolescent males. JAMA 1993;270:2057–64.
[60] Ginocchio RH, Veenstra DL, Connell FA, et al. The clinical and economic consequences of screening young men for genital chlamydial infection. Sex Transm Dis 2003;30:99–106.
[61] Kretzschmar M, Welte R, van den Hoek A, et al. Comparative model-based analysis of screening programs for Chlamydia trachomatis infections. Am J Epidemiol 2001;153: 90–101.
[62] Welte R, Kretzschmar M, van den Hoek JA, et al. A population based dynamic approach for estimating the cost effectiveness of screening for Chlamydia trachomatis. Sex Transm Infect 2003;79:426.
[63] Whittington WL, Collis T, Dithmer-Schreck D, et al. Sexually transmitted diseases and human immunodeficiency virus-discordant partnerships among men who have sex with men. Clin Infect Dis 2002;35:1010–7.
[64] Public Health—Seattle & King County. Sexually transmitted disease and HIV screening guidelines for men who have sex with men. Sex Transm Dis 2001;28:457–9.
[65] Cohen DA, Nsuami M, Etame RB, et al. A school-based Chlamydia control program using DNA amplification technology. Pediatrics 1998;101:E1.
[66] Cohen DA, Nsuami M, Martin DH, et al. Repeated school-based screening for sexually transmitted diseases: a feasible strategy for reaching adolescents. Pediatrics 1999;104: 1281–5.
[67] Bachmann LH, Lewis I, Allen R, et al. Risk and prevalence of treatable sexually transmitted diseases at a Birmingham substance abuse treatment facility. Am J Public Health 2000;90:1615–8.
[68] Mehta SD, Rothman RE, Kelen GD, et al. Unsuspected gonorrhea and chlamydia in patients of an urban adult emergency department: a critical population for STD control intervention. Sex Transm Dis 2001;28:33–9.
[69] Mehta SD, Rothman RE, Kelen GD, et al. Clinical aspects of diagnosis of gonorrhea and Chlamydia infection in an acute care setting. Clin Infect Dis 2001;32:655–9.
[70] Mehta SD, Rompalo A, Rothman RE, et al. Generalizability of STD screening in urban emergency departments: comparison of results from inner city and urban sites in Baltimore, Maryland. Sex Transm Dis 2003;30:143–8.
[71] Embling ML, Monroe KW, Oh MK, et al. Opportunistic urine ligase chain reaction screening for sexually transmitted diseases in adolescents seeking care in an urban emergency department. Ann Emerg Med 2000;36:28–32.
[72] Monroe KW, Weiss HL, Jones M, et al. Acceptability of urine screening for Neisseria gonorrhoeae and Chlamydia trachomatis in adolescents at an urban emergency department. Sex Transm Dis 2003;30:850–3.
[73] Lifson AR, Halcon LL, Hannan P, et al. Screening for sexually transmitted infections among economically disadvantaged youth in a national job training program. J Adolesc Health 2001;28:190–6.
[74] Judson FN, Miller KG, Schaffnit TR. Screening for gonorrhea and syphilis in the gay baths—Denver, Colorado. Am J Public Health 1977;67:740–2.
[75] Lister NA, Smith A, Tabrizi S, et al. Screening for Neisseria gonorrhoeae and Chlamydia trachomatis in men who have sex with men at male-only saunas. Sex Transm Dis 2003;30: 886–9.

[76] Rietmeijer CA, Yamaguchi KJ, Ortiz CG, et al. Feasibility and yield of screening urine for Chlamydia trachomatis by polymerase chain reaction among high-risk male youth in field-based and other nonclinic settings. A new strategy for sexually transmitted disease control. Sex Transm Dis 1997;24:429–35.
[77] Kahn RH, Moseley KE, Thilges JN, et al. Community-based screening and treatment for STDs: results from a mobile clinic initiative. Sex Transm Dis 2003;30:654–8.
[78] Parran T. Shadow on the land: syphilis. New York: Reynal & Hitchcock; 1937.
[79] Mertz KJ, Voigt RA, Hutchins K, et al. Findings from STD screening of adolescents and adults entering corrections facilities: implications for STD control strategies. Sex Transm Dis 2002;29:834–9.
[80] Marrazzo JM, White CL, Krekeler B, et al. Community-based urine screening for Chlamydia trachomatis with a ligase chain reaction assay. Ann Intern Med 1997;127:796–803.
[81] Schillinger JA, Dunne EF, Chapin JB, et al. Prevalence of Chlamydia trachomatis infection among men screened in 4 US cities. Sex Transm Dis 2005;32:74–7.
[82] Kent CK, Branzuela A, Fischer L, et al. Chlamydia and gonorrhea screening in San Francisco high schools. Sex Transm Dis 2002;29:373–5.
[83] Burstein GR, Waterfield G, Joffe A, et al. Screening for gonorrhea and chlamydia by DNA amplification in adolescents attending middle school health centers. Opportunity for early intervention. Sex Transm Dis 1998;25:395–402.
[84] Gaydos CA, Howell MR, Quinn TC, et al. Sustained high prevalence of Chlamydia trachomatis infections in female army recruits. Sex Transm Dis 2003;30:539–44.
[85] Crosby RA, DiClemente RJ, Wingood GM, et al. Associations between sexually transmitted disease diagnosis and subsequent sexual risk and sexually transmitted disease incidence among adolescents. Sex Transm Dis 2004;31:205–8.
[86] La Montagne DS, Patrick LE, Fine DN, et al. Re-evaluating selective screening criteria for Chlamydial infection among women in the U S Pacific Northwest. Sex Transm Dis 2004;31:283–9.
[87] Arcari CM, Gaydos JC, Howell MR, et al. Feasibility and short-term impact of linked education and urine screening interventions for Chlamydia and gonorrhea in male army recruits. Sex Transm Dis 2004;31:443–7.
[88] Whittington WL, Kent C, Kissinger P, et al. Determinants of persistent and recurrent Chlamydia trachomatis infection in young women: results of a multicenter cohort study. Sex Transm Dis 2001;28:117–23.
[89] Orr DP, Langefeld CD, Katz BP, et al. Behavioral intervention to increase condom use among high-risk female adolescents. J Pediatr 1996;128:288–95.
[90] Kjaer HO, Dimcevski G, Hoff G, et al. Recurrence of urogenital Chlamydia trachomatis infection evaluated by mailed samples obtained at home: 24 weeks' prospective follow up study. Sex Transm Infect 2000;76:169–72.
[91] Blythe MJ, Katz BP, Batteiger BE, et al. Recurrent genitourinary chlamydial infections in sexually active female adolescents. J Pediatr 1992;121:487–93.
[92] Golden MR, Whittington WL, Handsfield HH, et al. Impact of expedited sex partner treatment on recurrent or persistent gonorrhea or chlamydial infection: a randomized controlled trial. N Engl J Med 2005;352:676–85.
[93] Hu D, Hook EW III, Goldie SJ. Screening for Chlamydia trachomatis in women 15 to 29 years of age: a cost-effectiveness analysis. Ann Intern Med 2004;141:501–13.
[94] Oh MK, Cloud GA, Fleenor M, et al. Risk for gonococcal and chlamydial cervicitis in adolescent females: incidence and recurrence in a prospective cohort study. J Adolesc Health 1996;18:270–5.
[95] Fortenberry JD, Brizendine EJ, Katz BP, et al. Subsequent sexually transmitted infections among adolescent women with genital infection due to Chlamydia trachomatis, Neisseria gonorrhoeae, or Trichomonas vaginalis. Sex Transm Dis 1999;26:26–32.

[96] Brooks GF, Darrow WW, Day JA. Repeated gonorrhea: an analysis of importance and risk factors. J Infect Dis 1978;137:161–9.
[97] Brown ST, Wiesner PJ. Problems and approaches to the control and surveillance of sexually transmitted agents associated with pelvic inflammatory disease in the United States. Am J Obstet Gynecol 1980;138:1096–100.
[98] Judson FN, Wolf FC. Rescreening for gonorrhea: an evaluation of compliance methods and results. Am J Public Health 1979;69:1178–80.
[99] Dicker LW, Mosure DJ, Berman SM, et al. Gonorrhea prevalence and coinfection with chlamydia in women in the United States, 2000. Sex Transm Dis 2003;30:472–6.
[100] Bloomfield PJ, Steiner KC, Kent CK, et al. Repeat chlamydia screening by mail, San Francisco. Sex Transm Infect 2003;79:28–30.
[101] Sparks R, Helmers JR, Handsfield HH, et al. Rescreening for gonorrhea and chlamydial infection through the mail: a randomized trial. Sex Transm Dis 2004;31:113–6.
[102] Malotte CK, Ledsky R, Hogben M, et al. Comparison of methods to increase repeat testing in persons treated for gonorrhea and/or chlamydia at public sexually transmitted disease clinics. Sex Transm Dis 2004;31:637–42.
[103] Spencer JN. A critical piece by whatever name. Sex Transm Dis 2000;27:19–20.
[104] Rothenberg R. The transformation of partner notification. Clin Infect Dis 2002;35:S138–45.
[105] Engelgau MM, Woernle CH, Rolfs RT, et al. Control of epidemic early syphilis: the results of an intervention campaign using social networks. Sex Transm Dis 1995;22:203–9.
[106] Gunn RA, Harper SL. Emphasizing infectious syphilis partner notification. Sex Transm Dis 1998;25:218–9.
[107] Rosenberg D, Moseley K, Kahn R, et al. Networks of persons with syphilis and at risk for syphilis in Louisiana: evidence of core transmitters. Sex Transm Dis 1999;26:108–14.
[108] Rothenberg R, Kimbrough L, Lewis-Hardy R, et al. Social network methods for endemic foci of syphilis: a pilot project. Sex Transm Dis 2000;27:12–8.
[109] Kohl KS, Farley TA, Ewell J, et al. Usefulness of partner notification for syphilis control. Sex Transm Dis 1999;26:201–7.
[110] Jordon W, Tolbert L, Smith R. Partner notification and focused intervention as a means of identifying HIV-positive patients. J Natl Med Assoc 1998;90:542–6.
[111] Jordan W, Spring M. HIV focused intervention program. Presented at the Infectious Disease Society of America. Philadelphia, November 18–21, 1999.
[112] Golden MR, Hogben M, Handsfield HH, et al. Partner notification for HIV and STD in the United States: low coverage for gonorrhea, chlamydial infection, and HIV. Sex Transm Dis 2003;30:490–6.
[113] Golden MR, Whittington WL, Gorbach PM, et al. Partner notification for chlamydial infections among private sector clinicians in Seattle-King County: a clinician and patient survey. Sex Transm Dis 1999;26:543–7.
[114] Potterat JJ, Rothenberg R. The case-finding effectiveness of self-referral system for gonorrhea: a preliminary report. Am J Public Health 1977;67:174–6.
[115] Woodhouse DE, Potterat JJ, Muth JB, et al. A civilian-military partnership to reduce the incidence of gonorrhea. Public Health Rep 1985;100:61–5.
[116] Patel HC, Viswalingam ND, Goh BT. Chlamydial ocular infection: efficacy of partner notification by patient referral. Int J STD AIDS 1994;5:244–7.
[117] Oh MK, Boker JR, Genuardi FJ, et al. Sexual contact tracing outcome in adolescent chlamydial and gonococcal cervicitis cases. J Adolesc Health 1996;18:4–9.
[118] Fortenberry JD, Brizendine EJ, Katz BP, et al. The role of self-efficacy and relationship quality in partner notification by adolescents with sexually transmitted infections. Arch Pediatr Adolesc Med 2002;156:1133–7.
[119] van de Laar MJ, Termorshuizen F, van den Hoek A. Partner referral by patients with gonorrhea and chlamydial infection. Case-finding observations. Sex Transm Dis 1997;24:334–42.

[120] Committee on Prevention and Control of Sexually Transmitted Diseases, Institute of Medicine; Eng TR, Butler WT, editors. The hidden epidemic: confronting sexually transmitted diseases. Washington (DC): National Academy Press; 1997.
[121] Steiner KC, Davila V, Kent CK, et al. Field-delivered therapy increases treatment for chlamydia and gonorrhea. Am J Public Health 2003;93:882–4.
[122] Golden MR, Whittington WL, Handsfield HH, et al. Partner management for gonococcal and chlamydial infection: expansion of public health services to the private sector and expedited sex partner treatment through a partnership with commercial pharmacies. Sex Transm Dis 2001;28:658–65.
[123] Hogben M, McCree D, Golden MR. Patient-delivered partner therapy for sexually transmitted diseases as practiced by US physicians. Sex Transm Dis 2005;32(2):101–5.
[124] Ramstedt K, Forssman L, Johannisson G. Contact tracing in the control of genital Chlamydia trachomatis infection. Int J STD AIDS 1991;2:116–8.
[125] Kissinger P, Brown R, Reed K, et al. Effectiveness of patient delivered partner medication for preventing recurrent Chlamydia trachomatis. Sex Transm Infect 1998;74:331–3.
[126] Schillinger JA, Kissinger P, Calvet H, et al. Patient-delivered partner treatment with azithromycin to prevent repeated Chlamydia trachomatis infection among women: a randomized, controlled trial. Sex Transm Dis 2003;30:49–56.
[127] Kissinger P, Farley TA, Richardson-Alston G, et al. A comparison of three different strategies to treat partners of men with urethritis. Presented at the 15th International Society for Sexually Transmitted Disease Research Congress. Ottawa, Canada, July 27–30, 2003.
[128] Stekler J, Bachmann L, Brotman RM, et al. Concurrent sexually transmitted infections (STIs) in sex partners of patients diagnosed with selected STIs: implications for patient-delivered partner therapy. Clin Infect Dis 2005;40(6):787–93.
[129] Golden MR, Anukam U, Williams DH, et al. The legal status of patient-delivered partner therapy for sexually transmitted infections in the United States: a national survey of state medical and pharmacy boards. Sex Transm Dis 2005;32(2):112–4.
[130] Holmes KK, Johnson DW, Kvale PA, et al. Impact of a gonorrhea control program, including selective mass treatment, in female sex workers. J Infect Dis 1996;174(Suppl 2):S230–9.
[131] Wawer MJ, Sewankambo NK, Serwadda D, et al. Control of sexually transmitted diseases for AIDS prevention in Uganda: a randomised community trial. Rakai Project Study Group. Lancet 1999;353:525–35.
[132] Kaul R, Kimani J, Nagelkerke NJ, et al. Monthly antibiotic chemoprophylaxis and incidence of sexually transmitted infections and HIV-1 infection in Kenyan sex workers: a randomized controlled trial. JAMA 2004;291:2555–62.
[133] Rekart ML, Patrick DM, Chakraborty B, et al. Targeted mass treatment for syphilis with oral azithromycin. Lancet 2003;361:313–4.
[134] Pourbohloul B, Rekart ML, Brunham RC. Impact of mass treatment on syphilis transmission: a mathematical modeling approach. Sex Transm Dis 2003;30:297–305.
[135] Klausner JD, Wolf W, Fischer-Ponce L, et al. Tracing a syphilis outbreak through cyberspace. JAMA 2000;284:447–9.
[136] Centers for Disease Control and Prevention. Internet use and early syphilis infection among men who have sex with men—San Francisco, California, 1999–2003. MMWR Morb Mortal Wkly Rep 2003;52:1229–32.
[137] Kim AA, Kent C, McFarland W, et al. Cruising on the Internet highway. J Acquir Immune Defic Syndr 2001;28:89–93.
[138] McFarlane M, Bull SS, Rietmeijer CA. Young adults on the Internet: risk behaviors for sexually transmitted diseases and HIV(1). J Adolesc Health 2002;31:11–6.
[139] McFarlane M, Bull SS, Rietmeijer CA. The Internet as a newly emerging risk environment for sexually transmitted diseases. JAMA 2000;284:443–6.
[140] Klausner JD, Levine DK, Kent CK. Internet-based site-specific interventions for syphilis prevention among gay and bisexual men. AIDS Care 2004;16:964–70.

[141] Centers for Disease Control and Prevention. Using the Internet for partner notification of sexually transmitted diseases—Los Angeles County, California, 2003. MMWR Morb Mortal Wkly Rep 2004;53:129–31.
[142] Tomnay JE, Pitts MK, Fairley CK. Partner notification: preferences of Melbourne clients and the estimated proportion of sexual partners they can contact. Int J STD AIDS 2004;15: 415–8.
[143] Bull SS, Lloyd L, Rietmeijer C, et al. Recruitment and retention of an online sample for an HIV prevention intervention targeting men who have sex with men: the Smart Sex Quest Project. AIDS Care 2004;16:931–43.

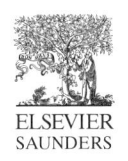

Behavioral Interventions—Rationale, Measurement, and Effectiveness

Jonathan M. Zenilman, MD

Division of Infectious Diseases, Johns Hopkins Bayview Medical Center, 4940 Eastern Avenue, B-3 North, Baltimore, MD 21224, USA

This article provides an overview for clinicians on the development and implementation of behavioral interventions for sexually transmitted diseases (STDs) and HIV infection. It includes a brief discussion of behavioral models and how these are used to develop intervention strategies, providing some examples in specific populations. One of the most vexing problems in behavioral research is evaluation because disease outcomes are relatively rare and behavioral outcomes are subject to bias. This article explores some new techniques and technologies for circumventing these issues, then presents case studies of population-based STD/HIV intervention programs, and concludes by addressing important political and structural challenges to STD/HIV prevention efforts. This article interdigitates with Dr. Aral's article on sexual behavior and Dr. Golden's article on new approaches to STD intervention found elsewhere in this issue.

Before the HIV epidemic, behavioral intervention for STDs typically consisted of distributing a pamphlet at the end of the patient encounter, with perhaps some additional advice on how to prevent reinfection. In retrospect, this approach is naïve, representing modest patient education/information but not behavioral intervention [1]. The past 25 years have been characterized by an enormous increase in knowledge of the interaction between sexual behavior and STD/HIV risk. This increase has been paralleled by an increase in understanding of the key determinants of risky sexual behavior, the development of sophisticated behavioral interventions for acute infectious diseases, and understanding of the intertwined relationships between risky sexual behavior, the social environment, and other comorbidities such as mental health disorders and illicit drug use.

E-mail address: jzenilm1@jhmi.edu

Challenges in developing behavioral interventions: assessment

Major challenges in designing and implementing intervention strategies include using appropriate assessment tools, defining an individual's or population's baseline status, and implementing an intervention [2–4]. These challenges became particularly evident early in the 1980s, when most intervention outcome assessments were made based on process measures. Process measures include programmatic outcomes that are related to level of program activity, such as number of pamphlets handed out, condoms distributed, individuals contacted, persons treated in clinic, and so forth. However, these types of measures do not yield any data relevant to outcomes or efficacy. The underlying public health question in these settings is: "Did the intervention work?"

A major challenge in developing effective behavioral prevention strategies is identifying appropriate outcome effectiveness measures [5]. For STD interventions, efficacy markers can include changes in self-reported behaviors, and biologic markers such as bacterial and viral STD incidence [6]. Behavioral and biologic markers each have their own advantages and disadvantages. Sexual behavior assessment and reporting are notoriously subject to ascertainment and reporting bias, and are also affected by the structure of questionnaires, the context and environment of the interview, and cultural factors. Biologic markers, although attractive, present other problems. For example, HIV incidence would be the ultimate measure of most interest in large behavioral intervention studies. However, incident HIV is a rare event, which if used exclusively as the evaluation tool would require sample sizes in the tens of thousands, even when evaluating interventions that are highly effective. In high-risk populations, such as individuals attending STD clinics, where incidence of gonorrhea and chlamydia is high, measuring incident bacterial STD is a potential approach. These approaches require careful longitudinal clinical and laboratory assessment to document that the incident infection was acquired during the evaluation period, and is not an asymptomatic infection that was present earlier ("prevalent infection"). Furthermore, even in the highest risk population, bacterial STDs affect only a few individuals, leading to type-2 measurement error [7]. For example, in Baltimore and other high-risk inner-city STD clinic populations, combined gonorrhea and chlamydia incidence at 3-month follow-up is typically 10% to 15% [8]. Although this is an extraordinarily high rate, under this scenario 85% of the individuals who did not get infected may be misclassified as "safe" but still be at substantial risk because of their underlying behaviors. Another drawback is that using biologic disease-related bacterial end points also requires substantial investment in laboratory resources [9]. Quality control of laboratory results is critically important, especially when dealing with field-based acquisition of samples and specimen transport. Even when using detection assays with high sensitivity and specificity, in populations where the prevalence is low the positive predictive value is consequently low (Bayes' conundrum), which has important implications for assay and intervention design. In these situations, confirmatory algorithms conceptually similar to those used in HIV testing may be an alternative approach.

Biologic factors also impact STD incidence. For example, STD risk can be impacted by host immunity. It has been hypothesized that the steep age-related declines in chlamydia in inner-city women after the teen-age years are caused by acquired host immunity resulting in protection from later exposures [10–12]. In contrast, persons who have HIV or other immune deficiencies may be at higher risk for herpes and HPV infection.

Assessment bias: self-reported measures

Behavioral questionnaires have traditionally focused on individual's risk behaviors, such as number of partners, lifetime partners, and recent sexual activity. However, STD risk factor analyses have found that individual-based risks for STDs have odds ratios no greater than three in most studies, and cannot fully explain STD rates in high-risk populations [13]. Network approaches, which study and evaluate an individual's sexual network (ie, who they have sex with), can inform the risk assessment, but the methods of obtaining these assessments are not standardized and are labor-intensive [14–16]. The network approach attempts to ascertain the qualitative aspects of the partners, which is missed in typical scalar analyses. For example, it is difficult to incorporate into the term the impact of a high-risk versus a low-risk partner. For example, is a partner who is a commercial sex worker more high risk as opposed to a partner who is in a monogamous relationship?

Although widely used, self-reported behavioral markers—especially those that report sexual and drug-using behaviors—are subject to reporting bias. Issues in behavioral reporting include validity and reliability [17]. Validity is the measure of the underlying accuracy of the data, whereas reliability is a measure of data reproducibility. Validity is the major concern in evaluating the effectiveness of intervention. In general, studies in various populations have shown that men may overreport the number of sexual partners, women may underreport the number of sexual partners, and condom use tends to be overreported. These factors substantially impact on understanding and measuring the effectiveness of interventions.

In evaluating interventions, what is the appropriate outcome measure? Does the intervention result in a biologic outcome reduction? In most, if not all, settings where biologic outcome events are rare, can a proxy behavioral indicator be used? For example, are STDs a valid biologic proxy for high-risk sexual behavior that would lead to HIV infection? Alternatively, if accurately reported, are sexual behaviors an adequate proxy for disease risk?

Behavioral markers are the easiest and most inexpensive. Despite the issues, there is consensus in the literature that self-reported behaviors can be used, but only in settings where methodology concerns are comprehensively addressed [9]. These approaches include improving validity from either live (ie, face-to-face) interviewers or using alternative, more accurate modes of data collection. Live interviewer–response validity can be improved through extensive training and even desensitization of interviewers, and continuous quality control monitoring during surveys. However, this approach is extremely labor-intensive and expensive. The alternative modes include self-administered written questionnaire, self-administered computerized questionnaire, such as the Audio Computer Assisted Self-Interview (A-CASI), or even telephone-administered questionnaires, such as T-CASI [17–20]. A-CASI uses a computerized questionnaire that is voice-administered directly to the subject; there is no human interviewer present. The underlying hypothesis is that individuals taking the computerized questionnaire will be less likely to have reporting/social desirability bias, thereby improving response validity. Studies in various population-based and clinical settings have demonstrated that A-CASI increases validity of self-reported drug use, same-sex partners, prior abortion, and rectal intercourse compared with interview-administered methods. Condom use in most settings is overreported because of the repeated intervention and public information campaigns that especially target reproductive age groups and persons at risk for HIV/STD [8,21].

Even after an intervention is developed, fielded, and evaluated, and even in phase 3 randomized clinical trials, there are critical translational issues. From a pragmatic standpoint, does a behavioral intervention and its intended outcome translate into a program that can be appropriately fielded? Effective translation may be impeded by lack of funding for implementation, lack of field-based support, or operational barriers in implementations. Examples of the latter are clinic-based interventions that require additional clinician or counselor time in clinic environments where service demand already exceeds supply. A counseling intervention would increase the time needed to serve each client, and even if adequately funded, there may be physical space constraints in most facilities.

There are several behavioral interventions that have been effective under clinical research conditions but have not been translated into effective programs. For example, the Centers for Disease Control and Prevention (CDC) funded Project RESPECT [22], which was a large phase 3 behavioral intervention study conducted from 1991 to 1995. Project RESPECT demonstrated that an enhanced counseling intervention, implemented as part of HIV counseling and testing, reduced high-risk behaviors (defined as unprotected intercourse) and biologic STD outcomes at longitudinal follow-up. The project was completed in 1995 and the summary intervention effectiveness paper was published in the *Journal of the American Medical Association* in 1998, which defined the Project RESPECT counseling method as the optimal standard of care in most public health settings. Nevertheless, Project RESPECT counseling methods have been implemented in only few clinics because the funding and commitment for infrastructure and training was never provided.

Sexual context impacts interventions

Epidemiologic risk assessment of STDs and other infectious diseases most frequently evaluates individual-based risk. A challenge in using STDs as intervention measures is that risk is also determined by environmental and contextual factors that are beyond the immediate sexual encounter situation, in particular the qualitative aspects not of the individual being assessed but of the sexual partners. For example, the risk profile of a partner may dictate an individual's STD risk independent of that individual's sexual behavior. The best examples of these cases are the high rates of STDs and HIV in monogamous women in sub-Saharan Africa and Asia [23], who had one lifetime sexual partner yet have high disease rates because of the risk profile of their husbands.

Behavioral models

When developing STD/HIV interventions, behavioral models are necessary for their design and evaluation [24–28]. Behavioral models are deterministic constructs of sexual behavior. These constructs are usually delineated in sequential steps, with each step being either an environmental factor, a behavioral attitude (eg, positive or negative attitude regarding condom use), subject-area knowledge, or a previous behavior. For STD research, risky behavior is a necessary precursor to disease acquisition. These elements are assembled in a logical framework, with the end result being a risky or preventative behavior.

Behavior models provide a deterministic basis and underlying rationale for intervention. They also provide a process for evaluation because the preceding key behavioral determinants to a behavior can also be measured. Defined as a multistep process, the behavioral models reveal logical points for intervention. For example, if a model posits that the key determinant of a behavior is the presence or absence of a specific attitude, then an intervention approach would be to change the underlying attitude. Evaluation methods would determine whether the intervention impacted the attitude, usually defined by before-and-after assessments. The evaluation framework can also determine the validity of the underlying behavioral model. For example, if the model just cited was valid, then changes in attitudes should result in changed behaviors. Behavioral models also facilitate multistep intervention approaches (synergy). In these approaches, interventions at multiple points of attack (eg, simultaneously impacting knowledge, attitudes, and other factors) should have an additive or even synergistic effect. Conceptually, a biomedical model analog would be cancer chemotherapy regimens, where drugs are active at multiple sites of the cell life cycle.

Beyond the scope of this paper, there are a number of major theories of behavior change that have been either adapted to HIV/STD prevention or developed for this purpose. These models include [27]:

- Health Belief Model
- AIDS-Risk Reduction Model
- Stages of Change Theory
- Theory of Reasoned Action
- Social Learning and Social Cognitive Theory
- Social Networks, Social Influence, and Peer Norms Theory
- Social-Structural Factors Theories
- Diffusion of Innovations Theories

All models have common elements, including the importance of preexisting attitudes as a key determinant for sexual behavior; the presence of structural/environmental factors that can promote, reinforce, or inhibit change (which may include media, religious beliefs, peer group effects, gender, and socioeconomic status); and knowledge, attitudes, and technical efficacy.

Behaviors do not occur in a social vacuum. Structural and environmental factors related to sexually transmitted infection (STI) control and prevention can affect an individual's ability to implement prevention behaviors, with the peer group often being most important. When developing an intervention, a common error is to focus changes on the individual level while ignoring whether the social or societal structure provides a supportive environment for STD/HIV behavior change.

Critical intervention components need to contain not only information but also motivation and skills. Successful interventions are characterized by extensive formative/qualitative research [29]. As of Semaan's 2002 review [30], there are only 12 relevant studies that were controlled. Seven of the 12 studies examined small group interventions, three investigated the effects of community-level approaches, and two considered individual-level interventions. Dichotomous effects were available for only six studies and continuous effects for only four studies. There were substantial problems with evaluating background risks: "Effects were so homogeneous among studies that no differences between groups can be statistically significant." [30]. Point estimates for effects were slightly more favorable among community-level interventions (odds ratio, 65; CI, 0.47–0.9) and among small group or individual-level interventions.

Celentano and colleagues [31] and Thai collaborators developed the best examples of a successful intervention program in the early 1990s to prevent HIV/STDs in the Royal Thai Army. At that time, HIV seroincidence in draftees was more than 4% per year and STD rates were high. The intervention approach included an individual-based component, but also structural changes. The individual-based components included skills building, increasing knowledge, condom skills training, and improved risk perception. This program was developed simultaneously with the 100% Condom Program in Thailand [32,33] that monitored brothels to ensure that condoms were used with all sex acts. The developers also recognized that the group dynamic in the Royal Thai Army field units was a critical part of high-risk sexual behavior with commercial sex workers. For example, soldiers in Royal Thai Army units based in rural areas were paid on a monthly basis. After payday there was a group dynamic that would involve binge drinking and en-masse visits to commercial sex workers. By staggering paydays across the 4 weeks of the month, stipulating interventions in the field units that built on the cohesion and group dynamic that is integral to army units, and implementing "buddy" systems to monitor condom use and safer sex practices among peers, the incidence of bacterial STDs and HIV dropped by 79%. A key feature is that safer sex became the peer and recognized norm.

Temporal sequence is also important to model development and interventions. The Stages of Change Theory [34] is a construct that was used in several interventions, including the widely reported Project RESPECT [35]. This model has been particularly attractive in intervention development because it divides a behavior into five steps: (1) *precontemplation* is before an individual is beginning to think of changing or adopting safer sexual behaviors, (2) *contemplation* is when an individual is considering a behavior change but not ready to act on it, (3) *preparation* is when an individual is actively considering changing behavior and is taking steps to actualize that behavior change ("ready for change"), (4) *action* is the process of changing behavior and moving toward a preventive behavior mode, and (5) *maintenance* is what is needed and imputed to maintain behavior change. This model describes sexual behavior change in a positive direction; regression is also possible when following a behavioral biomedical model, similar to the remission and relapse that one may see with other chronic diseases.

The Theory of Reasoned Action (TRA) [36] is another behavioral model with the underlying assumption that a person's beliefs toward a behavior lead to certain outcomes and move the attitude toward the behavior that is considered beneficial in an internal cost–benefit calculation rather than based on the societal and individual norms and potential contravening influences, resulting in a changed (or unchanged) intention followed by behavior change. Although this model has been largely supplanted by other behavioral models, the TRA provides a good example of how interventions are developed. Initial work involves understanding a population's sexual behavior risk in the context of the TRA. Intervention development then targets changing attitudes through various counseling interventions, and attempts to change societal norms through structural interventions. This type of approach can be combined with the Stages of Change Theory, as was done in Project RESPECT, with each stage resulting in a different "behavioral prescription" for the subject or client.

Intervention objectives

The objectives of behavioral interventions are to foster increases in knowledge, changes in attitudes, and adoption of safer behaviors. From a structural/ecologic standpoint, the objective is to develop environmental conditions that foster positive behavioral change. This change would include changing the peer norms, providing environmental supports (such as persistent messages or social supports outside the immediate environment), and increasing technical effectiveness (including training individuals in skills such as condom use, negotiating safer sex, or recognizing risky situations). Motivating individuals to adopt preventive behavior is important in many of the behavioral models. Motivation can be positively directed, such as self-esteem building, skills building, and preventing long-term consequences. Traditional approaches toward negative motivation, such as "safer behavior to avoid a risky outcome" [3] or fear tactics, have not been shown to be effective. One of the critical problems is that there are countervailing peer and societal pressures for adopting safer behaviors in many communities. These influences can include peer groups that are not safer-sex oriented, media that is promoting high-risk behaviors, or even religious groups that have policies against safer-sex education or condom use.

Project RESPECT

Project RESPECT was one large example of a behavioral intervention that was implemented in a field-based setting using a theoretical model bias [22]. Project RESPECT enrolled over 5000 individuals in a longitudinal intervention evaluation of STDs in the United States. There were three evaluable arms. An intensive intervention arm comprised enhanced counseling that involved one pretest session and three post-HIV test sessions with an individual counselor. The objective of the counseling was to change technical skills, attitudes, and perception of norms regarding condom use using the Theory of Reasoned Action and the Stages of Change models. The second arm had a similar objective to the first, but instead of multiple individual sessions, there was a single prevention counseling session that occurred as part of posttest counseling. The sessions focused in a more direct way on increasing perception of personal risk and on small achievable goals as opposed to overall cessation of risky behavior. Counseling was based on an interactive session, with the objective of making this translatable to clinic operating conditions. The third arm was the control arm, which represented the standard of care at the time of the study and used an educational message focused on safer sex STD prevention.

Project RESPECT had several important findings using behavior that measured either abstinence or 100% condom use. There was demonstrable evidence of efficacy at 3- and 6-month periods that appeared to be dose responses. When biologic measures (ie, incident STDs) were assessed, there was a similar dose response. In other words, the intervention arms demonstrated substantially increased effects compared with the control arm in many individuals having 100% condom-protected intercourse or abstinence only. However, the intervention effect decayed over time, particularly measurable in the biologic endpoints used. Incident STDs, specifically gonorrhea, syphilis, chlamydia, and trichomonas infections, were measured at each interval. At each study visit, there was demonstrable evidence between the control arm and the two intervention study arms. However, the accrual of STDs continued over the course of the study, and proportional difference between the intervention arms and the control arm decreased over time. Furthermore, there was no statistical difference between the two intervention arms, which demonstrated that a short-term intervention could be equally effective as a multiple-session intervention.

The study results were powerful, demonstrating that decreased risky sexual behavior can be induced by a behavioral intervention. However, concerns over the continued accrual of risky behavior over time posited the need for behavioral booster inventions. In preliminary results regarding the initial development of a booster intervention, Metcalf and colleagues [37] found that there was minimal difference between subjects who were exposed to a booster intervention and those who were not. These findings have been mirrored by other interventions in various population groups.

The limitation of Project RESPECT is that it was a large study conducted in STD clinics, which involve a nongeneralizable population. However, it does provide a conceptual and experiential basis to evaluate these issues. In a meta-analysis of all reported behavioral intervention trials through 2002, Semaan [27,38] concluded that:

- Most people who are at risk will change behavior.
- No program has eliminated risky behavior, and therefore residual risk is a major concern.
- Risk reduction is complex and often requires synergistic approaches.
- Overall, behavioral intervention experimental groups, mostly using motivational interviewing, had a self-reported effect of reducing risky behaviors over follow-up periods of 19% to 31%, similar to those found in Project RESPECT.

Nevertheless, the evaluated behavioral interventions have short follow-up periods, and even when successful have a number of limitations, including translation issues and research versus field conditions.

Several HIV behavioral interventions have been developed and studied, yet few have been translated into clinical practice. From the standpoint of the private practitioner, behavioral intervention is a counseling service and is not often reimbursable. Even in public clinics, such as those in which the interventions were studied, behavioral interventions have not been implemented as part of primary clinical practice largely because of the lack of funding provided for this procedure. Administratively, direct medical clinical services are more apt to be funded than behavioral intervention services. Funding for behavioral intervention services in 2005 and beyond, in an environment where resources for medical care and public health services are severely constrained, is a serious problem.

Interventions are often studied under conditions that are optimized for research purposes but often criticized for not being representative of real-world conditions. For example, the Project RESPECT intervention was studied only in individuals who were HIV tested and posttest counseled. Other studies have found that individuals who are at high risk may actually come for HIV testing, but would miss their posttest counseling appointments. For example, most persons tested in STD clinics for HIV are "opportunistically" tested (ie, they came primarily for their STD complaint). Posttest counseling rates in people who are HIV-negative where active follow-up is not performed are dismal [39]. Therefore, were the study participants actually individuals in a subgroup who would be at very low risk for intervention failure, and were they screened out by the criteria that required HIV posttest counseling?

Later large-scale intervention studies

DiClemente and colleagues [40] performed a large randomized controlled trial (RCT) in adolescent African American girls aged 14 to 18 years who were recruited at community health centers. The intervention group received four 4-hour sessions that used the Theory of Gender and Power. The intervention group had higher rates of consistent condom use (75% compared with 58%) and reduced numbers of new sex partners (2.7% compared with 7.4%) at 6 and 12 months, with some attrition at 12 months [41]. Overall condom use at 12 months increased 36% in the intervention group, including a 28% increase in women who put condoms on their partners. This study demonstrated that positive behavioral changes were achievable in inner-city, minority, adolescent populations. As a clinical trial, the intervention was performed with parental consent, demonstrating that parental accession to sexual risk-reduction efforts in their teens was not an issue. However, as with the other interventions, this required substantial infrastructure, staff training, and support.

Interventions in gay men

During the 1980s and 1990s [42], numerous studies demonstrated that risky behaviors in gay men can be reduced through various interventions, such as motivational counseling (either group or one-on-one) or interventions that target peer norms, such as the Peer Opinion Leader interventions [43,44]. Overall effectiveness of these interventions was 20% to 30% reductions; however, most studies did not have disease outcomes. The EXPLORE study was a large multicenter one-on-one intervention trial that targeted gay men, with over 4000 persons enrolled in six cities in the United States. The counseling was labor intensive, consisting of ten sessions followed by booster sessions. The Project RESPECT counseling model was used and included assessing situational factors, moods, sexual risk-taking, substance use/abuse, and other domains. In the intervention group, there was an 18% lower rate of HIV seroconversion, and similar rates of reduction of unprotected anal intercourse and serodiscordant unprotected anal intercourse, with more favorable estimates in the first 12 to 18 months. Nevertheless, although not mentioned specifically in the EXPLORE study, the results were clearly disappointing in that the intensive intervention resulted in only a modest effect. This fact may have been a response to the environment, as this study was performed during the late 1990s and early 2000s, precisely when there were major increases in high-risk behavior in the gay community [45].

Case studies: examples of successful programs and lessons learned

There are three successful examples of large-scale programs that incorporate behavioral interventions components and structural changes which contribute to reduction in rates of the targeted STDs. These examples include the Uganda Abstinence/Be Faithful/Use Condoms (ABC) Programs [46], the Thailand 100% Condom Use Program [33], and the US Syphilis Elimination Project [47,48] which targeted minority syphilis in the 1990s.

These programs have several common threads, including:

- Community and macro-scale political support: high-level political support within the community associated with a multisectoral response. In other words, the intervention message was being propagated at several different societal levels.
- Decentralized planning or implementation, or community buy-in: there was decentralized planning for behavioral intervention using multiplicity methods, including governmental agencies; nongovernmental organizations; workplace-directed, peer opinion leader interventions; and personal interventions. Community groups included traditional organizations, such as religious and social action groups, and nontraditional groups, such as organizations of persons who have

AIDS, commercial sex worker groups, and grassroots community groups.
- Social acceptance and avoidance of stigma: STDs and HIV disproportionately impact marginalized communities. In all of these cases, interventions were specifically directed at groups at highest risk, women, youth, or homosexual men, and there was specific emphasis placed on avoiding stigma.
- Combined prevention and clinical care and provision of STD screening and HIV counseling and testing [27,49,50]: the clinical components of these interventions include emphasis on control of STIs, provision of readily accessible health care, and promotion of HIV testing and counseling. Condom promotion and instruction on inappropriate use was also a part of all of these interventions.

This combination of factors results in essentially a "contextual" intervention. Multiple levels are impacted, including family, relationship, and community levels, which essentially results in an intangible individual effect. This could be considered in the same model as a "herd effect" for vaccine, although clearly resulting from different biologic and behavioral mechanisms. The environment provides support and structural changes that reinforce safer-sex behavior and interventions. No good theoretical models exist for identifying the impacts of these types of interventions.

Syphilis elimination

The US Syphilis Elimination Program [47,48,51] focused on African Americans and was a response to the syphilis epidemic of the early 1990s that severely impacted the minority community. Recognizing historical roots to the syphilis epidemic, the focus was on outreach—identifying and screening individuals who had poor access to health care. This involved substantial work on destigmatizing syphilis to the community, and direct involvement with community groups often in nontraditional health care prevention roles. The program included rapid ethnographic assessments, development of medical anthropology expertise to impact communities' grassroots efforts or to change the belief system for stigmatized diseases, and major increases in outreach screening. Outreach screening efforts have been made particularly in populations that do not access or are marginalized from the health care system. This effort includes offering screening and treatment services in community-based settings, jails, drug treatment centers, and mobile vans. Although the intervention did not target behavior per se, in an environment where behavioral change was being marketed aggressively as part of HIV transmission reduction and in communities where drug treatment was being actively promoted, it is unlikely that reduction in risk behaviors did not occur. From an ecologic standpoint, there was a 90% decrease in syphilis incidence in target groups [52].

Uganda Abstinence/Be Faithful/Use Condoms

The Uganda ABC Program [46] exemplifies country-level structural intervention. This was a multifaceted intervention program that included increased access to STD care, universal access to the comprehensive sex education and HIV prevention messages that begin in primary school, and target messages at the workplace, social meeting places, and even on public transportation. Furthermore, Uganda has demonstrated the role national leadership plays in promoting HIV and STD risk reduction. The data are quite compelling, with demonstrated reduction in median HIV antenatal prevalence, which peaked at 32% in Kampala in 1991, to less than 10% by 2003. National surveys demonstrated that the age of sexual debut increased by approximately 1 year during the 1990s with increases occurring initially in the urban areas. There was also a decline in premarital sexual intercourse and an increase in abstinence among women at least in the first part of the decade [53].

Most impressive was a large reduction in multiple sexual partnerships, particularly in urban areas among men and women during the period when the greatest decline in HIV incidence occurred. The decline stabilized in the latter half of the decade [53]. In a report on Africa prepared by Hearst and Chen [54] for the United Nations program on AIDS in 2003, the highest country-level rates of individuals reporting condom use at last sex (2001) were for Zimbabwe (69%) and Uganda (62%). However, condom use at last sexual intercourse is a complex variable, particularly confounded by long-term monogamous relationships in which individuals are less likely to use condoms. Condom use rates at last intercourse with a nonregular partner demonstrated substantial increases in both nations, particularly in the urban sample. In the urban areas, condom use at last sex with a noncohabiting partner increased from 62% to 81% between 1995 and 2000. These are specifically the individuals for whom education has been targeted because these casual relationships are the ones that are the most at risk for the spread of STDs. Changes similar to this were seen across sub-Saharan Africa, with the largest changes seen in Zambia and Kenya [54].

An interesting subtext of the Uganda ABC program success is recent criticism of condom use and the claims that the major advances were actually caused by increased abstinence. From a political standpoint, these claims have entered domestic and international politics to the point where the Uganda program paradoxically is being used as a justification for not recommending condom use. From a scholarly standpoint, Stoneburner and Low-Beer [55] reported, "Widespread support for condom distribution using social marketing (ie, commercial techniques to achieve social goals), voluntary testing and counseling, and improved treatment of STIs largely came after the initial decline in HIV incidence and prevalence." However, they also noted that many countries have failed in their leadership to communicate a credible message of alarm and advice. For example, in South Africa there is still confusion about the cause of AIDS and its threat, which contributes to denial and inaction.

Wilson [56], reporting in the *British Medical Journal*, found that

> Analysis of factors contributing to behavior change in Uganda and elsewhere is even more challenging than the reaffirmation of partner reduction......HIV prevention responses were rapid, endogenous, inexpensive and simple....they were based on the premises that communities, however disparate, have within themselves the resources and the capital to reverse this epidemic....they were locally led by gay leaders and activists in California, and by political, religious, and community leaders in Uganda.

HIV prevention programs promoted changes in community norms, thus creating enabling and protective environments long before the concept gained currency. They stressed simple messages and actions, and in doing so, achieved declines in HIV infection that preceded the growth in HIV services, including distribution of condoms and voluntary counseling and testing (CNT).

Despite the success [57], there was no decrease in the age of sexual debut. The data suggest increased condom use, but there are no data available on proper condom use (such as incidence of errors, and so forth). More recently, Blum [57] and Wawer and colleagues [58], reporting on Uganda cohorts, presented compelling data from careful population surveys that suggest that the age of sexual debut has not changed, and in fact, that much of the decrease attributable to abstinence is because of methodology issues and misclassification bias in surveys conducted in school-based settings and because of mortality caused by HIV. However, the criticisms of the Uganda data do not account for the definitions of abstinence in Uganda compared with those in the United States. Furthermore, the Uganda studies occur in the context of comprehensive, universal sex education available on the schools.

The Thai 100% Condom Program

The best examples of society-wide interventions were in Thailand. Cooperation between the Thai health ministry and brothel owners resulted in the 100% Condom Program, which was implemented in the mid-1990s [33]. This program, involving increased regulations of brothels, improved STI management, and the dissemination of HIV counseling and testing, resulted in decreases in HIV seroprevalence of over 80% between 1993 and 2000. Behavioral interventions in military communities were also widely implemented. Because of constriction, military access presented an opportunity to broadly impact the population. The military communities incorporated the best features of nongovernmental organization and grassroots intervention development and behavioral science based on peer opinion leaders and peer norms. Interventions were implemented at the small group (squad) level, incorporating skills development and integration into daily routines, and were systematically presented and reinforced continually on an interpersonal and environmental level [31,59]. The structural interventions included development of alternative activities for military personnel outside of alcohol and brothel use; the incorporation of the "buddy system" to encourage condom use when groups of soldiers went to the brothels; and the staggering of paydays to discourage the large group dynamic that incorporated alcohol use and unprotected brothel visits as part of a social activity. These interventions have been highly successful and now are incorporated by the World Health Organization's Western Pacific Region and other environments, including China, Cambodia, and Vietnam.

There are several consistent themes among these interventions [27,60]:

- No one magic bullet could be identified as the specific cause of decreased HIV/STD rates.
- Each intervention had a multifactor approach at different levels socially and structurally.
- Each intervention impacted behaviors that involved contact with core group members or high-risk activity and targeted these activities and groups. As such, the intervention did not become diluted in low prevalence/low incidence intervention populations. This feature should be counterbalanced by the concern that corporate targeting can result in stigma; therefore, stigma reduction should be incorporated as a key part of any intervention.
- Each intervention had a large condom promotion component. Condom use promotion is a highly complex variable that includes promoting condom use, appropriate use of condoms, condom failure rates, and partner selection. For example, in many situations, individuals may use condoms with high-risk partners, thereby actually resulting in an association between condom use and increased STD risk. Therefore, the increased risk would not be the result of condom use (or failure), but rather partner selection.
- Each intervention developed and implemented (sometimes by design, sometimes by chance) structural and ecologic changes that fostered the adoption of prevention practices. These changes included reducing stigma, the consistent use of a nonjudgmental approach, community support, confidentiality, and changing peer norms to promote adoption and maintenance. Increased access to medical services, especially reproductive health services, is a key component of the interventions.
- Each intervention had strong leadership at the political and public health levels that directly addressed the community. In summary, controversy in HIV prevention has primarily centered on abstinence versus condoms. Partner reduction has had an important role in

countries that have seen a decrease in HIV infection. Locally developed behavior change approaches are most effective in altering social norms. Abstinence, monogamy, and condom use should be promoted in an evidence-based, mutually supported way [57,61].

Challenges and problems

Condom use: criticism of condom promotion based on effectiveness

Since 2001, there has been increased criticism of condom promotion as a major form of STD prevention. Despite having a long history of being recommended and used for contraception and STD control, condoms actually lack formally and rigorously obtained clinical data demonstrating effectiveness. A large part of this problem is the fact that condom effectiveness is difficult to study, especially because study designs would require that all individuals at the minimum be counseled on standard public health practice, which is condom use. Paradoxically, it is unethical to conduct a trial where individuals are exposed to STIs without recommending use of condoms. Therefore, indirect methodologies have to be used, which present problems with selection and reporting bias. These concerns, combined with political pressure, resulted in a 2001 report published by the National Institutes of Health (NIH) [62,63] that reviewed condom efficacy. The report found that conclusive evidence (from clinical trials) existed to support efficacy claims for HIV and gonorrhea in men. The anticondom lobby has proposed that the lack of clinical trial evidence presupposes ineffectiveness.

One of the problems was that the NIH Panel Report was based on studies that were available up to June 2000. The studies followed stringent methodologies, including controlled trials. Another problem was that condom effectiveness could be underestimated because of social desirability bias or underestimating the effectiveness of proper use.

Results from other studies have become available since 2001. In terms of herpes transmission, Wald and colleagues [64] analyzed 528 monogamous HSP-2 discordant couples who had a condom use rate of 25%. The investigators found that condom use during more than 25% of the sexual acts was associated with a 92% reduction in HSP-2 risk for women. Later analysis in a subsequent clinical trial found that when condoms were used more than 65% of the time, there was partial protection for men.

Sanchez and colleagues [65] followed commercial sex workers in Lima, Peru who were evaluated monthly for STIs. In a large cohort, condom use rates were 20%. These women had a 62% reduction in the risk for acquiring gonorrhea and a 26% reduction in the risk for chlamydia infection. Crosby and colleagues [66,67] followed a group of African American adolescents (aged 14–18 years) and found that consistent condom use was associated with an 18% risk for STI compared with 30% in the nonusers. Finally, in the large Rakai, Uganda population-based cohort study, which followed 18,000 persons longitudinally as part of an HIV prevention intervention, there was a significant reduction in HIV incidence (relative risk of 0.37) and significant reductions in syphilis, gonorrhea, and chlamydia in the individuals who reported 100% condom use [68].

The Cochrane collaboration [69–71] reviewed HIV incidence and condom use in heterosexuals, found 13 cohorts of "always" condom users in the observational longitudinal studies, and estimated that overall effectiveness was 83% and as high as 94%. Many of the component studies were done early in the epidemic and so social support structures for condom use may not have been as extensive as they are at present. Therefore, more recent studies where condom use is much more socially acceptable and promoted may actually result in higher levels of effectiveness.

Challenges to parental notification laws

A key feature of public health–oriented prevention and control of STDs has been the development of comprehensive approaches. For teenagers, this includes providing reproductive health education, including the promotion of delayed intercourse, and services such as contraception and STD prevention to those who are sexually active. Abstinence-only programs have been vigorously promoted but are of questionable effectiveness [72]. As part of increasing restrictions on reproductive health, some states have adopted or are considering parental notification laws for adolescents requesting reproductive health services. These restrictions have the potential for enormous problems. A study of teenaged clients of family planning clinics in Wisconsin found that if parental notification was implemented, 59% would stop using all sexual health care services [73]. Franzini and colleagues [74] reviewed the impact of restrictive confidentiality laws in Texas and their economic and morbidity impact on teenagers. In January 2003, Texas required parental consent for teenagers younger than age 18 to receive contraceptives. Furthermore, Texas now requires health care providers to report the identity of all patients who are younger than age 17 who providers believe are sexually active to law enforcement, under the rationale that sexual contact with a person younger than age 17 is a criminal offense. The rationale of mandated parental involvement is that confidential services reserve the rights of parents and that regulation will decrease adolescent sexual activity. This contrasts with survey data suggesting that only 1% to 4% of girls report that they would stop having intercourse if their parents were notified. The estimated outcome of these policies in Texas would be an additional 8265 pregnancies, including 5378 births and 1654 terminations. From an STD standpoint, there would be an additional 2200 cases of chlamydia, 521 cases of gonorrhea, and approximately 500 cases of pelvic inflammatory disease, and overall total direct medical costs of $43 million.

Summary

Effective STD and HIV prevention requires synergism of individual-based prevention behaviors and societal/structural supports that will promote and maintain these behaviors. We should also expect the unexpected. STD rates in gay men have risen after effective prevention of HIV/STD in gay men and effective antiretroviral therapy. New drugs of abuse, such as methamphetamine ("crystal meth"), have induced risky sexual behaviors in gay and heterosexual communities. Economic dislocation in Eastern Europe has resulted in trafficking of commercial sex workers to Europe, the Mideast, and Asia, all with the potential for STD and HIV spread.

James Curran, formerly director of the HIV epidemiology and prevention effort at the CDC, has written:

> It is ironic that the two clearest examples of large-scale success in HIV prevention—reduction in HIV transmission in gay men in the United States and national declines in HIV incidence in Thailand—arise in societies/communities known in their own way for sexual openness....the openness in both communities provided the environment to make the powerful revolutionary changes needed. In Africa, the powerful voice of President Museveni of Uganda has also encouraged candor about sexual risk-taking and facilitated that nation's encouraging early success in reducing HIV prevalence...Unfortunately, most of the world remains unable or unwilling to deal frankly and consistently with sexuality despite the considerable risks of HIV infection in many communities. There is a worldwide sexual hangup hampering HIV prevention efforts [75].

References

[1] Higgins DL, Galavotti C, O'Reilly KR, et al. Evidence for the effects of HIV antibody counseling and testing on risk behaviors. JAMA 1991;266:2419–29.

[2] Bonell C, Imrie J. Behavioural interventions to prevent HIV infection: rapid evolution, increasing rigour, moderate success. Br Med Bull 2001;58:155–70.

[3] Darrow WW. Health education and promotion for STD prevention: lessons for the next millennium. Genitourin Med 1997;73:88–94.

[4] No time to lose: getting more from HIV prevention. Washington (DC): National Academy Press; 2001.

[5] Ku L, Sonenstein FL, Turner CF, et al. The promise of integrated representative surveys about sexually transmitted diseases and behavior. Sex Transm Dis 1997;24:299–309.

[6] Peterman TA, Lin LS, Newman DR, et al. Does measured behavior reflect STD risk? An analysis of data from a randomized controlled behavioral intervention study. Project RESPECT Study Group. Sex Transm Dis 2000;27:446–51.

[7] Zenilman JM, Yuenger J, Galai N, et al. Polymerase chain reaction detection of Y chromosome sequences in vaginal fluid: preliminary studies of a potential biomarker for sexual behavior. Sex Transm Dis 2005;32:90–4.

[8] Zenilman JM, Weisman CS, Rompalo AM, et al. Condom use to prevent incident STDs: the validity of self-reported condom use. Sex Transm Dis 1995;22:15–21.
[9] Pequegnat W, Fishbein M, Celentano D, et al. NIMH/APPC workgroup on behavioral and biological outcomes in HIV/STD prevention studies: a position statement. Sex Transm Dis 2000;27:127–32.
[10] Brunham RC, Nagelkerke NJ, Plummer FA, et al. Estimating the basic reproductive rates of Neisseria gonorrhoeae and Chlamydia trachomatis: the implications of acquired immunity. Sex Transm Dis 1994;21:353–6.
[11] Brunham RC, Kimani J, Bwayo J, et al. The epidemiology of Chlamydia trachomatis within a sexually transmitted diseases core group. J Infect Dis 1996;173:950–6.
[12] Zenilman JM, Yuenger J, Galai N, et al. Polymerase chain reaction detection of Y chromosome sequences in vaginal fluid: preliminary studies of a potential biomarker for sexual behavior. Sex Transm Dis 2005;32:90–4.
[13] Ellen JM, Aral SO, Madger LS. Do differences in sexual behaviors account for the racial/ethnic differences in adolescents' self-reported history of a sexually transmitted disease? Sex Transm Dis 1998;25:125–9.
[14] Aral SO, Hughes JP, Stoner B, et al. Sexual mixing patterns in the spread of gonococcal and chlamydial infections. Am J Public Health 1999;89:825–33.
[15] Aral SO. Sexual network patterns as determinants of STD rates: paradigm shift in the behavioral epidemiology of STDs made visible. Sex Transm Dis 1999;26:262–4.
[16] Potterat JJ, Rothenberg RB, Muth SQ. Network structural dynamics and infectious disease propagation. Int J STD AIDS 1999;10:182–5.
[17] Turner CF, Danella RD, Rogers SM. Sexual behavior in the United States 1930–1990: trends and methodological problems. Sex Transm Dis 1995;22:173–90.
[18] Turner CF, Ku L, Rogers SM, et al. Adolescent sexual behavior, drug use, and violence: increased reporting with computer survey technology. Science 1998;280:867–73.
[19] Gribble JN, Miller HG, Cooley PC, et al. The impact of T-ACASI interviewing on reported drug use among men who have sex with men. Subst Use Misuse 2000;35:869–90.
[20] Metzger DS, Koblin B, Turner C, et al. Randomized controlled trial of audio computer-assisted self- interviewing: utility and acceptability in longitudinal studies. HIVNET Vaccine Preparedness Study Protocol Team. Am J Epidemiol 2000;152:99–106.
[21] Ellish NJ, Weisman CS, Celentano D, et al. Reliability of partner reports of sexual history in a heterosexual population at a sexually transmitted diseases clinic. Sex Transm Dis 1996;23:446–52.
[22] Kamb ML, Fishbein M, Douglas JM Jr, et al. Efficacy of risk-reduction counseling to prevent human immunodeficiency virus and sexually transmitted diseases: a randomized controlled trial. Project RESPECT Study Group. JAMA 1998;280:1161–7.
[23] Gangakhedkar RR, Bentley ME, Divekar AD, et al. Spread of HIV infection in married monogamous women in India. JAMA 1997;278:2090–2.
[24] Neumann MS, Johnson WD, Semaan S, et al. Review and meta-analysis of HIV prevention intervention research for heterosexual adult populations in the United States. J Acquir Immune Defic Syndr 2002;30(Suppl 1):S106–17.
[25] Johnson WD, Semaan S, Hedges LV, et al. A protocol for the analytical aspects of a systematic review of HIV prevention research. J Acquir Immune Defic Syndr 2002;30(Suppl 1):S62–72.
[26] Hedges LV, Johnson WD, Semaan S, et al. Theoretical issues in the synthesis of HIV prevention research. J Acquir Immune Defic Syndr 2002;30(Suppl 1):S8–14.
[27] Des Jarlais DC, Semaan S. HIV prevention research: cumulative knowledge or accumulating studies? An introduction to the HIV/AIDS prevention research synthesis project supplement. J Acquir Immune Defic Syndr 2002;30(Suppl 1):S1–7.

[28] Diclemente R, editor. Preventing AIDS. Theories and methods of behavioral interventions. New York: Plenum; 1994.
[29] Stephenson JM, Imrie J, Sutton SR. Rigorous trials of sexual behaviour interventions in STD/HIV prevention: what can we learn from them? AIDS 2000;14(Suppl 3): S115–24.
[30] Stephenson JM. Systematic review of hormonal contraception and risk of HIV transmission: when to resist meta-analysis. AIDS 1998;12:545–53.
[31] Celentano DD, Bond KC, Lyles CM, et al. Preventive intervention to reduce sexually transmitted infections: a field trial in the Royal Thai Army. Arch Intern Med 2000;160: 535–40.
[32] Nelson KE, Celentano DD, Eiumtrakol S, et al. Changes in sexual behavior and a decline in HIV infection among young men in Thailand. N Engl J Med 1996;335:297–303.
[33] Rojanapithayakorn W, Hanenberg R. The 100% condom program in Thailand. AIDS 1996; 10:1–7.
[34] Prochaska JO, DiClemente CC, Norcross JC. In search of how people change. Applications to addictive behaviors. Am Psychol 1992;47:1102–14.
[35] Malotte CK, Jarvis B, Fishbein M, et al. Stage of change versus an integrated psychosocial theory as a basis for developing effective behaviour change interventions. The Project RESPECT Study Group. AIDS Care 2000;12:357–64.
[36] Fishbein M, Hennessy M, Kamb M, et al. Using intervention theory to model factors influencing behavior change. Project RESPECT. Eval Health Prof 2001;24: 363–84.
[37] Metcalf CA, Malotte CK, Douglas JM Jr, et al. Efficacy of a booster counseling session 6 months after HIV testing and counseling: a randomized, controlled trial (RESPECT-2). Sex Transm Dis 2005;32:123–9.
[38] Semaan S, Kay L, Strouse D, et al. A profile of US-based trials of behavioral and social interventions for HIV risk reduction. J Acquir Immune Defic Syndr 2002;30(Suppl 1): S30–50.
[39] Erbelding EJ, Chung S, Zenilman JM. Following-up for HIV test results: what limits return in an STD clinic population? Int J STD AIDS 2004;15:29–32.
[40] Wingood GM, Scd, DiClemente RJ. Application of the theory of gender and power to examine HIV-related exposures, risk factors, and effective interventions for women. Health Educ Behav 2000;27:539–65.
[41] DiClemente RJ, Wingood GM, Harrington KF, et al. Efficacy of an HIV prevention intervention for African American adolescent girls: a randomized controlled trial. JAMA 2004;292:171–9.
[42] Elwy AR, Hart GJ, Hawkes S, et al. Effectiveness of interventions to prevent sexually transmitted infections and human immunodeficiency virus in heterosexual men: a systematic review. Arch Intern Med 2002;162:1818–30.
[43] Kelly JA, Murphy DA, Sikkema KJ, et al. Randomised, controlled, community-level HIV-prevention intervention for sexual-risk behaviour among homosexual men in US cities. Community HIV Prevention Research Collaborative. Lancet 1997;350:1500–5.
[44] Kelly JA, Kalichman SC. Behavioral research in HIV/AIDS primary and secondary prevention: recent advances and future directions. J Consult Clin Psychol 2002;70: 626–39.
[45] Koblin B, Chesney M, Coates T. Effects of a behavioural intervention to reduce acquisition of HIV infection among men who have sex with men: the EXPLORE randomised controlled study. Lancet 2004;364:41–50.
[46] Beyond slogans: lessons from Uganda's ABC experience. Issues Brief (Alan Guttmacher Inst) 2004;2:1–4.
[47] Gayle HD, Counts GW. Syphilis elimination: a unique time in history. J Am Med Womens Assoc 2001;56:2–3.

[48] St Louis ME, Wasserheit JN. Elimination of syphilis in the United States. Science 1998;281: 353–4.
[49] Sangani P, Rutherford G, Wilkinson D. Population-based interventions for reducing sexually transmitted infections, including HIV infection. Cochrane Database Syst Rev 2004;(2):CD001220.
[50] Aral SO, Padian NS, Holmes KK. Advances in multilevel approaches to understanding the epidemiology and prevention of sexually transmitted infections and HIV: an overview. J Infect Dis 2005;191(Suppl 1):S1–6.
[51] Centers for Disease Control and Prevention. Syphilis Elimination Effort Toolkit. Available at: http://www.cdc.gov/std/SEE/default.htm. Accessed March 30, 2005.
[52] Centers for Disease Control and Prevention. Primary and secondary syphilis–United States, 2002. MMWR Morb Mortal Wkly Rep 2003;52:1117–20.
[53] Uganda Ministry of Health. AIDS in Africa during the 1990s. Uganda. Kampala: Uganda AIDS Commission; 2003.
[54] Hearst N, Chen S. Condom promotion for AIDS prevention in the developing world: is it working? Available at: http://www.usp.br/nepaids/condom.pdf. Accessed March 30, 2003.
[55] Stoneburner RL, Low-Beer D. Population-level HIV declines and behavioral risk avoidance in Uganda. Science 2004;304:714–8.
[56] Wilson D. Partner reduction and the prevention of HIV/AIDS. BMJ 2004;328:848–9.
[57] Blum RW. Uganda AIDS prevention: A, B, C and politics. J Adolesc Health 2004;34:428–32.
[58] Wawer MJ, Gray R, Serwadda D, et al. Declines in HIV prevalence in Uganda: not as simple as ABC. Presented at the 12th Conference on Retroviruses and Opportunistic Infections. Boston, March 30, 2005.
[59] Celentano DD, Nelson KE, Lyles CM, et al. Decreasing incidence of HIV and sexually transmitted diseases in young Thai men: evidence for success of the HIV/AIDS control and prevention program. AIDS 1998;12:F29–36.
[60] Des Jarlais DC, Padian N. Strategies for universalistic and targeted HIV prevention. J Acquir Immune Defic Syndr Hum Retrovirol 1997;16:127–36.
[61] Shelton JD, Halperin DT, Nantulya V, et al. Partner reduction is crucial for balanced "ABC" approach to HIV prevention. BMJ 2004;328:891–3.
[62] Workshop summary: scientific evidence on condom effectiveness for sexually transmitted disease (STD) prevention. National Institutes of Health. Herndon, June 12–13, 2000.
[63] Holmes KK, Levine R, Weaver M. Effectiveness of condoms in preventing sexually transmitted infections. Bull World Health Organ 2004;82:454–61.
[64] Wald A, Langenberg AG, Link K, et al. Effect of condoms on reducing the transmission of herpes simplex virus type 2 from men to women. JAMA 2001;285:3100–6.
[65] Sanchez J, Campos PE, Courtois B, et al. Prevention of sexually transmitted diseases (STDs) in female sex workers: prospective evaluation of condom promotion and strengthened STD services. Sex Transm Dis 2003;30:273–9.
[66] Crosby RA, DiClemente RJ, Wingood GM, et al. Value of consistent condom use: a study of sexually transmitted disease prevention among African American adolescent females. Am J Public Health 2003;93:901–2.
[67] Crosby RA, DiClemente RJ, Wingood GM, et al. Identification of strategies for promoting condom use: a prospective analysis of high-risk African American female teens. Prev Sci 2003;4:263–70.
[68] Ahmed S, Lutalo T, Wawer M, et al. HIV incidence and sexually transmitted disease prevalence associated with condom use: a population study in Rakai, Uganda. AIDS 2001; 15:2171–9.
[69] Wilkinson D, Rutherford G. Population-based interventions for reducing sexually transmitted infections, including HIV infection. Cochrane Database Syst Rev 2001;(2): CD001220.

[70] Kennedy GE, Peersman G, Rutherford GW. International collaboration in conducting systematic reviews: the Cochrane Collaborative Review Group on HIV Infection and AIDS. J Acquir Immune Defic Syndr 2002;30(Suppl 1):S56–61.
[71] Sangani P, Rutherford G, Wilkinson D. Population-based interventions for reducing sexually transmitted infections, including HIV infection. Cochrane Database Syst Rev 2004;(2):CD001220.
[72] Bruckner H, Bearman P. After the promise: The STD consequences of adolescent virginity pledges. J Adolesc Health 2005;36:271–8.
[73] Reddy DM, Fleming R, Swain C. Effect of mandatory parental notification on adolescent girls' use of sexual health care services. JAMA 2002;288:710–4.
[74] Franzini L, Marks E, Cromwell PF, et al. Projected economic costs due to health consequences of teenagers' loss of confidentiality in obtaining reproductive health care services in Texas. Arch Pediatr Adolesc Med 2004;158:1140–6.
[75] Curran JW. Reflections on AIDS, 1981–2031. Am J Prev Med 2003;24:281–4.

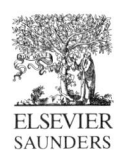

Index

Note: Page numbers of article titles are in **boldface** type.

A

Abstinence
 in genital herpes management, 436

Abuse
 sexual
  childhood
   sexual behavior effects of, 306–307

Antiviral therapy
 in genital herpes management, 436–437

Attitude(s)
 sexual behavior effects of, 304–305

B

Bacterial STDs
 prevention and control of
  innovative approaches to, **513–540**. See also *Sexually transmitted diseases (STDs), bacterial, prevention and control of, innovative approaches to.*

Bacterial vaginosis, **393–401**. See also *Vaginosis, bacterial.*

Behavior(s)
 sexual. See *Sexual behavior.*

Behavioral interventions
 in bacterial STDs prevention and control, 514–520

C

Cancer
 cervical
  screening for, 447–452

CDC. See *Centers for Disease Control and Prevention (CDC).*

Centers for Disease Control and Prevention (CDC), 352

Cervical cancer
 screening for, 447–452

Cervical HPV infection
 oncogenic, **439–458**. See also *Human papillomavirus (HPV) infection, cervical.*

Cervicitis
 mucopurulent, **333–349**. See also *Mucopurulent cervicitis (MPC).*

Cervix
 anatomy and physiology of, 333–335

Chlamydia trachomatis
 detection of
  new specimen types for, 371–372
 vaccines for, 478

Chlamydial infection
 clinical overview of, 283
 epidemiology of, **283–288**
  assessment of
   challenges to, 283
  in special populations
   estimates of, 285–286
 microbiology of, 283
 nucleic acid amplification tests for, **368–375**. See also *Nucleic acid amplification tests, for chlamydia.*
 prevalence of
  population-based estimates of, 283–285
 reported cases of, 287
 screening for
  in males
   in bacterial STDs prevention and control, 522
 surveillance for, 287
 symptoms of, 287

Cluster tracing
 in bacterial STDs prevention and control, 524, 527

Condom(s)
 in genital herpes management, 436

564 INDEX

Counseling
    for patients with genital HPV infection, **467–472.** See also *Genital HPV infection, counseling for patients with.*
    for patients with genital HSV infection, **459–476.** See also *Genital HSV infection, counseling for patients with.*
    risk-reduction
        in STD management in MCOs, 502–503
Culture(s)
    for gonorrhea, 376

D

Demography
    sexual behavior effects of, 300–305
Direct smear examination
    for gonorrhea, 375–376

E

Expectation(s)
    sexual behavior effects of, 304–305

F

Fluoroquinolone(s)
    mechanisms of action of, 354–357
    Neisseria gonorrhoeae resistant to, **351–365.** See also *Neisseria gonorrhoeae, fluoroquinolone-resistant.*

G

Genital HPV infection
    counseling for patients with, **467–472**
        external genital warts and, 472
        key messages in, 470–471
        partners and, 472
        pregnancy-related, 472
        special considerations in, 471–472
    described, 467
    educational challenge of, 469–470
    psychosocial aspects of, 467–469
Genital HSV infection. See also *Herpes simplex virus (HSV) infection, genital.*
    counseling for patients with, **459–467**
Genital warts
    external
        in genital HPV infection
            counseling for patients with, 472

GISP. See *Gonococcal Isolate Surveillance Project (GISP).*
Gonococcal Isolate Surveillance Project (GISP), 352
Gonorrhea
    clinical overview of, 288
    epidemiology of, 288–290
    in special populations
        estimates of, 289
    microbiology of, 288
    nucleic acid amplification tests for, **375–379.** See also *Nucleic acid amplification tests, for gonorrhea.*
    prevalence of
        population-based estimates of, 288
    reported cases of, 289–290
    surveillance for, 289–290

H

Herpes simplex virus (HSV) infection
    barriers to dialogue about, 460–461
    genital
        counseling for patients with, **459–476**
            asymptomatic shedding in, 466
            determination of length of infection in, 465–466
            importance of, 466–467
            in asymptomatic patients who test positive, 466
            psychosocial adjustment and, 463–465
        described, 427–428, 459–460
        diagnosis of
            disclosure of, 435–436
        diagnostic tests for
            characteristics of, 430
            damaging effects of, 434
            during pregnancy, 433–434
            in general population, 434
            in high-risk patients, 432–433
            in partners, 432
            reliability of, 430–431
            serologic assays, 430–432
        identification of, 429
        management of, **427–438**
            antiviral therapy in, 436–437
            condoms in, 436
            selective abstinence in, 436
        medical importance of, 428
        problems associated with, 428–429

transmission of
  management of, 435
  talking with patients about, 461–463
  vaccines for, 482–485
Herpes simplex virus (HSV) infection type 2
  in HIV acquisition, 417–419
Herpes simplex virus (HSV) type 2
  in HIV prevention, 421–422
  in HIV spread, 417
  in HIV transmission, 419
  in outcomes of intervention trials for STDs, 419–421
  treatment of
    impact on HIV progression, 422–423
Hierarchy
  sexual behavior effects of, 305
Homosexual men
  STDs in
    in Western Europe and U.S., **311–331.** See also *Sexually transmitted diseases (STDs), in homosexual men, in Western Europe and U.S.*
HPV infection. See *Human papillomavirus (HPV) infection.*
HSV infection. See *Herpes simplex virus (HSV) infection.*
Human immunodeficiency virus (HIV) infection
  acquisition of
    HSV type 2 in, 417–419
  prevention of
    HSV type 2 in, 421–422
  progression of
    HSV type 2 treatment impact on, 422–423
  spread of
    HSV type 2 in, 417
  transmission of
    HSV type 2 in, 419
Human immunodeficiency virus (HIV)/STDs interactions
  developments in, **415–425**
Human papillomavirus (HPV) infection
  cervical
    epidemiology of, 439–447
    natural history of, 439–447
    oncogenic, **439–458**
    screening for, 447–452
  diagnostic tests for, 452–453
  vaccines for, 479–482
Hybridization

probe
  for gonorrhea, 376

I

Infection(s). See also specific types.
  sexually acquired
    in women
      Mycoplasma genitalium as, 407–408
Internet-based interventions
  in bacterial STDs prevention and control, 532

M

Managed care organizations (MCOs)
  STD care in, **491–511.** See also *Sexually transmitted diseases (STDs), treatment of, in MCOs.*
  types of, 492
Mass treatment
  in bacterial STDs prevention and control, 529–532
Mental health
  sexual behavior effects of, 306–307
Microbicide(s)
  in bacterial STDs prevention and control, 520–521
MPC. See *Mucopurulent cervicitis (MPC).*
Mucopurulent cervicitis (MPC), **333–349**
  causes of, 337–340
  controversy related to, 344
  defined, 335–337
  epidemiology of, 335–337
  management of, 342–344
    future efforts related to, 344
  nonchlamydial nongonococcal, 340–342
Mycoplasma genitalium
  as sexually acquired infection in women, 407–408
  PID due to, **407–413.** See also *Pelvic inflammatory disease (PID), causes of.*

N

Neisseria gonorrhoeae
  fluoroquinolone-resistant, **351–365.** See also *Fluoroquinolone(s).*
    clinical significance of, 357–360
    determinant mechanisms in, 354–357
    epidemiology of, 357–360

Neisseria gonorrhoeae (*continued*)
    future directions in, 360–361
    prevalence of, 351–353
    treatment of
        principles in, 353–354
    nucleic acid amplification tests for, 375
    vaccines for, 478–479

Nucleic acid amplification tests
    development of, 367–368
    for chlamydia, **368–375**
        confirmation of positive tests, 372
        epidemiologic effects of, 373–375
        future of, 378–379
        inhibitors of, 369–370
        PCR, 368
        professional organizations recommendations, 373
        strand displacement amplification, 368
        transcription mediated amplification, 368–369
    for gonorrhea, **375–379**
        cost-effectiveness studies in, 377
        cultures, 376
        diagnostic specimen pooling in cost savings due to, 377–378
        direct smear examination, 375–376
        future of, 378–379
        partnering in, 378
        pelvic examination in, 377
        probe hybridization, 376
        sample of, 376–377

P

Parental notification laws
    behavioral interventions for STDs and challenges to, 557

Partner therapy
    expedited
        in bacterial STDs prevention and control, 527–529

Patient education
    in STD management in MCOs, 502–503

PCR. See *Polymerase chain reaction (PCR)*.

Peer referral
    in bacterial STDs prevention and control, 524, 527

Pelvic examination
    in gonorrhea detection, 377

Pelvic inflammatory disease (PID)
    causes of, **407–413**

Mycoplasma genitalium, **407–413**
    described, 408–410
    management of, 410–411

PID. See *Pelvic inflammatory disease (PID)*.

Polymerase chain reaction (PCR)
    for chlamydia, 368

Pregnancy
    genital HPV infection during, 472
    genital HSV infection during diagnostic tests for, 433–434

Probe hybridization
    for gonorrhea, 376

Project RESPECT, 548–550

Q

Quality of care
    of STDs in MCOs, 495

R

Risk-reduction counseling
    in STD management in MCOs, 502–503

S

Selective mass treatment
    in bacterial STDs prevention and control, 529–532

Sexual abuse
    childhood
        sexual behavior effects of, 306–307

Sexual behavior
    changes in attitudes effects on, 304–305
    changes in expectations effects on, 304–305
    changes in structure of marriage and family effects on, 304
    changes in values effects on, 304–305
    childhood sexual abuse effects on, 306–307
    demographic effects on, 300–305
    global socio-political and economic structure effects on, 299–300
    hierarchy effects on, 305
    mental health effects on, 306–307
    modern day influences on, **297–309**
    technology effects on, 305–306

Sexually acquired infections
    in women
        Mycoplasma genitalium as, 407–408

INDEX 567

Sexually transmitted diseases (STDs)
  bacterial
    prevention and control of
      innovative approaches to, **513–540**
        behavioral interventions, 514–520
        case-finding– and treatment-related, 521–532
        cluster tracing, 524, 527
        expedited partner therapy, 527–529
        female screening in medical care settings, 521
        in unconventional locations, 522–523
        Internet-based interventions, 532
        male chlamydial screening, 522
        mass treatment, 529–532
        microbicides, 520–521
        peer referral, 524, 527
        rescreening, 523–524
  behavioral interventions for, **541–562**
    behavioral models in, 545–548
    case studies, 551–556
    challenges of, 556–557
    development of
      challenges in, 542–543
    large-scale intervention studies, 550–551
    objectives of, 548
    parental notification laws related to
      challenges to, 557
    problems associated with, 556–557
    Project RESPECT, 548–550
    sexual context impact on, 545
    syphilis elimination, 552
    Thai 100% Condom Program, 554–556
    Uganda ABC Program, 553–554
  health transition related to, 298
  in homosexual men
    in Western Europe and U.S.
      epidemiology of
        changes in, 312–315
      increase in, **311–331**
        biologic factors in, 315–317
        demographic trends and, 317
        high-risk sexual behavior and, 317–320
        psychosocial contexts and, 322–325
        reasons for, 315–325
        sexual marketplace and, 320–322
  intervention trials for
    outcomes of
      HSV type 2 in, 419–421
  prevalence of, 491–492
  risk factors for
    assessment bias in, 543–545
  sexual behavior and, **297–309**. See also *Sexual behavior*.
  treatment of
    in MCOs, **491–511**
      case reporting in, 503–504
      clinical practice guidelines in, 494–495
      described, 493–494
      diagnostic testing in, 498–501
      literature review methods in, 493
      management of exposed sex partners, 504–505
      patient education in, 502–503
      quality of care, 495
      risk assessment in, 495–497
      risk-reduction counseling in, 502–503
      screening in, 498–501
      study of, 493–506
        discussion of, 505–506
        results of, 493–505
      types of, 501–502
  vaccines for
    acceptability of, 485
    Chlamydia trachomatis, 478
    future directions in, 485–486
    HSV, 482–485
    human papillomavirus, 479–482
    Neisseria gonorrhoeae, 478–479
    progress in, **477–490**

Sexually transmitted diseases (STDs)/HIV interactions
  developments in, **415–425**

Stages of Change Theory, 547

STDs. See *Sexually transmitted diseases (STDs)*.

INDEX

Strand displacement amplification for chlamydia, 368

Syphilis
  elimination of
    behavioral interventions for, 552

T

Thai 100% Condom Program, 554–556

Theory of Reasoned Action, 548–549

Transcription mediated amplification for chlamydia, 368–369

Trichomoniasis, **387–393**
  clinical manifestations of, 388–390
  clinical overview of, 290
  complications of, 388–390
  diagnosis of, 390–392
  epidemiology of, 290–291, 387–388
  in special populations
    estimates of, 291
  microbiology of, 290
  prevalence of
    population-based estimates of, 291
  treatment of, 392–393

2001 Bethesda System, 444–445

U

Uganda Abstinence/Be Faithful/Use Condoms (Uganda ABC Program), 553–554

V

Vaccine(s)
  for STDs, **477–490**. See also *Sexually transmitted diseases (STDs), vaccines for.*

Vaginosis
  bacterial, **393–401**
    complications of, 396–399
    diagnosis of, 399–400
    epidemiology of, 393
    pathophysiology of, 393–396
    treatment of, 400–401

Value(s)
  sexual behavior effects of, 304–305

W

Wart(s)
  genital
    external
      in genital HPV infection
        counseling for patients with, 472

Changing Your Address?

Make sure your subscription changes too! When you notify us of your new address, you can help make our job easier by including an exact copy of your Clinics label number with your old address (see illustration below.) This number identifies you to our computer system and will speed the processing of your address change. Please be sure this label number accompanies your old address and your corrected address—you can send an old Clinics label with your number on it or just copy it exactly and send it to the address listed below.

We appreciate your help in our attempt to give you continuous coverage. Thank you.

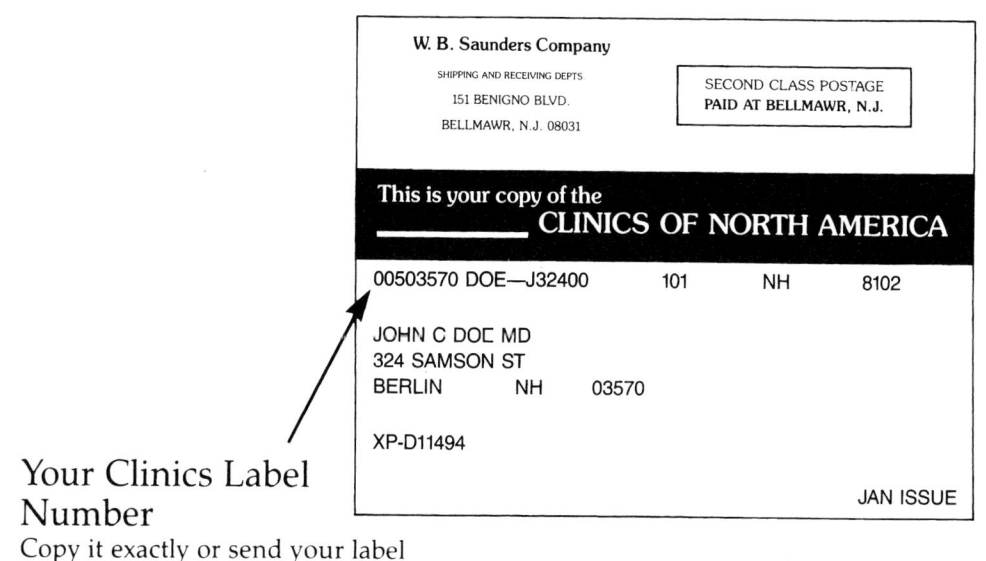

```
┌─────────────────────────────────────────────────────────────┐
│  W. B. Saunders Company                                     │
│     SHIPPING AND RECEIVING DEPTS.    ┌──────────────────┐   │
│        151 BENIGNO BLVD.             │ SECOND CLASS POSTAGE │
│        BELLMAWR, N.J. 08031          │ PAID AT BELLMAWR, N.J.│
│                                      └──────────────────┘   │
├─────────────────────────────────────────────────────────────┤
│  This is your copy of the                                   │
│  _____ CLINICS OF NORTH AMERICA                     │
│                                                             │
│  00503570 DOE—J32400          101       NH       8102       │
│                                                             │
│  JOHN C DOE MD                                              │
│  324 SAMSON ST                                              │
│  BERLIN        NH      03570                                │
│                                                             │
│  XP-D11494                                                  │
│                                                   JAN ISSUE │
└─────────────────────────────────────────────────────────────┘
```

Your Clinics Label Number

Copy it exactly or send your label along with your address to:
W.B. Saunders Company, Customer Service
Orlando, FL 32887-4800
Call Toll Free 1-800-654-2452

Please allow four to six weeks for delivery of new subscriptions and for processing address changes.

YES! Please start my subscription to the **CLINICS** checked below with the ❏ first issue of the calendar year or ❏ current issues. If not completely satisfied with my first issue, I may write "cancel" on the invoice and return it within 30 days at no further obligation.

Please Print:

Name _____

Address _____

City _____ State _____ ZIP _____

Method of Payment

❏ Check (payable to **Elsevier**; add the applicable sales tax for your area)

❏ VISA ❏ MasterCard ❏ AmEx ❏ Bill me

Card number _____ Exp. date _____

Signature _____

Staple this to your purchase order to expedite delivery

❏ **Adolescent Medicine Clinics**
  ❏ Individual $95
  ❏ Institutions $133
  ❏ *In-training $48

❏ **Anesthesiology**
  ❏ Individual $175
  ❏ Institutions $270
  ❏ *In-training $88

❏ **Cardiology**
  ❏ Individual $170
  ❏ Institutions $266
  ❏ *In-training $85

❏ **Chest Medicine**
  ❏ Individual $185
  ❏ Institutions $285

❏ **Child and Adolescent Psychiatry**
  ❏ Individual $175
  ❏ Institutions $265
  ❏ *In-training $88

❏ **Critical Care**
  ❏ Individual $165
  ❏ Institutions $266
  ❏ *In-training $83

❏ **Dental**
  ❏ Individual $150
  ❏ Institutions $242

❏ **Emergency Medicine**
  ❏ Individual $170
  ❏ Institutions $263
  ❏ *In-training $85
    ❏ Send CME info

❏ **Facial Plastic Surgery**
  ❏ Individual $199
  ❏ Institutions $300

❏ **Foot and Ankle**
  Individual $160
  Institutions $232

❏ **Gastroenterology**
  ❏ Individual $190
  ❏ Institutions $276

❏ **Gastrointestinal Endoscopy**
  ❏ Individual $190
  ❏ Institutions $276

❏ **Hand**
  ❏ Individual $205
  ❏ Institutions $319

❏ **Heart Failure (NEW in 2005!)**
  ❏ Individual $99
  ❏ Institutions $149
  ❏ *In-training $49

❏ **Hematology/ Oncology**
  ❏ Individual $210
  ❏ Institutions $315

❏ **Immunology & Allergy**
  ❏ Individual $165
  ❏ Institutions $266

❏ **Infectious Disease**
  ❏ Individual $165
  ❏ Institutions $272

❏ **Clinics in Liver Disease**
  ❏ Individual $165
  ❏ Institutions $234

❏ **Medical**
  ❏ Individual $140
  ❏ Institutions $244
  ❏ *In-training $70
    ❏ Send CME info

❏ **MRI**
  ❏ Individual $190
  ❏ Institutions $290
  ❏ *In-training $95
    ❏ Send CME info

❏ **Neuroimaging**
  ❏ Individual $190
  ❏ Institutions $290
  ❏ *In-training $95
    ❏ Send CME info0

❏ **Neurologic**
  ❏ Individual $175
  ❏ Institutions $275

❏ **Obstetrics & Gynecology**
  ❏ Individual $175
  ❏ Institutions $288

❏ **Occupational and Environmental Medicine**
  ❏ Individual $120
  ❏ Institutions $166
  ❏ *In-training $60

❏ **Ophthalmology**
  ❏ Individual $190
  ❏ Institutions $325

❏ **Oral & Maxillofacial Surgery**
  ❏ Individual $180
  ❏ Institutions $280
  ❏ *In-training $90

❏ **Orthopedic**
  ❏ Individual $180
  ❏ Institutions $295
  ❏ *In-training $90

❏ **Otolaryngologic**
  ❏ Individual $199
  ❏ Institutions $350

❏ **Pediatric**
  ❏ Individual $135
  ❏ Institutions $246
  ❏ *In-training $68
    ❏ Send CME info

❏ **Perinatology**
  ❏ Individual $155
  ❏ Institutions $237
  ❏ *In-training $78
    ❏ Send CME inf0

❏ **Plastic Surgery**
  ❏ Individual $245
  ❏ Institutions $370

❏ **Podiatric Medicine & Surgery**
  ❏ Individual $170
  ❏ Institutions $266

❏ **Primary Care**
  ❏ Individual $135
  ❏ Institutions $223

❏ **Psychiatric**
  ❏ Individual $170
  ❏ Institutions $288

❏ **Radiologic**
  ❏ Individual $220
  ❏ Institutions $331
  ❏ *In-training $110
    ❏ Send CME info

❏ **Sports Medicine**
  ❏ Individual $180
  ❏ Institutions $277

❏ **Surgical**
  ❏ Individual $190
  ❏ Institutions $299
  ❏ *In-training $95

❏ **Thoracic Surgery (formerly Chest Surgery)**
  ❏ Individual $175
  ❏ Institutions $255
  ❏ *In-training $88

❏ **Urologic**
  ❏ Individual $195
  ❏ Institutions $307
  ❏ *In-training $98
    ❏ Send CME info

*To receive in-training rate, orders must be accompanied by the name of affiliated institution, dates of residency and signature of coordinator on institution letterhead. Orders will be billed at the individual rate until proof of resident status is received.

© Elsevier 2005. Offer valid in U.S. only. Prices subject to change without notice. **MO 10808 DF4184**

Order your subscription today. Simply complete and detach this card and drop it in the mail to receive the best clinical information in your field.

NO POSTAGE
NECESSARY
IF MAILED
IN THE
UNITED STATES

BUSINESS REPLY MAIL
FIRST-CLASS MAIL   PERMIT NO 7135   ORLANDO FL

POSTAGE WILL BE PAID BY ADDRESSEE

PERIODICALS ORDER FULFILLMENT DEPT
ELSEVIER
6277 SEA HARBOR DR
ORLANDO FL 32821-9816